Susanne Steinbock
2111 Woodbourne Ave
Lou. Ky. 40205
454-3831

Ambulatory Pediatrics for Nurses

Ambulatory Pediatrics for Nurses

Marie Scott Brown, R.N., Ph.D.
Assistant Professor of Nursing
Pediatric Nurse Practitioner Program
University of Colorado, Denver

Mary Alexander Murphy, R.N., M.S.
Assistant Professor of Nursing
Pediatric Nurse Practitioner Program
University of Colorado, Denver

McGRAW-HILL BOOK COMPANY

A Blakiston Publication

New York St. Louis San Francisco
Auckland Düsseldorf Johannesburg Kuala Lumpur
London Mexico Montreal New Delhi Panama
Paris São Paulo Singapore Sydney Tokyo Toronto

NOTICE

Medicine is an ever-changing science. As new research and clinical experience broaden our knowledge, changes in treatment and drug therapy are required. The editors and the publisher of this work have made every effort to ensure that the drug dosage schedules herein are accurate and in accord with the standards accepted at the time of publication. The reader is advised, however, to check the product information sheet included in the package of each drug he or she plans to administer to be certain that changes have not been made in the recommended dose or in the contraindications for administration. This recommendation is of particular importance in regard to new or infrequently used drugs.

Ambulatory Pediatrics for Nurses

5 6 7 8 9 0 D O D O 7 9 8

This book was set in Times Roman by Rocappi, Inc. The editors were Cathy Dilworth, Sally Barhydt Mobley, and Matthew Cahill; the cover was designed by Joseph Gillians; the production supervisor was Charles Hess.
The drawings in Chapter 4 were done by Dorothy Merkel Alexander.
R. R. Donnelley & Sons Company was printer and binder.

Library of Congress Cataloging in Publication Data

Brown, Marie Scott.
Ambulatory pediatrics for nurses.

"A Blakiston publication."
Includes bibliographies.
1. Pediatric nursing. I. Murphy, Mary Alexander, joint author. II. Title.
[DNLM: 1. Ambulatory care—Nursing texts. 2. Pediatrics—Nursing texts.
WY159 B879a]
RJ245.B78 610.73'62 74-26972
ISBN 0-07-008290-1

To my parents,
who knew all about
ambulatory pediatrics
30 years ago

Marie

To my husband, Jim,
with affection

Mary

Contents

Preface

The scientific approach to the care of basically well children is in its infancy. Although both physicians and nurses have been attempting to fill this need for many years, they have had little well-researched literature available to them. Only in very recent times have investigators begun to look carefully at vision screening, hearing screening, common problems of childhood, and minor ailments such as diaper rash and colic. Yet these are the problems which most frequently concern parents and children and which, if not approached correctly at the beginning, can become major difficulties in family life. Careful attention to these problems is at the very heart of preventive, or ambulatory, pediatrics. This book is an attempt to synthesize the information developed from the newly emerging scientific interest in preventive pediatrics and to make it available to all nurses working with nonhospitalized children. We feel strongly that preventive pediatrics is where the nurse can make the most significant contribution.

Nurses have not always played a role in ambulatory pediatrics; seldom have they done so in outpatient and clinic settings, and almost never with the private sector of the population. Public health nurses have always been expected to provide such care but were handicapped in doing so because their education usually included little, if any, of the proper background, and it was not easy to find the necessary information in either the medical or nursing literature. Consequently, the preventive part of pediatrics, even in the field of public health, was often either ignored or based on intuitive rather than scientific information. Primarily because of the pediatric nurse practitioner movement of the last ten years, ambulatory pediatrics has become an increasingly important part of good nursing care and basic nursing education.

The history of the authors' interest in this field dates back to 1965 when they became involved in one of the first pediatric nurse practitioner programs at the University of Colorado. The idea at that time was experimental. In general, it was felt that there needed to be some changes in the delivery of health care to children in ambulatory settings. There were some obvious inconsistencies in the system as it was then. Private pediatricians, for instance, spent approximately 60 percent of their time in well-child care and management of minor illnesses such as diaper rash, colic, and similar important but minor problems. There was a demand for this type of care, and physicians provided it. Yet in their education in medical school, internship, and residency, they had usually received very little training in these areas. Nurses, on the other hand, had had three or four years of education, frequently a bachelor's degree, and certainly a great deal of specialized knowledge. Yet when nurses worked in ambulatory pediatrics, they generally spent the majority of their time doing clerical, receptionist, and nurse's aide duties—what has been called the "deprived role of the nurse in outpatient pediatrics." Everyone in this system suffered. Physicians spent most of their time doing things they had not been trained to do and frequently did not enjoy doing; nurses used very little of their nursing skills; and patients were caught in the system.

The primary goal of the pediatric nurse practitioner program was to improve this situation by expanding the traditional skills of the nurse in ambulatory care. Nurses were already capable of "physical assessment." With a little extra education, they could easily perform a "physical examination." They had an excellent foundation in normal growth and development and in counseling. With some additional knowledge in specific areas of well-child management, they could give primary health care to children.

This was the idea behind the pilot project in which the authors took part in 1965. The idea met some initial resistance but has gradually been accepted enthusiastically by the majority of nurses, physicians, and patients. Physicians are freed to give the type of medical care for which they are trained. Nurses are able to utilize their skills more fully, and patients are receiving care from someone educated specifically for and interested primarily in well-child management and care of minor illnesses.

After spending some years as pediatric nurse practitioners, the authors returned to the University of Colorado to begin teaching the program to other nurses. Over the years the program has grown and improved. The one great lack in the course has been a textbook written specifically for nurses concerning ambulatory care in pediatrics. There is also no handbook on the subject for public health nurses or nurses working in outpatient pediatric departments or in physicians' offices. For these reasons we have attempted to compile in this book the material we feel is essential to the nursing role in ambulatory pediatrics. We hope this material will serve not only as a text for pediatric nurse practitioner programs but also as a reference for all nurses working with children in ambulatory care settings and for schools of nursing which are now incorporating this body of knowledge into their undergraduate and graduate curriculums.

This text provides the most current information on such topics as hearing, vision, speech, developmental, and laboratory screening tests; information about applied growth and development that is useful in counseling parents; some of the newest advances in the growing field of perinatology; and the basics of well-child management, including in-depth material on nutrition, immunizations, safety, and other aspects of ambulatory pediatrics. The authors believe that this text with its companion, *Pediatric Physical Diagnosis for Nurses,* will supply all the information necessary for the nurse working in preventive pediatrics.

Marie Scott Brown
Mary Alexander Murphy

Ambulatory Pediatrics for Nurses

Chapter 1

History Taking

INTRODUCTION

Just as the physical examination is a tool, so is the health history. Taking a history is also, however, an art that must be learned, and the history must be used appropriately and evaluated carefully. Basically, history taking is the gathering of some verbal information about the patient, although it includes many other things as well. Every time the nurse speaks with the patient she is gathering information. Given enough time, anyone could obtain all the information needed about one patient, but the trick is to get that same amount of information within the 30-minute visit. Thus, it is important to learn to take a good, precise, detailed history in a limited amount of time. This chapter will discuss the health history—its purpose, value, some of the information that should be included, some problems that arise, and some different methods of recording the findings.

PURPOSE AND VALUE

Any work-up on a child contains five basic components: a verbal gathering of information (history taking), a look at the child (physical examination), interpretation of all laboratory findings, an impression based on all the objective and subjective information gathered, and a plan of action including both counseling and interpretation of this information to the patient. Although these five categories can be discussed separately, they are, in reality, closely intermeshed. The examiner may begin to take some history, but stop to talk about a problem the mother wants to discuss immediately; during the physical examination questions may also arise which need an immediate answer. It is impossible to postpone all the counseling until the end of the visit.

Every work-up contains all five components, but certain types of examinations may place heavier emphasis on certain components. It is a mistake however, to leave out any of them entirely. For example, when a nurse does only a physical examination, she receives a very small part of the information necessary. If the examination shows a bump on his leg, such questions as: Does it hurt? When did it appear? Have you ever had one before? Does anyone else in the family have one? go unanswered. Without this kind of information it is hard to reach an accurate conclusion. On the other hand, if during the history the mother mentions that the child has a pain in his big toe, after the examiner has asked some further questions about the pain, it is important to then actually examine the toe before reaching any conclusions or offering any suggestions. Often, after performing one part of the work-up, the examiner thinks she has a good idea of what is going on, only to have the entire picture change as more information is gathered.

There are several reasons for taking a history and using it appropriately. In the process of taking the information, the examiner and patient begin to establish a relationship with some trust. The mother comes to the clinic seeking some help, and the examiner seems concerned and capable of giving help. To know what kind of help is needed, the examiner must diagnose the problem. In taking the history, certain problems may arise that need discussion and perhaps a solution; in this way, the history facilitates education of the mother. The history may also point out areas that in the future may become problems; this allows preventive care to be initiated early, minimizing or avoiding the upcoming trouble.

While the actual history may be a list of questions asked by the examiner and answered by the patient, the art of history taking means applying the questions to each patient and child individually. The way the questions are asked, which questions are asked, and the examiner's facial expressions, body gestures, and relaxed attitude all aid in obtaining the total picture of what is happening to the child. A history is much more than a sheet of facts—it tells the story of this child's life.

KINDS OF INTERVIEWS

There are several kinds of interviews to fit different times, places, and needs. The well-child interview is the one most frequently done by nurses and pediatricians. It usually includes an initial complete history and follow-up histories on subsequent visits. These histories are usually fun to take, since the mother and child are doing well and all the nurse need do is affirm that all is going well.

The problem interview is also common. In this instance the child is brought to the clinic because of some immediate problem (either physical or emotional) and the entire visit may be limited to factors relating to that problem. With this situation the nurse has several alternatives: (1) take a brief history and decide that the problem is so severe that the child needs to see a physician immediately, (2) take a brief history and decide that the problem is something she can handle without a complete work-up, or (3) take a brief history and decide that the child also needs a complete work-up and proceed to handle the problem after finishing the complete work-up. Whether the nurse handles the problem herself or refers the child on, she must always check to see where the child is getting care and make arrangements for some continued care. It is important not only to treat the presenting symptom but to provide for the total care needed by the child. Occasionally the child's presenting problem is not the most important problem, but only the excuse for seeking help for another problem. But if the interviewer does not take time to elicit the real problem, the parent may return again and again with some minor complaint or instead give up entirely on using the health system as a helping organization.

Once a problem has been identified, the nurse may hold a therapeutic interview. Sometimes the value of talking is underestimated. If previous visits have isolated the problem, the nurse and mother, or nurse and child, or all three may need some time to discuss what is happening and why the patient thinks it is happening and to explore some possible solutions. These are frequently the problems for which there is no fast, simple cure. There is a tendency to refer all problems of lengthy duration on to someone else, and in severe situations this is needed, but many times the nurse, with the help of a consultant, is in a better position to handle the situation herself.

There are also information-getting and information-giving interviews. Some information can be obtained only by asking. It should be remembered that every question asked during the history should have some purpose in the patient's care—either for present or for future use. For example, it may be important to know the financial status of the family if the nurse thinks the child may need an expensive allergenic diet. Or it may be important to inquire as to the number of bedrooms the family has before suggesting that the parents move the newborn out of their bedroom. If the family is living in a one-room apartment in the father's parent's home, it is ludicrous to suggest a separate bedroom for the baby; the nurse only sets herself up as an idealistic, impractical resource person. The information-giving interview is also important. It is sometimes easy to hedge on giving advice, but if a mother asks a question, she deserves an answer. If the question requires more information (obtained through more detailed questions during the history and a look at the child), the examiner must tell the mother that more information is needed and then come back to the question later in the interview. If the examiner does not know the answer to the question, it is best to tell the mother that she does not know but will find out. Sometimes during the visit the nurse simply looks up the information or asks the appropriate person and returns to the examining room with the answer. Other times, the answer requires more time and must be put off until the next visit or a telephone call at a later date. But it is unwise to bluff a response and hope the patient will not know the difference. She will know, and any trust relationship will be destroyed.

APPROACHES TO HISTORY TAKING

The entire history should be considered from the viewpoint of both the interviewer and the interviewee. If the interviewer is relaxed and unhurried, the patient will generally relax and become more comfortable. Privacy should be provided for the session, since no one likes to discuss his personal problems before an audience. If the examiner wishes to record some of the information as it is discussed, the note taking should be casual and not overly zealous. The patient may not wish every word recorded. The examiner must be warm, friendly, nonjudgmental, responsive, and courteous. The nonverbal communication displayed by facial expressions may serve as a clue influencing the patient to change his story to please the nurse, rather than relate the real situation. It is important for the examiner to know what the patient thinks was said, rather than what was actually said.

The setup for the interview will depend on the age of the child. The infant is usually content to sit on his mother's lap while the examiner talks with the mother about the child. The toddler may wish to sit on his mother's lap or play with a few toys on the floor. The school-age child needs his own chair to sit on, and the examiner may take some history from the mother and some from the child. The nurse should be spontaneous, enthusiastic, and friendly, using simple words that the child can understand. The examining room should contain some furniture to fit the child's small size—a small chair, steps to the examining table, etc. Bright colors, pictures, and mobiles also help. Some hardy, colorful toys in the box or drawer help the child to relax during the talking part and can give the examiner a lot of information about the child's coordination and motor activity.

METHODS OF INTERVIEWING

There are several ways of obtaining information from the patient. A printed form may be handed to the mother (see Example 5 at the end of this chapter) with instruction to fill in the blanks and no more history obtained. This is rather limited and can give a stereotyped view of the patient. The examiner may use direct questioning and expect direct, short answers in return. Examples of direct questions would be: "How old are you?" "Did you eat an egg for breakfast this morning?" "Did you have prenatal care?" The most effective, but most difficult, way to obtain the information is to ask the parent or child to tell his story as he sees it—an indirect method of questioning. The nurse simply fills in the gaps and gives gentle direction to obtain the information needed. Such phrases as "Tell me about . . . ," "What do you remember about . . . ," and "How was your . . ." leave the patient free to tell the situation from his viewpoint. No one is a purist, and most interviews contain elements of all three methods of questioning. The patient may be presented with a printed form, which is reviewed by the nurse as she asks more direct questions and finally helps direct the patient to a more specific detailed personal account of the problems.

RECORDING

The information must not only be gathered but also be written into some organized form that can be used later by the same examiner or understood by others. Everyone develops his own method of what should be written, but a write-up should never be as short as "11/12/75—Bean in, Bean out" for the child who had a bean removed from his external ear canal, or as long as the 10- to 15-page write-ups that beginning medical and nurse practitioner students do when they are first learning. Some practitioners feel that nothing should be written during the work-up—the nurse talks with the mother and child, does the examination and any indicated counseling, and does the charting only after the family has left. Others feel they need to begin the recording during the interview partly because of the time pressure and partly so that they will not forget important information. A stack of unfinished charts at the end of the day will not be recorded correctly. Probably a combination of some writing during the interview and some just talking is most comfortable and efficient. Note taking should not be so vigorous as to make the mother uncomfortable or so long that the flow of the conversation is stopped. With practice the nurse learns to judge how much space to leave for more detail later and which words to jot down as she goes. A history is not written out in complete sentences and paragraphs, but in outline form with headings, short phrases, and key words.

The information gathered during the work-up may be organized and written up according to the standard system or to the newer problem-oriented system. The standard system divides information into several large areas, such as chief complaint and past history, and comes to the final conclusion, labeled an impression or diagnosis. The newer problem-oriented system, which was developed by Dr. Lawrence L. Weed, gathers the basic information and divides it into problems. The record includes a problem list which changes as old problems are solved and new ones added. Examples of both the standard and problem-oriented systems are given at the end of this chapter.

PROBLEMS

It must be remembered that not every interview runs smoothly. Problems are frequent. No two people interview the same way, and one nurse will not interview two different patients the same way. Frequently there is a language barrier; sometimes it is the difficulty of two different languages, but more often the barrier is more subtle, and although both nurse and mother are speaking English, there is no communication. Most mothers are subdued and eager to please in the nurse's office and will nod and smile appropriately even when they do not understand the instructions being given. Very few mothers are courageous enough to say that what the nurse is saying does not make any sense to them. The nurse may have to clarify words for the mother and ask the mother to clarify words for her; for instance, does the mother really know what "decongestant" means, and what does the mother mean when she says her child is "spoiled"? The nurse also needs to gauge the reliability of the informant. The history of a nontalking infant that is brought in by a babysitter, aunt, or grandmother is very difficult to evaluate. On the other hand, the mother who works all day may not have some of the necessary information either.

Sometimes the problem of the work-up lies with the patient; other times it is the fault of the examiner. Most often it is due to a poor interaction between the two. At the end of the day the nurse is tired, and may not be as observant and careful as she was in the beginning. Sometimes a nurse just does not hit it off with a particular patient. No one says that every examiner has to like every patient. However, if the nurse sees the friction coming and knows she cannot give good care to a patient, she should ask someone else to see the child for her. Often cues are missed and important questions skipped because of a poor relationship. At times the nurse may be glib when the patient is deadly serious. The mother who states, "Oh, I don't think I can stand him anymore," may not be joking and certainly does not need the answer, "You're doing just fine." Sometimes the nurse meets her own objectives, but fails to meet the child's or parent's. If this is discovered early, there may be time for correction; if not, the family may give up trying to get help from the health care system. Fortunately with most of these problems everyone is given a second chance. Some families may come only once, but more frequently if the mother and child know the nurse is concerned, they will return, and with time, and a growing relationship, some of the initial problems may be resolved. It is never pleasant to fail, but if the failure teaches and makes one a better practitioner, the next patient reaps those benefits.

INFORMATION TO BE INCLUDED IN THE HISTORY

Up to this point the discussion has concentrated on some general background knowledge that is needed in interviewing patients and taking a health history. This section will focus on some of the specific information needed for a history. The following headings and questions are those traditionally utilized.

CHIEF COMPLAINT: Why is the child attending clinic today? (Generally the answer is a simple statement in the mother's own words, i.e., "Well-child care," "Cold," "Earache.")

PRESENT ILLNESS: What signs and symptoms of illness is the child showing? (It is best to list the symptoms in order of appearance. Sometimes specific questions must be asked, i.e., Is the child coughing? When? What kind? How much? Does the child have diarrhea? When? What kind? How much? For how long?) How is the child acting otherwise? (How is his or her appetite? Bowels? Fluid intake? Sleep? Activity?) Has the child been exposed to others with illness? (Anyone in the family? Relatives? Friends? School? What type of illness was it?) What kind of treatment has the mother been giving? (Has she sought medical care before? Any medications? Any procedures?)

PAST HISTORY: ***Birth*** *Prenatal* How was the mother's health during her pregnancy with this child? Where did she receive her prenatal care and for how many months of the pregnancy? Did she have any infections? During what month? Did she have any illnesses? During which month, and how were they treated? Did she have any accidents? When and how was she treated? Was she taking medications during the pregnancy? What kind and why? At what point during pregnancy? What is her blood type? The child's father's blood type? Does she know the child's blood type? Did she have any x-rays during her pregnancy? Was she on any special diet during the pregnancy? How nutritional was her diet? Was she hospitalized during her pregnancy? When and for what reasons? How many living children does she have? Was either she or her doctor worried about this pregnancy for any reason? Did the pregnancy last 9 months? (A report of the baby coming less than 2 weeks early or late is usually not significant unless accompanied by a history of low birth weight or neonatal problems.)

Natal How long was the labor and were there any problems? What type of delivery was it? What kind of anesthesia was used, and were there any problems? (Such questions as: Did the baby come headfirst? Did the doctor use forceps? are often helpful in eliciting this information.) Where was the baby born? What was the baby's birthweight? What was the baby's condition at birth? Did the baby cry? Was the baby blue? Did the baby need oxygen?

Postnatal Did the baby have any problems during the stay in the nursery? What was the length of the baby's hospital stay? Did the mother and infant come home together? Did the baby have jaundice? Was the baby ever cyanotic or blue? Were there any feeding problems during the hospitalization? Did the baby develop any rashes? How much weight did the baby lose?

Allergies Is the child allergic to any foods? To any medications? To any insects? To any animals? At any seasons? If so, describe what happens with these allergies. Does the child ever break out in rashes? Does the mother know why?

Accidents Has the child ever had an accident? If so, was it in the car? At home? At school? At the babysitter's? Can the mother describe what happened? What was the treatment? What was the child's reaction? Any residual?

Illnesses Has the child had any infections? When? Where? What treatment? What follow-up? Has the child had any childhood diseases? Measles? Rubella? Roseola? Mumps? Chickenpox? Whooping cough?

Operations Has the child ever had any operations? When? For what condition? Where? What was the outcome?

Hospitalizations Has the child ever spent any time in a hospital? For what reason? Where? Is this condition resolved? Any residual?

Immunizations Has the child had any immunizations? Which kinds? Any reactions? Any boosters? (Usually a written record is the most accurate source of this information.) Has the child been tested for tuberculosis? How? When? What was the result? Has the child ever had x-rays?

FAMILY HISTORY: ***Family Members*** What is the mother's age and state of health? What is the father's age and state of health? Are there any siblings? What ages and what sex? State of health? (A diagram is often used to show this. A circle indicates a female, and a square indicates a male; a horizontal line indicates a marriage, and a vertical line indicates a descendant. A dotted circle or square indicates that the individual is deceased. An X indicates the patient with whom this particular history is concerned. The diagram on page 9 shows a maternal grandfather and paternal grandmother deceased, a maternal grandmother and paternal grandfather alive, two parents alive, one brother, and one sister alive, and one brother deceased.)

Family Diseases Within the immediate family, including both sets of grandparents and first aunts and uncles, are any of the following conditions present: EENT: Are there any nose bleeds? Sinus problems? Glaucoma? Cataracts? Myopia? Strabismus? Any other problems with their

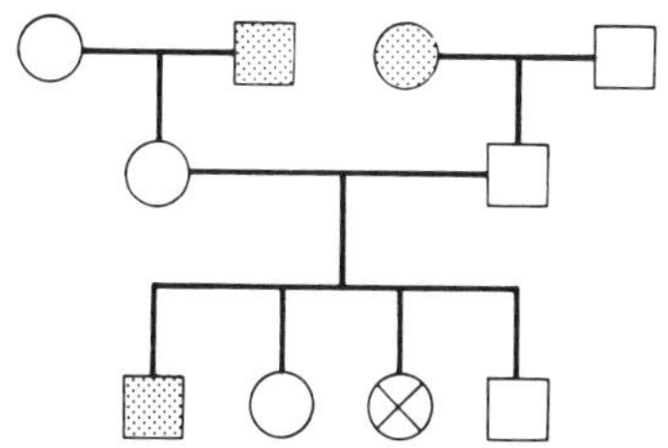

eyes, ears, nose, or throat? Cardio-Resp.: Is there any tuberculosis? Asthma? Hay fever? Hypertension? Heart murmurs? Heart attacks? Strokes? Anemia? Rheumatic fever? Leukemia? Pneumonia? Emphysema? Any other problems with heart or lungs? GI: Does anyone have ulcers? Colitis? Any other problems with stomach or intestines? GU: Does anyone have kidney infections? Bladder infections? Skeletal-Muscular: Are there any congenital dislocated hips? Muscular dystrophy? Arthritis? Club feet? Any other problems with bones or muscles? Neuro: Does anyone have convulsions? Mental retardation? Mental problems? Comas? Epilepsy? Senses: Is anyone deaf? Blind? Chronic: Does anyone have diabetes? Congenital anomalies? Cancer? Tumors? Thyroid problems? General: Are there any other medical problems in the family that the patient thinks are important?

Social Where does the family live? In a house? Apartment? Room? How large? Is there a yard? Are there stairs? Does anyone live with the family? Grandparents? Aunts? Uncles? Friends? What is the financial situation of the family? Does the father work? Does the mother work? What are their occupations? If no one works, how are they living? Is there any outside help? Babysitters? Day-care centers? Schools? What is the general relationship of the family members? Do they seem to be a happy family? Chaotic family? Sad family? Depressed family? Violent family?

REVIEW OF SYSTEMS: EENT: Does this child have persistent nosebleeds? Frequent streptococcal sore throats? Frequent colds? (more than four a year?) Pneumonia? Frequent earaches? Do the child's eyes ever cross? Do they tear excessively? Cardio-Resp: Does the child have any trouble breathing? Running? Finishing a 3- to 4-oz. bottle without tiring? Does the child turn blue? GI: Does the child have any problems with diarrhea? Constipation? Bleeding around the rectum? Bloody stools? Pain? Vomiting? GU: Does the child have a straight, strong urinary stream, or does the urine just dribble out? Urinary frequency? Is there any pain? Bleeding? If an older girl, does she menstruate? How often? Any problems? Neuro: Has the child ever had a convulsion? A fainting spell? Tremors? Twitches? Blackouts? Dizzy spells? Frequent headaches? Skeletal: Has the child ever broken any bones? Had any sprains? Complained of pain in the joints, swelling, or redness around the joints? Senses: Does the child see well? Hear well? Does the child seem clumsy? Can the child see the blackboard from where he or she sits in the classroom? Is the child always falling or walking into doors?

HABITS: ***Eating*** Is the child's appetite good? Poor? Varied? If on formula, what kind, how much, how is it mixed, and how frequently? How much does the child take in a 24-hour period? What kinds of foods does the child eat? Meat? Fruits? Vegetables? Cereals? Juices? Eggs? Sweets? Milk? Snacks? How often? What size portions? How many times a week or day does the child eat each of these? Does the child feed herself or himself? Does the child use a cup? Spoon? Knife? Fork? Is the child messy? Does the child sit with the rest of the family? Does the child take vitamins? What kind? How often? How much?

Bowels What are the child's bowel patterns? Frequency? Consistency? Color? Any discomfort? Is the child toilet-trained? Is toilet training planned? When? Any problems? If the child is toilet-trained, does he or she have accidents? If so, are they during the day or night? How often? Are they frequently associated with emotional upsets?

Sleep When does the child go to bed? Wake up? Does the child awaken during the night? How often? What happens? What does the mother do? Any nightmares? Night terrors? Does the child take naps? When? For how long? Where does the child sleep? How many hours does the child sleep in a 24-hour period? When awake, is the child alert? Or does the child seem to need more sleep than he or she is getting?

Development How does the child compare with his or her siblings? Quicker to learn? Slower to learn? When did the child first sit? Stand? Roll over? Talk? Walk? What kinds of activities does the child do now? What is the child doing that is new since the last visit? What grade is the child in? Does the child like school? Does the child have playmates? What does the child like to do in school? What does the child like to play?

Some of the questions asked when taking a complete history need to be modified for specific ages, and some areas would need more detail if problems were encountered. But generally if the nurse covers these seven areas, she has a good idea of which topics need more expansion and detail. The nurse must also decide which of these areas need to be discussed at every visit, which must be investigated at regular intervals, and which can be covered only once. Certainly once the birth history has been taken and no problems appear, there is no reason to repeat that material every visit. However, the habits of the child change from visit to visit, sometimes from day to day, and this may be an important area to include in every history. The review of systems can easily change, but usually it will take a longer period of time for significant change to appear. Thus the nurse may decide to routinely take a review of systems once a year rather than monthly or weekly. She must go through each category and fit it into her routine for giving good, comprehensive health care to her patients.

HISTORY OF AN ILLNESS

As the nurse moves into the care of sick children, she enters a large, nebulous, often undefined area binding nursing and medicine. There are some very definite limits within this area, but they are often difficult to define, and some nurses can find themselves being pushed into practicing medicine. Every state legally defines the activity of nursing, and institutions employing nurses allow certain activities within that realm. Generally nurses may not write prescriptions or perform certain procedures (e.g., surgery, spinal taps) on their own. There are some things nurses can do independently, and additional activities they can do in conjunction with and under the supervision of a physician. Within the area of sickness the nurse must know her limits, the expectations of her employing agency, and her resources.

Another problem concerns the differential diagnosis versus a list of symptoms, which represent two entirely different thinking processes. Until the last few years doctors worked diligently at finding the proper label for the proper disease. When the patient was seen, it was important to define the condition in one word—"diabetes," "hypertension," "hepatitis," etc. But with the newer methods of recording which emphasize the symptom and dealing with each symptom, the single label may become less important. Generally nurses are responsible for the list of symptoms and not the differential diagnosis, and they should use care to stay within this limitation unless they have additional training in differential diagnosis. It can be harmful to the patient to attempt doing a limited differential diagnosis. Thus the nurse is responsible for reporting that the patient has rales in the upper left lung, clear nasal discharge, watery eyes, inflamed throat, and bilateral red tympanics. The doctor may lump all those signs under one heading of lobar pneumonia, bronchitis, upper respiratory tract infection, allergy, brucellosis, tuberculosis, or other conditions that he has considered. The damage is done when the nurse thinks those symptoms must indicate an upper respiratory tract infection, when indeed it may be the rare case of brucellosis that presents with those symptoms.

In most clinic settings the nurse will work out some procedures with her physician for handling patients. There should be some agreement on what are minor illnesses, how she can treat them, and when or if the doctor wants to see each patient. There will always be the child who comes in as a well child but is found to have inflamed, deformed tympanics or the child who presents with the chief complaint of a cold and turns out to have jaundice and possible hepatitis. But if the nurse has a good working relationship with the doctor, problems should be minimal and the patient should receive very good, comprehensive care.

The original history data form needs little modification to include the history of the present illness. Generally the illness is listed as a problem, e.g., "Problem 2, Cold," and a new section is added under the subjective heading: Present Illness. This is more clearly seen in the examples at the end of the chapter.

In covering the material under this heading, some questions need to be asked generally, and other questions should be asked in specific situations. In general there are five areas to gather information about: (1) how long ago the child was entirely well, (2) symptoms of this condition, (3) habits found with this condition, (4) exposures, and (5) treatment.

It is important to know when the child was well last to ascertain whether the present illness is a slow, chronic process or a sudden, acute episode. The information should be recorded as 3 days ago or 1 week ago, not as Thursday or Monday or Tuesday since the next person reading the chart will not know on what day of the week the chart was written.

The progress of the condition is recorded as a progression of symptoms and the types of symptoms present. Some mothers can tell the examiner in an orderly, detailed way; others need some guidance and prodding. The examiner should ask about the child's condition 3 days ago, 2 days ago, yesterday, today, this morning, and this afternoon. The examiner may have to ask whether certain conditions were present—coughing, diarrhea, constipation, vomiting, earache, stomachache, pain, etc.—and what is bothering the mother the most—the coughing at night, the pain, the noneating.

It is important to find out about the child's general habits since the condition appeared. How is the child's appetite? How are the child's bowels? Is the child sleeping? What is his or her level of activity? The child who is eating as usual, having no bowel problems, sleeping through the night, and playing or going to school as usual is probably not as ill as the one who is not eating, is having diarrhea, is waking at night with a cough, and is refusing to go to school.

Exposures can be another clue to the condition. The examiner should ask whether the child has recently been exposed to anyone showing similar symptoms or streptococcal infections, childhood diseases (measles, mumps, chickenpox, etc.), viral infections, etc. Is anyone else in the immediate family ill, and if so, how are they ill? Are those members having the same symptoms or the same progression of illness, and what has been the outcome?

It is vital to find out what kind of treatment the child has received so far. What has the mother been doing for the condition? Has the child been seen by another nurse or doctor? How much and how often has the child been taking any medications and have they seemed to work?

The questions asked when seeing a sick child will vary with some conditions such as rashes, pain, diarrhea, and colds. The American Academy of Pediatrics has made up a list of such questions to fit certain situations (see Table 1-1).

Table 1-1 Suggested Questions for Interviewing

Identification of problem	To be seen by M.D. if:	Home treatment and follow-up
Specific guidelines for medical factors applicable to abdominal pain		
Where is the pain? How does the child react to the pain: 1. Is it constant or does it come and go? 2. Is it related to feeding? 3. Does it interrupt sleep? 4. Does it cause him to cry out? 5. Does he favor any one position? 6. Is he walking and standing normally? How does the child describe the pain? Is he constipated, having diarrhea, or passing a lot of gas? Has he vomited? Does he have a sore throat, cold, or cough? Is he urinating normally? Does he have a fever? Does his abdomen feel tense or rigid? Has he been hit in the abdomen? Could he have strained abdominal muscles? Has he been upset or anxious about anything recently?	Child is under 4 years and has no symptoms of an infection. Pain is severe, constant, localized, and causing child to cry out or double up. Abdomen feels tense and rigid. There are any urinary problems. There is abdominal pain following trauma to the abdomen.	Nothing by mouth except ginger ale or Seven-Up. Warm tub bath. If suspicious of "pain" on a "tension" basis, talk with mother to try to identify the problem. Plan follow-up call in a few hours. Observe for signs of change; instruct mother to call back immediately if child's condition worsens.

The following examples of the complete history of an illness indicate the type of information elicited in comprehensive interviewing. Examples of both the standard system of recording and the problem-oriented system are used.

Example 1 Complete history recorded according to the standard system
Female, 6 weeks old   height: 22 in.   weight: 9 lbs, 8 oz.
H.C.: 36.5 cm

CHIEF COMPLAINT: Well-child care

Table 1-1 Suggested Questions for Interviewing *(Cont'd)*

Identification of problem	To be seen by M.D. if:	Home treatment and follow-up
Specific guidelines for medical factors applicable to colds and coughs		
Cough? 1. Is it dry or loose? 2. When does child cough most? 3. Does it wake him from sleep? Is child breathing any differently than normally? 1. faster? 2. harder? 3. shallower? 4. retracting? 5. noisy? 6. grunting? Any signs of earache or sore throat? What does the nasal discharge look like? How is child sucking (if infant)? Does child have a fever? Does child have any allergies?	Afebrile with cold, then fever 3–4 days later. Cough wakes child when asleep. Significant changes in breathing pattern. Child less than 3 years with cold and temperature for 2–3 days without improvement. Thick, foul-smelling, or bloody-colored nasal discharge.	Nose drops with instructions for use as specified by M.D. Decongestants (dosage as specified by M.D.) Cough syrup (type and dosage, specified by M.D.) Vaporizer or cool steam or shower. Ear bulb syringe to clear infant's nose before feeding. Postural drainage (nasal discharge). Elevate head of bed with books or blocks (for breathing). Position infant on stomach to increase drainage from nose. Be sure house is not too warm and/or dry. If allergy suspected, follow up with mother and plan medical follow-up with M.D. If child is less than 3–4 years, plan telephone follow-up with mother because of the incidence of colds as presenting signs of streptococcal infection in this age group. Give mother specific changes in condition which should be reported immediately.

PAST HISTORY: ***Birth*** *Prenatal* G_1 P_1 A_0 Followed at Denver General Hospital clinic from 3d to 9th month. No infections, illnesses, hospitalizations, x-rays, or accidents during the pregnancy. No medications except vitamins and iron. Both she and the baby's father have Rh positive blood types. Normal diet except slight sodium restrictions during the final trimester.

Specific guidelines for medical factors applicable to diarrhea

If infant, review feeding practices. When did diarrhea start? What does it look like? How many stools in 24 hours? How large are they? Does he have cramps? Does he have a fever? Has he vomited? What has he had to eat and drink? Is he urinating normally? Does skin or tongue look dry? Eyes sunken? Is he thirsty? Drinking fluids well?	There is blood in the stools. More than 12–15 diarrhea stools per day, or smaller number but large quantity (in infant). Signs of dehydration (skin, tongue, eyes, thirst, scant urine). Diarrhea for more than 48 hours, with no improvement.	If related to infant feeding, review practices. Nothing by mouth for 2–4 hours. Then, ginger ale or Seven-Up until diarrhea stops. Progress diet slowly. Antispasmodics (as prescribed by M.D.). Watch for dehydration. If actually only "loose" stools: 1. Give no fruit. 2. Reduce bulk. 3. Give cottage cheese. 4. Keep diet bland. Have mother report back if diarrhea fails to improve in 48 hours or if it recurs. If other problems, refer to specific problem guideline.

Specific guidelines for medical factors applicable to earache

Does he have a fever? Does he have a cold or sore throat? Has he had one in the past week? Is there or has there been any drainage from the ear? What does it look like? How much does the ear hurt? Constantly? On and off? Associated with swallowing? Is there any itchiness and/or a burning sensation associated with the discomfort? Has he been doing a lot of swimming? Does he complain when you touch the ear? Is there any swelling around the ear? Exposure to mumps?	Suspicion of otitis media: 1. Sudden, acute, severe discomfort 2. Drainage from ear 3. Discomfort when the ear is touched 4. Mild complaints of ear discomfort associated with temperature over 101°F for 24 hours. Suspicion of external otitis 1. Presence of itching and/or a burning sensation. 2. Discomfort when ear is touched. 3. Child has been doing a lot of swimming.	External heat. Aspirin or similar compound at dosage for age specified by M.D. Decongestant at dosage for age specified by M.D. Exempt, narcotic codeine-containing cough mixtures at dosage for age specified by M.D. No swimming. Watch temperature. If other problems, refer to specific problem guidelines.

Table 1-1 Suggested Questions for Interviewing ***(Cont'd)***

Identification of problem	To be seen by M.D. if:	Home treatment and follow-up
Specific guidelines for medical factors applicable to fever		
How long has he had fever? How much? Constant or periodic? Does he have an earache or is he rubbing or pulling at his ear? Does he have a sore throat, cold, or cough? Is he nauseated or has he vomited? Does he have a stiff neck? Can he bend his chin to his chest? Is he urinating normally? Any burning or pain? Has he had any diarrhea? Does he have any rash? Has he ever had a febrile convulsion?	There is fever of 101–102°F for 3 days without explanation. Neck is stiff. Low grade, but unexplained, fever for 5 days.	Aspirin or similar compound at dosage for age specified by M.D. Keep child in cool environment. Push fluids. Sponge for temperature over 103°F. Phenobarbital if the child has had a previous convulsion at dosage specified by M.D. Watch for change. Report back. If problem is more specific, refer to applicable problem guideline.
Specific guidelines for medical factors applicable to rashes		
Where did it first occur? Has it spread? To where? What does it look like? 1. Color? 2. Flat or raised, blisterlike? 3. Is it weeping? 4. Is it crusted? 5. Is it scabbed? Does it itch? Does child have a fever? Does he have enlarged glands? Does he have a sore throat? Does he have any other signs of illness? Is he allergic to anything? 1. Any new clothes? 2. Any new foods? 3. Any new detergent, bleach, or rinse agent being used? 4. Has he been playing in the woods? Is his neck stiff? Can he touch his chin to his chest? Has he ever had a rash like this before?	Presence of stiff neck. Presence of enlarged glands and/or sore throat. Rash is present and child sounds "really sick." Rash sounds like a childhood disease and mother wants definite diagnosis.	If common communicable disease, teach management, complications to watch for, incubation period, and follow with mother. If allergy is suspected: 1. Remove allergen. 2. Give antihistamine (dosage specified by M.D.). 3. Give baths with soothing agent, e.g., baking soda, corn starch. 4. Apply external lotion, e.g., calamine lotion, to suppress itch. 5. Follow up as indicated for further work-up. If child seems well except for rash, have mother call back next day.

Specific guidelines for medical factors applicable to sore throat		
Does he have a fever? Are the glands in his neck enlarged and/or tender? Have you looked at his throat? Any white patches? Is his throat sore just in the morning or continuously? How much is his appetite affected? Any liquids or foods in particular he is refusing? Does he have a cold? Earache? Coughs? Does he have a stomachache? Has he had any nausea or vomiting? Diarrhea? Has he had a lot of sore throats? Streptococcal infections? Does he have any rash? Does he have any open sores?	Suspicion of streptococcal throat: 1. Severe sore throat causing decrease in appetite. 2. Enlarged lymph glands. 3. Presence of white patches in throat or petechiae on palate. 4. Temperature over 102°F. 5. Child acts "miserable." 6. Indication of rash on body. 7. Indications of skin infection. History of susceptibility to sore throats, even if symptoms are mild.	Push bland fluids, e.g., tonic, water, popsicles, gelatin desserts. Soothing, coating substance, e.g., syrup, honey. Add humidity to room and keep room cool but comfortable. If other problems, refer to specific problem guidelines.

Natal Labor with caudal lasted 5 hours. Her husband was able to be with her for most of the time. Baby delivered vertex without forceps. Baby born at DGH. Birth weight 7 lbs, 5 oz. and was 40 weeks gestation by physical and mother's dates. Baby cried spontaneously and did not need oxygen. Apgar was 7 and 9.

Postnatal Nursery stay uneventful with mother and infant going home after 3 days. Infant exhibited slight jaundice on 3d and 4th days, but no cyanosis or rashes. Baby lost 3 oz. during first week, but regained birth weight by 12 days. Breast feeding was initiated in the hospital and went well; baby was hungry and sucked well and the breasts were well conditioned.

Allergies No allergic reactions to foods, medications, insects, animals, or seasons.

Accidents Baby has never had an accident.

Illnesses Baby had a slight upper respiratory infection at 4 weeks and was treated by her mother with a cold steam vaporizer and no medications

Table 1-1 Suggested Questions for Interviewing ***(Cont'd)***

Identification of problem	To be seen by M.D. if:	Home treatment and follow-up
Specific guidelines for medical factors applicable to vomiting		
When has child vomited? How much? How often? Type and color of vomitus? Is vomiting forceful? If infant, review feeding practices. Is child nauseated? Retching? Is child coughing? Breathing normally? What did he eat or drink before this started? Have you made any recent changes in his diet? Could he have eaten any poisonous substance or any medicines? Does he have gas? Diarrhea? Stomach pains? Does he have a fever? Is he urinating normally? Is he very thirsty? Irritable? Twitchy? Do skin or tongue look dry? Are eyes sunken?	Forceful vomiting in infant under 3 months. Signs of dehydration (skin, tongue, eyes, thirst, scant urine). Ingestion of poison or medication. Blood in vomitus. Associated, severe abdominal pain. Frequent and constant vomiting. Duration of more than 24 hours with no improvement.	If related to infant feeding, review practices. No fluids or solids for 2–4 hours. Coca Cola syrup every 15 minutes six times. Ginger ale or Seven-Up in small quantities frequently. No solids or milk for 24 hours. Start progressing diet 24 hours after last vomiting. If medication is indicated, consider suppository. Watch for dehydration. Antiemetic (as prescribed by M.D.). Have mother call back if no progress in 2–4 hours. Have mother call in daily for instructions if vomiting is of concern. Give mother specific guideline of change in condition which should be reported immediately. If other problems, refer to specific problem guideline.

Printed by permission of the American Academy of Pediatrics, *Standards of Child Health Care,* Evanston, Ill.: American Academy of Pediatrics, 1972, pp. 47–54.

after consulting with the nurse by phone. No further problems. She has not had any childhood diseases.

Operations Baby has never spent the night in the hospital after being discharged at birth.

Immunizations None.

FAMILY HISTORY: ***Family Members*** Mother—25 years, good health. Father—27 years, good health.

Family Diseases EENT: No nose bleeds, sinus problems, glaucoma, or cataracts. Mother has myopia and father has hyperopia. No strabismus. CR: No tuberculosis, hay fever, hypertension, heart murmurs, strokes, anemia, rheumatic fever, or leukemia. Maternal grandfather had asthma. Paternal aunt died of pneumonia. GI: No ulcers or colitis. GU: No kidney infections or bladder infections. MS: No arthritis or club feet. Maternal aunt had cogenitally dislocated hip. No muscular dystrophy. Neuro: No convulsions, mental retardation, mental problems, comas, or epilepsy. SS: No deafness or blindness. Chronic: No diabetes, congenital anomalies, cancer or tumors.

Social Family of three lives in small, two-bedroom house with a basement and back yard. Father works days as a dishwasher, and mother stays home with infant. Many relatives in town who visit, and offer to babysit. Both parents seem happy and able to enjoy infant. Father getting used to handling baby and will help with some care. Good mother-child relationship.

REVIEW OF SYSTEMS: EENT: No persistent nosebleeds, streptococcal sore throats, frequent colds, pneumonia, or earaches. Intermittent horizontal strabismus. Cardio-Resp: No trouble breathing, no turning blue, and no choking on mucous. Does not seem to tire easily. GI: No problems with diarrhea, constipation, bloody stools, pain, or vomiting. Burps well. No colic. GU: Mother has observed infant void: straight, strong stream seen. No problems with frequency, pain, bleeding, or strong odors. Neuro: Infant has had no seizures or blackouts. Mother observed that lower jaw occasionally trembles but only when crying. Skeletal: No broken bones, sprains, strains, or joint problems. Senses: Mother reports responses to light, movement, and sound and feels child is seeing and hearing.

HABITS: ***Eating*** Infant taking both breasts every 3½ to 4 hours. Empties both sides, sucks well, and is having no problems with burping. Feedings last about 15 to 20 minutes. Mother's nipples nontender and not cracked. Mother feels it is too early to begin solids. Takes 2 oz. water every 24 hours.

Bowels Bowels move 3 to 4 times every 24 hours; soft, yellow, formed stools. No pain or bleeding.

Sleep Sleeps 4 to 5 hours per night with occasional 8-hour night. Short naps during morning, afternoon, and evening. Sleeping in crib beside parent's bed. Sleeps 18 to 21 hours every 24 hours.

Development Mother feels baby is doing more and beginning to notice more of her surroundings. Beginning to smile spontaneously and responsively; looks at mother during feedings; content to watch mobile over bed for short periods of time; will lift head off bed to turn to other side. Cooing.

PHYSICAL EXAMINATION: Total explanation of physical findings would be written into this area.

IMPRESSION: Healthy 6-week-old female infant.

ADVICE: (1) First DPT and trivalent polio given. (2) Explained usual reactions and types of immunizations given. Discussed use of Tylenol. (3) Discussed feeding—how to handle sudden increase in appetite which sometimes occurs around 6th week. Recommended waiting on solids and supplemental bottles. (4) Discussed baby's sleeping in parents' room. Mother happy with situation for present and thinking of moving infant after 10 weeks. (5) Discussed some normal growth and development—trembling chin normal in newborn, what to expect in next few weeks.

PLAN: Return to clinic in 4 weeks for second DPT and polio, check feeding pattern, discuss addition of cereal, inquire about sleeping pattern.

Example 2 Complete history recorded according to the problem-oriented system
Female, 4 years old height: 41 in. weight: 36 lbs

PROBLEM 1: Well-child care (first visit)

DATA BASE: ***Subjective:*** 4-year-old girl

PAST HISTORY: ***Birth*** *Prenatal* Mother's second pregnancy. From her 3rd to 9th month she was followed at Denver General Hospital clinic. She had a kidney infection during the pregnancy. Her doctor placed her on vitamins and iron tablets for the entire pregnancy. Both she and the baby's father have Rh positive blood types. She followed her normal diet except for slight sodium restrictions during the final trimester. She has had no abortions or miscarriages.

Natal Labor lasted 5 hours. Her husband was able to be with her most of the time. She received a caudal anesthetic and the baby was delivered by vertex. Baby born at DGH. Birth weight 7 lbs, 5 oz. She cried spontaneously and did not need oxygen.

Postnatal Nursery stay uneventful with mother and infant going home after 3 days. Infant exhibited slight jaundice on 3rd and 4th days, but no cyanosis or rashes. She lost 3 oz. during first week. Breast feeding was initiated in hospital and went well; baby was hungry and sucked well.

Allergies No allergic reactions to medications, insects, animals, or seasons. Breaks out in fine, macular, itchy rash 12 hours after eating tomatoes.

Accidents None.

Illnesses Chickenpox at 2½ years. Rubella at 3 years.

Operations Tonsils removed at 3½ years. Stayed in hospital 1 night; no adverse reactions.

Immunizations DPT 1—1/1969, DPT 2—2/1969, and DPT 3—3/1969 (given by private pediatrician in Kansas City). DPT booster—3/1970 (given at Colorado General Hospital clinic). Trivalent polio—1/1969, trivalent polio—2/1969, and trivalent polio—4/1969 (given by private pediatrician in Kansas City). Trivalent polio booster—5/1970. Tine test—7/1969 (negative; given at Colorado General Hospital clinic). Measles-rubella-mumps vaccine—6/1972.

FAMILY HISTORY ***Family Members*** Mother—30 years, good health, father—35 years, back problems treated at work clinic, siblings: Jane—3 years, good health, John—6 years, partially deaf, attends special school.

Family Diseases No nose bleeds, sinus problems, glaucoma or cataracts. No tuberculosis, hypertension, heart murmurs, strokes, anemia, rheumatic fever, asthma, leukemia, or pneumonia. Mother has hay fever in springtime. No ulcers or colitis. Mother had kidney infections with each pregnancy and is still being seen in UTI clinic for recurring problem. No arthritis, club feet, or congenitally dislocated hips. No convulsions, mental retardation, mental problems, comas, or epilepsy. No diabetes, cancer, or tumors. Older sibling partially deaf; maternal aunt totally deaf from birth.

Social Family of five live in small, two-bedroom house with no basement and tiny yard. Father works nights as trainman and sleeps during day. Mother home with children. Family struggles to keep within a budget; recreational activities limited. Father becoming more interested in helping with children as they get older.

REVIEW OF SYSTEMS: ENT: No persistent nosebleeds, frequent colds or earaches. Had five streptococcal throat infections year of tonsillectomy. Cardio-Resp: No trouble breathing, no turning blue, and no choking. Keeps up with other children; runs stairs. GI: No problems with diarrhea, constipation, bleeding, bloody stools, pain, vomiting, encopresis. GU: No problems with frequency, pain, bleeding, enuresis. Neuro: No convulsions, fits, seizures, blackouts, dizzy spells, epilepsy. Skeletal: Broke right middle finger in fall from tricycle in 1970. No complaints of joint pain or swelling. Senses: Mother feels she hears and sees; no vision or hearing testing ever done.

HABITS: ***Eating*** Good appetite. Eats most foods. Eats cereal, milk, fruit, vegetables, and meat daily. Eats eggs 4 to 5 times per week. Likes snacks of fruit, cookies, juices, candy.

Bowels Mother unsure of pattern since child goes by herself and rarely complains of problems. No recent diarrhea or constipation. Toilet trained since early 3s.

Sleep Generally in bed by 8 or 9 and up by 6:30 or 7. Will sometimes take short nap in afternoon. Sleeps in top bunk bed in children's bedroom. No problems with nightmares or night terrors.

Development Friendly, outgoing little girl who gets along well with most people. Has several girl friends on block. Knows her name, can dress herself, can count to 5 and is looking forward to school next year.

OBJECTIVE: Weight, 36 lbs; height, 41 in.

Physical Examination (Total explanation of physical findings would be written into this area.)

ASSESSMENT: ***Impression*** Healthy 4-year-old.

Therapeutic DT booster and polio booster given. DDST done. Hct. done. Urinalysis done. Vision tested—normal. Hearing tested—normal.

Education (1) Discussed eating and snacking—limit candy intake and watch tooth brushing. (2) Discussed getting ready to go to school—learning to cross streets, tie own shoes, knowing home address and phone number, etc. (3) Return to clinic in 1 year for health check—all screening, check on school readiness.

Example 3 History of an illness recorded according to the standard system
Male, 5 years old   height: 43½ in.   weight: 42 lbs
temperature: 37°C

CHIEF COMPLAINT: Cold and fever.

PRESENT ILLNESS: Child well until 3 days ago. Then began sneezing and complaining of scratchy throat. 2 days ago: Nose began to drip clear drainage; occasional dry, tickly cough; fever of 37.5°C. Yesterday: Nose continued to drip; cough more frequent and wetter; coughing during day and night; fever of 37.3°C. Today: Nose dripping continually and base becoming reddened and sore; continual wet, gurgly cough, nonproductive; no fever. Child no longer complaining of sore throat; no complaints of earache, stomachache, pain anywhere, diarrhea, constipation, or vomiting. Child's appetite less, but he is eating and asking for extra fluids. He was sleeping well until 2 nights ago when coughing woke him twice. Activity about the same except for taking an afternoon nap which he usually does not do.

EXPOSURES: Mother recovering from cold and cough of last week. No one else ill at home. No complaints of schoolmates having any contagious diseases.

TREATMENT: Aspirin 5 gr every 4 hours during fever. None given today. Robitussin cough medicine 1 tsp every 4 hours for cough. Last dose 1½ hours ago. Cold mist vaporizer running in his room since last night. Giving extra juices, pop, water.

HABITS: ***Eating*** Appetite generally good. Likes most foods and trying some new foods at preschool lunches. Drinks 2 to 4 glasses of milk per day; eats eggs 4 to 5 times a week; generally eats meat, fruits, vegetables, and cereal daily. Taking one-a-day vitamins.

Bowels Normal; one movement per day. No problems.

Sleep Usually in bed by 8:30 and up by 7:00. Generally does not take afternoon nap. Sleeps in own bed in bedroom shared with older brother.

Development Attending preschool two blocks from home. Had problems starting, but is now enjoying. Goes half a day and walks by himself. Can dress himself; helps some around the house. Plays with several neighborhood children.

PHYSICAL EXAMINATION: Physical examination showing extra attention to areas concerned with present illness.

ASSESSMENT: ***Impression*** Normal 5-year-old with runny nose and cough.

ADVICE: (1) Since lungs clear, ears normal, and no fever, encourage mother to continue present treatment. (2) May go to school if he feels like it. (3) Throat culture taken. (4) May apply small amounts of Vaseline to base of nose for rawness.

PLAN: Return to clinic if child becomes worse (fever, earache, any pain, change in activity, etc.) or in 1 week for regular well-child care—complete history including R.O.S., family and social history, Hct. urinalysis, vision and hearing screening.

Example 4 History of an illness recorded according to the problem-oriented system
Male, 5 years old height: 43½ in. weight: 42 lbs temperature: 37°C BP: 99/65, P: 85, R: 20

PROBLEM 2: Cold and fever

DATA BASE: ***Subjective*** 5-year-old boy

ILLNESS: Child well until 3 days ago; then began sneezing and complaining of scratchy throat. 2 days ago: Nose began to drip clear drainage, occasional dry, tickly cough; fever of 37.5°C. Yesterday: Nose continued to drip; cough more frequent and wetter; coughing during day and night; fever of 37.3°C. Today: Nose dripping continually and base becoming raw; continual wet, gurgly cough, nonproductive; no fever. Child no longer complaining of sore throat; no complaints of earache, stomachache, pain anywhere, diarrhea, constipation, or vomiting. Child's appetite less, but he is eating and asking for extra fluids. He was sleeping well until 2 nights ago when coughing woke him twice. Activity about the same except for taking an afternoon nap which he usually does not do. Continues to go to school.

OBJECTIVE: Temperature: 37 °C, height: 43 ½ in., weight: 42 lbs, BP: 99/65. Physical examination showing extra attention to areas concerned with present illness would be recorded in this area.

HABITS: ***Eating*** Appetite generally good. Likes most foods and trying some new foods at preschool lunches. Drinks 2 to 4 glasses of milk per day; eats eggs 4 to 5 times a week; generally eats meat, fruits and vegetables, and cereal daily. Taking one-a-day vitamins.

Bowels Normal, one movement per day. No problems.

Sleep Usually in bed by 8:30 and up by 7:00. Generally does not take afternoon nap. Sleeps in own bed in bedroom shared with older brother.

Development Attending preschool two blocks from home. Had problems starting but is now enjoying. Goes half a day and walks by himself. Can dress himself; helps some around the house. Plays with several neighborhood children.

ASSESSMENT: Normal 5-year-old with runny nose and cough.

PLAN: ***Diagnostic*** Throat culture done.

Treatment Aspirin 5 gr every 4 hours during fever. None today. Robitussin cough medication 1 tsp every 4 hours for cough. Cold mist vaporizer running in his room since last night. Encouraged fluids.

Educational May go to school if he feels like it. Safety around a vaporizer. Return to clinic if child becomes worse, or in 1 week for Problem 1, regular well-child care.

The following history forms are used in the pediatric outpatient department at Colorado General Hospital. These forms are completed by the parents or the adolescent patient, and provide a starting point for the examiner, who reviews the material and uses it as a basis for building the remainder of the history.

Example 5 History form for a child from birth through 5 years

---

The pediatric clinic at Colorado General can provide either short-term emergency care or long-term continuous care. If your child is under the care of a private doctor or a convenient health clinic, we do not want to interfere with or duplicate the care you are receiving there.

My child usually gets his care at ______________________________ and his last physical examination was ______ months or ______ years ago.

I am here for this visit only and my child receives his care elsewhere.
Yes _____ No _____
If your answer to the above question is Yes, there is no need to go any further with this questionnaire.

If you would like your child cared for in a private doctor's office or a public health facility more convenient to you, please ask to speak with one of the public health nurses.

If your child is not receiving care elsewhere and you want him to get his care here, you can help us take better care of him by answering the following questions:

If your child is over 3 years old, is he/she too sick today to have his eyes checked? Yes _____ No _____

Is he/she too sick today or are you too rushed for us to test how he/she is developing? (approximately 15 minutes) Yes _____ No _____

I. *Pregnancy and Birth* *Circle One (1)*

1. Did you have any illnesses during your pregnancy? .... No Yes
2. Did you carry him/her for a full 9 months? .... Yes No
3. Where was your baby born? _____________
4. How much did he/she weigh at birth? _____ lbs _____ oz.
5. Did your baby have any trouble starting to breathe? .... No Yes
6. Did your baby have any trouble in the hospital? .... No Yes
7. Did your baby go home with you when you left the hospital? .... Yes No
8. How long did he/she stay in the hospital? _____ days

II. *Feeding and Digestion*

1. Did your baby have severe colic or any unusual feeding problems during the first three (3) months of life? .... No Yes
2. If on vitamins, what kind and how much? ______________________
3. If still on formula, which one do you use? _____
4. Is your child's appetite usually good? .... Yes No
5. Do any foods bother him/her? .... No Yes
6. Does he/she often have diarrhea or runny bowels? .... No Yes

III. *Baby Shots, Tests, and Development*

Has your child had:

1. A scar from smallpox vaccination? .... Yes No Year _____
2. All three of his/her DPT shots? .... Yes No Booster ___

3. All three doses of polio vaccine by mouth? .. Yes No Booster ___
4. Measles shot? .... Yes No
5. Skin test for TB? .... Yes No When ____
6. Rubella (German measles) shot? .... Yes No
7. Mumps shot? .... Yes No
8. Did your child sit alone before 7 months of age? .... Yes No
9. Did your child walk alone before 15 months of age? .... Yes No
10. Did your child say any words by 1½ years of age? .... Yes No
11. Is he/she as quick in learning as your other children? .... Yes No

IV. *Allergies*

Has your child had:

1. Eczema or hives? .... No Yes
2. Wheezing or asthma? .... No Yes
3. Allergies or reactions to any medicines or injections such as penicillin? .... No Yes
4. Does he/she have a constant cold, hay fever or sinus trouble? .... No Yes

V. *Family-Social History*

1. Are both parents in good health? .... Yes No
2. Are there any other members of your child's immediate family (brothers, sisters, parents, grandparents, aunts, uncles) with a serious health problem (mental or physical)? .... No Yes
   List each problem and who has it
   ____
3. How many people live in your home? Children_____ Adults_____
4. With whom does the child live? (circle one)
   Both parents Mother Father
   Legal guardian Other______________
5. Does anyone help you take care of your child on a regular basis? .... No Yes

VI. *Infections, Illnesses, and Other Problems*

Has your child:

1. Had *more* than six (6) colds or throat infections each year? .... No Yes
2. Had *more* than three (3) ear infections? .... No Yes
3. Had any trouble hearing? .... Yes No When_____
4. Had his/her hearing tested? .... Yes No When_____
5. Had any trouble seeing? .... No Yes
6. Had his/her eyes tested? .... Yes No When_____

7. Had any trouble with his/her teeth? .... No Yes
8. Seen a dentist recently? .... Yes No When_____
9. Had any trouble passing his/her urine? .... No Yes
10. Ever had a convulsion or fit or fainting spell? .. No Yes
11. Circle any of the following that your child has had: 3-day measles
    10-day measles Chicken pox
    Mumps Whooping cough
    Pneumonia
12. Had other diseases?________________
    Had to stay in the hospital overnight? .... No Yes
    Age_____ Hospital________________
    Reason________________________

VII. *Accidents*

1. Has your child had any serious accidents? ... No Yes
   Burns_____ Poisoning_____ Cuts needing a doctor_____ Broken bones_____
2. Does your child use seat belts and/or a safety chair in your car? .... Yes No
3. Do you know how to prevent infant smothering or choking? .... Yes No
4. Do you have firearms (loaded or unloaded) in your home? .... No Yes

VIII. *Behavior and Discipline*

1. Is he/she more difficult to raise than your other children? .... No Yes
2. What is the most effective way of disciplining your child? (circle) Spanking
   Sending to room
   Taking privileges away
   Other________________________
3. Are you concerned about any of the following? (circle which ones) Bad temper
   Will not mind Holds his breath
   Jealous Sleep problems
   Thumb sucking Nail biting
   Speech problems
   Cannot toilet train
   Very shy
   Does not pay attention
   Overactive Slow to learn
   Eats dirt or paint

Reviewed by________________________________

Printed by permission of Dr. Burris Duncan, Colorado General Hospital.

Example 6 History form for a child from 6 through 12 years

The pediatric clinic at Colorado General Hospital can provide either short-term emergency care or long-term continuous care. If your child is under the care of a private doctor or a convenient health clinic, we do not want to interfere with or duplicate the care you are receiving there.

My child usually gets his care at ______________________ and his last physical examination was _____ months or _____ years ago.

I am here for this visit only and my child receives his care elsewhere.
Yes_____ No_____
If your answer to the above question is Yes, there is no need to go any further with this questionnaire.

If you would like your child cared for in a private doctor's office or a public health facility more convenient to you, please ask to speak with one of the public health nurses.

If your child is not receiving care elsewhere and you want him to get his care here, you can help us take better care of him by answering the following questions:

I. *Pregnancy and Birth* *Circle one (1)*

1. Did you have any illnesses during your pregnancy? .... No Yes
2. Did you carry him/her for a full 9 months? .... Yes No
3. Where was your baby born?______________
4. How much did he/she weigh at birth?
_____lbs _____oz.
5. Did your baby have any trouble starting to breathe? .... No Yes
6. Did your baby have any trouble in the hospital? .... No Yes
7. Did your baby go home with you when you left the hospital? .... Yes No
8. How long did he/she stay in the hospital?
_____days

II. *Baby Shots, Tests, and Development*
Has your child had:

1. A scar from smallpox vaccination? .... Yes No Year_____
2. All three of his/her DPT shots? .... Yes No Booster____
3. All three doses of polio vaccine by mouth? .. Yes No Booster____
4. Measles shot? .... Yes No
5. Skin test for TB? .... Yes No When_____
6. Rubella (German measles) shot? .... Yes No
7. Mumps shot? .... Yes No

8. Did your child sit alone before 7 months of age? .... Yes No
9. Did your child walk alone before 15 months of age? .... Yes No
10. Did your child say any words by 1½ years of age? .... Yes No
11. Is he/she as quick in learning as your other children? .... Yes No

III. *Allergies*

Has your child had:

1. Eczema or hives? .... No Yes
2. Wheezing or asthma? .... No Yes
3. Allergies or reactions to any medicines or injections such as penicillin? .... No Yes
4. Does he/she have a constant cold, hay fever, or sinus trouble? .... No Yes

IV. *Accidents*

1. Has your child had any serious accidents? ... No Yes
   Burns_____ Poisoning_____
   Cuts needing a doctor_____
   Broken bones_____
2. Does your child use seat belts and/or a safety chair in your car? .... Yes No
3. Does your child know how to swim? .... Yes No
4. Do you have firearms (loaded or unloaded) in your home? .... No Yes

V. *Family-Social History*

1. Are both parents in good health? .... Yes No
2. Are there any other members of your child's immediate family (brothers, sisters, parents, grandparents, aunts, uncles) with a serious health problem (mental or physical)? .... No Yes
   List each problem and who has it:__________
   ____
3. How many people live in your home?
   Children_____ Adults_____
4. With whom does the child live? (circle one)
   Both parents Mother Father
   Legal guardian Other______________
5. Does anyone help you take care of your child on a regular basis? .... No Yes

VI. *Infections, Illnesses, and Other Problems*

Has your child:

1. Had *more* than six (6) colds or throat infections each year? .... No Yes

2. Had *more* than three (3) ear infections? .... No Yes
3. Had any trouble hearing? .... No Yes
4. Had his/her hearing tested? .... Yes No When_____
5. Had any trouble seeing? .... No Yes
6. Had his/her eyes tested? .... Yes No When_____
7. Had any trouble with his/her teeth? .... No Yes
8. Seen a dentist recently? .... Yes No When_____
9. Had any trouble passing his/her urine? .... No Yes
10. Ever had a convulsion or fit or fainting spell? .. No Yes
11. Circle any of the following that your child has had: 3-day measles 10-day measles
    Chicken pox Mumps
    Whooping cough Pneumonia
12. Had other diseases?____________________
13. Had to stay in the hospital overnight? .... No Yes
    Age_____ Hospital____________________
    Reason______________________________

VII. *Behavior and Discipline*

1. What school does your child attend?__________
   Grade_____
2. Does your child get along well in school? ..... Yes No
3. Have you met with the teacher? .... Yes No
4. Is the teacher worried about any problems? . No Yes
5. Does your child get along well with other children? .... Yes No
6. What is the most effective way of disciplining your child? (circle) Spanking
   Sending to room Taking privileges away
   Other______________________________
7. Are you concerned about any of the following? (circle which ones)
   Bad temper Will not mind
   Holds his breath Jealous
   Sleep problems Thumb sucking
   Nail biting Speech problems
   Cannot toilet train Wets bed
   Very shy Does not pay attention
   Overactive Slow to learn
   Eats dirt or paint

Reviewed by____

Printed by permission of Dr. Burris Duncan, Colorado General Hospital.

Example 7 History form for a child from 13 through 18 years

The pediatric clinic at Colorado General can provide either short-term emergency care or long-term continuous care. If you are under the care of a private doctor or a convenient health clinic, we do not want to interfere with or duplicate the care you are receiving there.

I usually get my care at ______________________ and my last physical examination was _____ months or _____ years ago.

I am here for this visit only and I receive my care elsewhere. Yes_____ No_____

If your answer to the above question is Yes, there is no need to go any further with this questionnaire.

I am too sick today to have my vision and hearing checked.
Yes_____ No_____

If you would like to get your care in a private doctor's office or a public health facility more convenient to you, please ask to speak with one of the public health nurses. If you are not receiving your care elsewhere and you want to get your care here, you can help us with your care by answering the following questions.

I. *Medical* — *Circle One (1)*

A. *Immunizations*

Do you have your immunization records with you today? .... No Yes
If not, please bring them on your next visit.

1. Did you get your DPT immunizations as an infant? .... Yes No
2. Date of last tetanus booster______________
3. Have you had the oral polio vaccine? .... Yes No
4. Have you had a tuberculin skin test in the past year? .... Yes No
5. Do you have a smallpox scar? .... Yes No
6. Have you had the German measles (rubella) vaccine? .... Yes No
7. Have you had German measles? .... Yes No
8. Have you had the measles (rubella) vaccine? . Yes No
9. Have you had measles (7-day)? .... Yes No
10. Have you had the mumps vaccine? .... Yes No
11. Have you had mumps? .... Yes No

B. *Past History*

1. Have you ever been hospitalized for illness or operations? .... No Yes
   Age_____ Hospital______________
   Reason______________________
2. Any other prolonged or serious illness? .... No Yes

3. Do you have any allergy (hives, wheezing, asthma, hay fever)? .... No Yes
4. Have you ever had a reaction (rash, hives, breathing difficulty) to any medicines or injections such as penicillin? .... No Yes
5. Are you taking any medicines now? .... No Yes
   If so, which ones?________

C. *Family History*
1. Are both your parents in good health? .... Yes No
2. Are there any other members of your immediate family (brothers, sisters, parents, grandparents, aunts, uncles) with a serious health problem (mental or physical)? .... No Yes
   List each problem and who has it:________
   ____
3. How many people live in your home? Children____ Adults____
4. With whom do you live? (circle one)
   Both parents Mother Father
   Legal guardian Other________
5. Do your parents get along well with each other? .... Yes No
6. Do you feel that your parents understand your problems? .... Yes No
7. Any long-term separations of the family? .... No Yes
8. Do you feel your parents (circle one)
   Are too strict Are too old fashioned
   Do not care
   Favor your brothers and sisters over you
   Are fair
9. Could things be better at home? .... No Yes

D. *Accidents*
1. Have you ever had any serious accidents? ... No Yes
   Burns____ Poisoning____
   Cuts needing a doctor____
   Broken bones____
2. Do you use seat belts in your car? .... Yes No
3. Do you know how to swim? .... Yes No
4. Are firearms (loaded or unloaded) kept in your home? .... No Yes

E. *Review of Systems*
1. Do you have any of the following complaints? (circle which ones)
   Headaches Dizzy spells Convulsions
   Difficulty hearing Blurred or double vision
   Sinus trouble Seizures

2. Do you wear glasses?_____ How long?_____
3. Last time you had your eyes checked______
4. Do you have swollen glands of the neck or under the arms? .... No Yes
5. Have you had pneumonia more than two times? .... No Yes
6. Do you get short of breath before other members of your class do? .... No Yes
7. Do you smoke?_____ How many packs per day?_____
8. Do you have a chronic cough? .... No Yes
9. Do you have a heart murmur? .... No Yes
10. Do you have (circle) Chest pain Abdominal pain Constipation Diarrhea Frequent vomiting
11. Have you ever had hepatitis (yellow eyes or skin)? .... No Yes
12. Have you had joint pain or swelling of joints? . No Yes
13. Have you ever had a kidney infection? .... No Yes
14. Does it burn when you pass your urine (water)? .... No Yes
15. Do you get up at night to urinate (pass water)? .... No Yes
16. Do you ever wet the bed? .... No Yes
17. Have you had venereal disease (VD)? .... No Yes
18. Do you have any questions about venereal disease? .... No Yes
19. Have you had recurrent fevers? .... No Yes
20. Do you have problems with acne? .... No Yes
21. Do you have problems with your teeth? .... No Yes
22. Are you tired in the morning when you get up? .... No Yes

II. *Individual Patterns*

1. What grade are you in?_____ Are you satisfied with your grades? .... Yes No
2. Do you miss more than 3 days of school each month? .... No Yes
3. Is something slowing your progress at school? .... No Yes
4. Do your teachers pick on you? .... No Yes
5. Is school (circle) A drag A means to an end Meaningless Worthwhile
6. What do you plan to do when you graduate?
____
7. Do you make friends easily? .... Yes No

8. Do you often feel left out? .... No Yes
9. Do things get on your nerves easily? .... No Yes
10. Do you feel that you are a nervous person? . No Yes
11. Do drugs make you feel better? .... No Yes
    Which ones?________________________
12. Do you take drugs when you are alone? .... No Yes
13. Would you like to learn more about the prevention of pregnancy? .... No Yes

For Girls Only

1. Have you had your first period?_____ At what age?_____
2. Would you like to learn more about periods? No Yes
3. Do you have cramping with your periods? .... No Yes
4. Are your periods regular? .... Yes No
5. Are you taking the "pill"? .... No Yes
6. Would you like more information about the "pill"? .... No Yes

Printed by permission of Dr. Burris Duncan, Colorado General Hospital.

BIBLIOGRAPHY

Garrett, Annette: *Interviewing: Its Principles and Methods,* New York: Family Service Association of America, 1970.

Golden, Phyllis, and Barbara Russell: "Therapeutic Communication," *American Journal of Nursing,* vol. 69, no. 9, September 1969, pp. 1928–1930.

Green, Morris, and Julius Richmond: *Pediatric Diagnosis,* Philadelphia: Saunders, 1962, pp. 3–12.

——— and Robert J. Haggerty: *Ambulatory Pediatrics,* Philadelphia: Saunders, pp. 110–118.

Hurst, Willis J., and H. Kenneth Walker: *The Problem-oriented System,* New York: Medcom, 1972.

Korsch, Barbara M., Barbara Freemon, and Vida Negrete: "Practical Implications of Doctor-Patient Interaction Analysis for Pediatric Practice," *American Journal of Diseases of Children,* vol. 121, February 1971, pp. 110–114.

Silver, Henry K., C. Henry Kempe, and Henry B. Bruyn: *Handbook of Pediatrics,* California: Lange, 1972, pp. 1-4.

Shulman, J. L.: *Management of Emotional Disorders in Pediatric Practice,* Chicago: Year Book, 1970, pp. 109–125.

Weed, Lawrence L.: "Medical Records That Guide and Teach," *New England Journal of Medicine,* Mar. 14 and 21, 1968, pp. 593-600 and 652–657.

Chapter 2

Neonatology

Certainly an important part of ambulatory pediatrics for nurses is an in-depth knowledge and understanding of the neonate. Ideally, the nurse will begin her care of the child during the gestational period, but if this is impossible, it is important to make every attempt to begin with the newborn in the delivery room or as soon as possible after birth. Even if the nurse is unable to follow the infant's gestational development, she should at least be aware of the importance of the period and the various influences that make their impact during this time. The mother's (and father's) health and circumstances from pregestation through delivery are of utmost importance to the health and well-being of the newborn child. In spite of the increased amount of time and research that have in recent years been devoted to the growing field of perinatology, surprisingly little is known about these influences. This chapter will discuss some of what is known, particularly concerning possible influences which may prove detrimental to the child's health.

FACTORS AFFECTING THE CHILD'S HEALTH

Genetic Defects

At the moment of conception itself some important aspects of the child's health are determined that can lay down the foundations for certain problems that will display themselves in the newborn nursery. Both chromosomes and genes are determined at this time, and defects in either can cause serious problems. Chromosomal abnormalities of any type, whether translocations, deletions, or trisomies, can result in various problems, often of a severe nature. Sometimes these abnormalities will be detectable at birth (e.g., trisomies E, D, and G; cri-du-chat syndrome; and Down's syndrome). Other times they may be more easily missed in the newborn period, but will show up later (this may be the case, for instance, with Turner's or Klinefelter's syndromes). Defects in the genetic material itself can also occur and result in such important problems as galactosemia and PKU.

Blood Group Incompatibilities

The blood group is also determined at the moment of conception; this may or may not pose a potential problem for the infant. In general, mother's blood will remain separate from that of the infant, but there are some times at which there may be a small amount of mixture. This is most common during the actual delivery, particularly if oxytoxics are used or if manual removal of the placenta is necessary. Even with such mixture, no problem is created unless an incompatibility exists between the child's and the mother's blood types.

About two-thirds of these incompatibilities will be of an ABO type. The most common type of ABO incompatibility is that in which the mother's blood type is O and the infant's is either A or B. In such a situation, a woman with type O blood has already formed antibodies to blood types A and B, and so no previous sensitization is necessary; the first time there is any mixing between her blood and her baby's, a reaction can occur. For this reason, a first baby is commonly affected. The same mechanism is possible if mother's blood type is A and her infant's is B (or vice versa), although these situations are less common. An ABO incompatibility is generally much less severe than an Rh incompatibility and, in addition, may provide some protection against an Rh incompatibility.

Most of the remaining blood group incompatibilities arise from differences in the Rh factor between mother and infant (there are a few other rare types of incompatibilities such as those involving the Duffy and Kell factors, but the principle is basically the same). Rh incompatibilities exist only when the mother is Rh negative and the infant is Rh positive. Although the Rh-negative woman normally does not secrete antibodies against the Rh factor, she will do so if her blood has at any time in the past been exposed to the Rh factor. Usually this will be caused by a previous pregnancy in which the infant was Rh positive and there was some blood exchange during the last trimester or, more likely, during delivery. It is also possible, although less likely, that she may have been sensitized by a previous abortion or blood transfusion or even by vitamin K shots that were processed from blood and given to newborns in the 1940s. In such a situation in which the mother's blood does contain antibodies against the Rh factor, these antibodies may react against the baby's Rh antigen if he is Rh positive. The result will be destruction of the infant's red blood cells, causing both an anemia and an excess of bilirubin (the breakdown product from the destroyed red blood cells). The bilirubin in turn results in a clinically visible jaundice, and more importantly, in kernicterus; this is erythroblastosis fetalis. The best approach to this problem is prevention, and the administration of RhoGam to the mother within 72 hours after birth should prevent an unsensitized woman from becoming sensitized. It is important that this be given after all Rh-incompatible births and all abortions of an Rh-negative woman. If a woman has already been sensitized, it is important that she be followed closely with frequent blood titers to measure any Rh antibodies she may have formed. Once a titer becomes positive for such antibodies, amniocentesis will usually be necessary. The withdrawn amniotic fluid must be studied for concentrations of bilirubin, and the physician then must weigh the dangers presented by the erythroblastosis against those which would be presented by prematurity should the pregnancy be interrupted. At times when the bilirubin has reached dangerous levels but the infant is still too premature to deliver, the physician may decide to do an intrauterine transfusion. Generally this decision will be determined by how far along the pregnancy is and how severe the concentration of bilirubin is.

At birth, an infant born from a sensitized pregnancy must be monitored closely. Assessment includes close observation for increase of jaundice as well as frequent laboratory determinations of bilirubin. Although the severely threatened infant may be jaundiced within 30 minutes after birth, it is more common for the jaundice to appear within 24 to 36 hours. High levels of unconjugated bilirubin (i.e., indirect reacting bilirubin) accompanied by reduced albumin-binding capacity is an indication for intervention. These tests will be more completely discussed later in this chapter. Intervention may be in the form of phototherapy (unconjugated bilirubin exposed to intense fluorescent lights decomposes in the skin and reduces the level of serum bilirubin). Although some controversy about this treatment exists, the objections are primarily hypothetical and long term, and there is as yet not enough evidence to evaluate them completely. In more severe situations, intervention may be in the form of exchange transfusion. In some places, phenobarbitol is being used as a therapy, but this method is still in the experimental stage.

Health of the Mother

Infectious Diseases Another important influence on the newborn's health is the health of the mother during her pregnancy. It appears that in general, diseases of the mother are likely to have ill effects on the fetus. Some specifics are known about certain diseases which adversely affect the baby, but there are many more about which little is known. Infections during pregnancy are a prime concern, and mothers will frequently ask just what effect various infections will have on the unborn child. Much has been written in the lay literature about certain infections, and it is something pregnant women are likely to be quite concerned about. In general, viral diseases appear to be more dangerous to the fetus than bacterial diseases. Presumably, this is due to the fact that a virus is smaller than a bacteria and more likely to pass through the placental barrier. Some specific viruses have been studied in great detail. Concerning others less is known.

Certainly rubella or German measles is the best-known viral infection of pregnancy. Actually, in this country most women who are now of childbearing age had rubella when they were children and are now immune, and thus cannot transport the virus to their children. However, about 10 to 20 percent of the women in this age group show no rubella antibodies; that is, they are susceptible to the infection. All pregnant women should have a blood test done to determine whether they are susceptible to rubella. If the test shows an antibody concentration of over 1:10, the woman is generally considered protected. It is important that this information be clearly explained to the mother, since many women are concerned about this but fail to ask any direct questions. If a woman is not protected, it is important that she know this also, both in order to try to avoid such exposure during the first 3 months and also so that she may have the opportunity to decide whether she wants to receive the vaccine postpartum (with the understanding that she take precautions to ensure that she does not become pregnant for 3 months after receiving the vaccine). Of susceptible pregnant women who are infected with rubella in the 1st month of pregnancy, about 33 to 50 percent will infect their infants. If not infected until the 2nd month, only 25 percent will transmit the infection. If not infected until the 3rd month, only 9 percent of the infants will be involved, and if the mother is not infected until the 4th month, only about 4 percent of the fetuses will suffer. The infections which are transmitted to the infant during the first trimester tend to be the most severe and result in various neonatal problems, most often in congenital heart disease, cataract formation, glaucoma, babies who are small for gestational age and who have splenomegaly and hepatomegaly as well as microencephaly and other neurological difficulties. Babies who are infected during the 4th month are more likely to suffer from hearing defects.

Cytomegalovirus infection (CID) is another virus transmitted either transplacentally or through the ascending route from the cervix. In this situation, the mother is usually asymptomatic and the disease is pinpointed only because of the virus excretion in her urine. However, many normal women and some normal newborns also excrete the virus in their urine. Cytomegalovirus disease can cause symptoms of jaundice, splenomegaly, and hepatomegaly, as well as problems such as microcephaly, chorioretinitis, and brain calcification, although the severity of the disease ranges from asymptomatic carriers to fatality. Lab studies which isolate the virus in the urine or in the IgM fraction of the blood or which show brain calcification may be helpful in establishing the diagnosis. There is no treatment for this disease.

Maternal infection with herpes virus can also cause problems in the neonate. There are two distinct types of herpes virus. Type 1 is the kind most commonly found in the lesions of the lips and gums of older children and adults. It is almost always found above the waist. Type 2, on the other hand, usually occurs on the cervix, vagina, and external genitalia. This is the type which poses the problem for the neonate, who can be infected by the ascending route or through direct contact during the birth process. It can occur in systemic form in the newborn, in which case it is about 96 percent fatal; or it can occur in more specific areas, most commonly in the skin, eye, central nervous system, or all three areas. In this form, the disease is 25 percent fatal and neurological sequelae occur in 50 percent of the survivors. Neurological symptoms may consist of convulsions, floppiness, and bulging fontanelle. Vesicles all over the body will be found in about 33 percent of these babies, and fever will also occur in about a third of them. Splenomegaly and jaundice are other symptoms. These symptoms may be present at birth or may appear in 3 to 4 weeks.

A protozoan disease which can also be quite devastating to the fetus is toxoplasmosis. This can be transmitted from an infected, but usually asymptomatic, woman to her unborn child. Although the newborn may also appear asymptomatic for the first few weeks after birth, the child may then develop a variety of symptoms including anemia, petechiae, ecchymosis, and neurological symptoms such as coma, convulsions, micro- or hydrocephaly, and hypotonia. In the infant this is an extremely serious situation with a 12 percent mortality rate. The majority of infants surviving it exhibit rather severe problems.

Syphilis, a spirochete, must also be considered among the infectious diseases of the mother which can affect the infant. This organism will not cross the placenta for the first 16 to 18 weeks of gestation, and if a VDRL reveals its presence, treatment of the mother before that time will prevent difficulties in the infant. If it is not treated or if the woman contracts syphilis after this time period, it will cross the placenta causing serious problems in the newborn. These babies are usually small for gestational age, exhibit hepatosplenomegaly, and may have snuffles and lesions on the skin and mucous membranes. Often the placenta appears large and boggy. Dark-field examination of the placental or cord tissues will reveal the spirochete.

Little is actually known about bacterial infections although it is generally believed that they are less damaging to the infant than viral infections. Gonorrhea is a bacterial disease which can cause blindness if it infects the infant's eyes during the birth process. This was at one time a frequent cause of blindness, but since the advent of silver nitrate, the incidence has been greatly decreased. Silver nitrate, although more irritating to the eyes, appears to be more efficient than the various antibiotic ointments used in some hospitals. It is possible that difficulty with this problem may increase with the current increase in numbers of home deliveries.

Noninfectious Diseases Certain noninfectious diseases of the mother may also have strongly detrimental effects on the newborn. Diabetes in a woman can significantly complicate a pregnancy. Her infant is likely to be large for gestational age, with the associated problems of hypoglycemia and sometimes a more difficult delivery. Prematurity with its accompanying hyaline membrane disease is also more likely, as is renal vein thrombosis, hypocalcemia, and hypobilirubinemia. The more severe the maternal disease, the more severe the problems for the newborn; the most significant aspect of the maternal disease is how much vessel involvement is present. Gestational diabetes (the phenomenon in which a woman spills sugar into her urine only while she is pregnant) is less detrimental to the infant, but is not innocuous. Maternal endocrine problems such as hypothyroidism, hyperthyroidism, and hyperparathyroidism, as well as circulatory disturbances such as rheumatic or congenital heart disease and chronic hypertension which compromises the placental transfer will also jeopardize the health of the infant. Glomerulonephritis, which increases the chances of prematurity, as well as conditions such as supine hypotension, hemorrhage, pneumonia, anemia, and uncontrolled epilepsy, which decrease the oxygen supply, might also be listed here.

Maternal Nutrition The question of maternal nutrition has really not been adequately researched. It would certainly seem that lack of specific important nutrients would affect the growth of the infant and that general malnutrition would result in the infant being small for gestational age, with all the problems that implies. One study done during World War II showed that although malnutrition resulted in lower fertility, the infants that were born did not seem to be affected.

Maternally Ingested Drugs Drugs can certainly be another important factor in the prenatal environment. It is a well-known fact that babies of heroin addicts and even those of mothers on methadone go through withdrawal shortly after birth. Many other maternally ingested drugs are also known to affect the baby, and there are probably many more about which we know very little. Table 2-1 is a list of drugs currently known to affect the fetus.

Other Other maternal characteristics and habits are also important. Age must be considered; a woman over 35 or under 16 has greatly increased chances of neonatal morbidity and mortality. A pregnancy in which the woman weighs less than 100 lbs or more than 200 lbs is also more likely to run into difficulty, as is one in very high altitudes or in which the mother is a heavy cigarette smoker. Previous pregnancy experience is an excellent

Table 2-1 Maternally Ingested Drugs Which Affect the Fetus

Maternal medication	Effects on fetus and newborn
Drugs to control epilepsy	Low levels of coagulation factors II, VII, IX, and X
Vitamin K analogues in excess	Hemolysis and kernicterus
Bishydroxycoumarin (Dicumarol)	Hemorrhage
Ethyl biscoumacetate (Tromexan)	Hemorrhage
Sodium warfarin (Coumadin)	Hemorrhage
Salicylates in large amounts	Neonatal bleeding
Sulfonamides	Kernicterus
Nitrofurantoin (Furadantin)	Hemolysis in susceptible fetuses, kernicterus
Tetracyclines	Inhibition of bone growth; staining of deciduous teeth
Potassium iodide	Goiter
Propylthiouracil	Goiter
Methimazole (Tapazole)	Goiter
Ammonium chloride	Acidosis
Reserpine	Stuffy nose; obstructed breathing
Morphine or heroin chronically	Addiction; withdrawal symptoms
Androgens	Masculinization
Some progestins	Masculinization
Tolbutamide (Orinase)	Neonatal hypoglycemia
Chlorothiazide	Thrombocytopenia
Quinine	Thrombocytopenia
Cephalothin (Keflin)	Positive direct Coombs test

Source: Louis Hellman and Jack Pritchard, *William's Obstetrics,* New York: Appleton-Century-Crofts, p. 343 (Table 2). By permission.

predictor of the success of a current pregnancy. Women with a history of previous premature labor, previous neonatal death or anomaly, more than six previous pregnancies, any previous fertility problems, or any other type of prior pregnancy or delivery problems are at a significantly increased risk for the present pregnancy. Various workers have attempted to "risk" pregnancies by assigning varying values to certain of these factors, adding them up, and then assigning them to a high-, low- or medium-risk category. (See Tables 2-2 and 2-3.)

Assessing Infant Health before Birth

Recent advances in laboratory techniques have resulted in a greatly increased ability to assess the well-being of the infant before birth. It is important for the nurse working in this area to be aware of some of these techniques and how to interpret them. Analysis of amniotic fluid can be extremely useful. It is possible to obtain samples of amniotic fluid as early as 12 weeks, and in general, the procedure of amniocentesis is quite safe, although such rare complications as abortion, maternal hemorrhage, fetal hemorrhage, fetal puncture, and infection have been reported. The most

Table 2-2 Neonatal Morbidity Risk

	Risk based on antenatal information only, percent risk	Risk based on antenatal, intrapartum, and immediate condition of newborn, percent risk
Previous neonatal death	8.1	
Previous low-birth-weight infant	5.1	
Mother's age less than 17 years	6.0	
Incompetent cervix	32.5	
Placenta previa, abruptio, antepartum hemorrhage	31.0	
Attempted abortion, suicide, drug intoxication	13.8	
Prolapsed cord	17.1	
Breech position	13.5	
Other labor complications*	27.2	23.8
Abnormal presentation at delivery	24.6	10.7
Maternal diabetes	40.7	33.3
Rh and other isoimmunization	39.4	34.5
Abdominal/major surgery, accident, antepartum	30.5	14.0
Premature rupture of membranes	27.6	12.3
Toxemia	22.4	14.0
Amniocentesis	7.8	6.6
Multiple gestation	7.2	−8.5
Prenatal care:		
None	9.4	4.2
1–3 visits	7.6	3.8
4–7 visits	4.4	3.0
more than 8 visits	1.3	2.2
Fetal distress	11.5	5.2
Cesarean section	10.5	5.5
Other delivery complications		10.4
Mother's age more than 30 years		2.7
Male infant		1.8
Active resuscitation, delivery room		8.3
		Birth weight–gestional age morbidity score (from chart) × .78 ☐
	Total ☐	Total ☐

* Induction, pit stimulation, uterine inertia, contracted pelvis. Based on UCMC liveborn data, July 1, 1966 to June 30, 1968.

Source: Dr. Lulu Lubchenko, University of Colorado Medical Center.

Table 2-3 Neonatal Mortality Risk*

Variable	Score
Constant	−12
Birth weight, grams	
500 or less	686
501-1,000	611
1,001-1,250	364
1,251-1,500	144
1,501-2,000	75
2,001-2,500	14
2,501-3,500	7
3,501-4,000	0
4,001 or more	14
Gestational age, weeks	
27 or less	217
28–29	80
30–31	44
32–33	22
34–35	7
36–39	2
40–41	0
42–43	5
44 or more	7
Unknown	7
Mother's age over 40	23
Previous neonatal death	175
Fetal deaths (more than 2)	13
Condition at birth	
Good (Apgar 8–10)	0
Fair (Apgar 5–7)	6
Poor (Apgar 0–4)	95
Toxemia	22
Fetal distress	9
Multiple birth	−49
Endotracheal aspiration or positive pressure resusitation	14
Total	

* Encircle the scores which apply and add to get neonatal death score.
Source: Dr. Lulu Lubchenko, University of Colorado Medical Center.

common laboratory study done on amniotic fluid is an assessment of the level of bilirubin. Bilirubin levels normally peak at about 16 to 20 weeks and then gradually drop. Bilirubin should be completely gone from the amniotic fluid by 36 weeks. In certain situations, such as the case of an Rh-jeopardized infant, the level may continue to rise.

Estriols, a form of estrogen, are currently the focus of much research. Estriols are normally present in large amounts in maternal urine toward the end of pregnancy. Twenty-four-hour values are expected to fall in the range of 12 to 50 mg/ml. Very low levels alert the physician to fetal distress. A level of 7 to 12 is usually assumed to predict trouble in the postnatal period, while levels of 1 to 7 indicate possible trouble during the actual labor and delivery. A level below 1 indicates fetal death in utero. Monitoring of estriols is particularly useful in diabetes, toxemia, hypertension, and postmaturity. Levels will sometimes be depressed in the presence of a small-for-gestational-age infant or an infant with congenital anomalies and failure to thrive. There are times when estriol levels are depressed for no apparent reason. Estriol levels are not good indicators for all types of fetal distress, however: Rh sensitization, eclampsia, renal problems, and certain drugs can result in damage to the fetus which is not reflected in the estriol levels.

The creatinine level is another important laboratory study during pregnancy, and it will be discussed more fully under the description of gestational aging. In general, unless there is a maternal renal system problem, a level of 1.8 to 2.0 indicates that the fetus is 36 or more weeks. A lecithin sphingomyelin ratio is important for the same purpose—establishing gestational age—and it too will be discussed later in this chapter.

There are other less frequently utilized studies of amniotic fluid. DAO (diamine oxidase) quantification is sometimes used in a manner similar to the estriol determination. It is possible to study amniotic fluid for Barr bodies when it is important to discover the sex of the unborn child. This is probably most useful in situations when a sex-linked disease like hemophilia is a possibility, and an abortion might be desired if the child were male. Biochemical studies for certain diseases like galactosemia and G_6PD as well as analysis for bilirubin levels and certain viral studies are also possible.

Labor and Delivery

Drugs Certain factors during the actual labor and delivery are also important influences on the health of the newborn. Drugs received by the mother during labor and delivery are of much interest, although a great deal is still unknown about them (Table 2-4). Apparently all drugs commonly used for pain relief during labor cross the placental barrier, and most of them can be shown to result in some depression of the baby. Any measures useful in helping the mother with nonmedicinal relief of pain (e.g., certain breathing techniques, interpersonal support, hypnotism, acupuncture) must surely be of great benefit to the newborn. Barbiturates, although not actually pain relievers, do help to allay apprehension and are sometimes used during

Table 2-4 Drugs Received during Labor and Delivery Which Affect the Fetus

Drug	Effects
*Barbiturates**	
Long-acting (Phenobarbital)	Neonatal respiratory depression
Intermediate-acting (Amobarbital)	Neonatal respiratory depression
Short-acting (Secobarbital, Pentobarbital)	Less neonatal depression
Ultra-short-acting (Thiopental)	Less neonatal depression
*Tranquilizers**	
Chlorpromazine (Thorazine)	Hazard of maternal hypotension and secondary fetal hypoxia; no appreciable depressant action on the fetus and neonate
Promethazine (Phenergan) Perphenazine (Trilafon) Prochlorperazine (Compazine) Hydroxyzine (Atarax, Vistaril) Meprobamate (Miltown, Equanil) Methylpentynol (Dormison) Benzodiazepines (Chlordiazepoxide, Diazepam); used in toxemia	No appreciable depressant action on fetus and neonate
Reserpine	Nasal congestion with respiratory distress, excessive secretions, lethargy, bradycardia
Hypnotics and sedatives	
Chloral hydrate	No evidence of effects on fetus and neonate
Ethyl alcohol	Respiratory depression (?), hypoglycemia (?)
Paraldehyde	If given in large doses to mother, may cause respiratory depression or drowsiness of infant
Thalidomide	Phocomelia
Belladonna derivatives	
Atropine	Tachycardia, mydriasis
Scopolamine	Mydriasis, slight depressant action on infant
Narcotics (dose and time interval between administration and delivery are important in neonatal depression)	
Morphine Heroin Methadone Meperidine (Demerol) Alphaprodine (Nisentil) Levorphanol (Dromoran) Codeine	All have respiratory depressant action

* Barbiturates and some tranquilizers may potentiate the depressant effects of inhalation agents and narcotics.

Table 2-4 Drugs Received during Labor and Delivery Which Affect the Fetus *(Cont'd)*

Drug	Effects
Narcotic antagonists	
Nalorphine (Nalline) Levallorphan (Lorfan)	May have respiratory depressant action
Gaseous and volatile anesthetics	
Chloroform	No appreciable effect on newborn
Ether	Neonatal depression directly related to depth and duration of maternal anesthesia
Cyclopropane	Respiratory depression of the newborn
Nitrous oxide	No effect if oxygen concentration is adequate
Trichlorethylene (Trilene)	Some respiratory depression of the newborn
Halothane (Fluothane)	Maternal hypotension with possible fetal hypoxia
Local anesthetics	
Lidocaine (xylocaine) and others	Direct injection into fetus, intoxication; indirect effects—maternal hypotension with possible fetal hypoxia
Skeletal muscle relaxants (neuromuscular blocking agents)	
Curare	No direct effect on the infant
Succinylcholine chloride (Anectine)	Effect on infant (?)
Gallamine triethiodide (Flaxedyl)	May affect the infant

Source: Sophie H. Pierog and Angelo Ferrara: *Approach to the Medical Care of the Sick Newborn,* St. Louis: Mosby, 1971, p. 208; compiled from A.W. Brann, Jr. and J.M. Montalvo: *Pediatrics Clinics of North America,* vol. 17, 1970, p. 851; S.N. Cohen and W.A. Olson: *Pediatrics Clinics of North America,* vol. 17, 1970, p. 835; E.V. Cosmi and G. Marx: *Anesthesiology,* vol. 30, 1969, p 238; F.W. Hehre, R. Hook, and E.H. Hon: *Anesth. Analg.,* vol. 48, 1969, p. 909; G. Marx and L.R. Orkin: *Physiology of Obstetric Enesthesia,* Springfield, Ill.: Charles Thomas, 1969; F. Moya and V. Thorndike: *American Journal of Obstetrics and Gynecology,* vol. 84, 1962, p. 1778; W.L. Nyhan: *Journal of Pediatrics,* vol. 59, p. 1, 1961.

the early stages of labor. All types, whether long-acting like phenobarbital, intermediate-acting like amobarbital, short-acting like secobarbital and pentabarbital, or ultra-short-acting like thiopental, cross the placenta, and it is important to give them long enough before delivery that their effect has worn off by the time the infant is born. There is no antidote to neonatal depression caused by barbiturates, and artificial respiration will be necessary for such babies. The American Academy of Pediatrics suggests limiting barbiturates given to mothers to 1½ gr phenobarbital or secobarbital by mouth or rectum early in labor. This dose is useful as a sedative only; other drugs must be used if analgesics are necessary. For analgesia, the academy mentions morphine and demerol in as small a dose as possible for effective relief of pain. It must be consistent, they mention, with the "pain threshold, the state of health and size of the mother, the maturity and condition of the fetus, as well as the advancement of labor."

Anesthetics are of two basic types: local and general. General anesthesia is certainly more likely to affect the infant. It is delivered either as a gas by mask or as a liquid by IV and reaches the baby in about 2 minutes. The longer and deeper the anesthesia, the more depressed the infant. The Academy of Pediatrics ranks the depressive characteristics of the frequently used anesthetics in this order, starting from the least potent: nitrous oxide, ethylene, cyclopropane, ether, trichloroethylene (Trilene) and chloroform. The academy further states that there is only one indication for deep anesthesia and that is uterine spasm. In this case ether or chloroform will probably be necessary, and preparations must be made immediately for artificial ventilation of the baby, who will be born with respiratory depression.

Regional anesthesia consists of either a local infiltration of the pudendal nerve or spinal anesthesia. Unless an anesthetist is present, there are far safer methods of pain relief. The two main danger signs encountered with these agents are hypotension and convulsions. In either case oxygen must be given, since a decreased oxygen level is available to the baby in these circumstances. In hypotension, the nurse should also raise the mother's legs and lower her head; sometimes rolling her onto her left side is also useful, since the weight of the pregnant uterus may be blocking the aortic blood flow. With convulsions a small amount of barbiturates is also given intravenously. There are two basic types of local anesthetics: esters and amides. Esters such as procaine have the disadvantage of poor penetration of maternal tissues but may be better for the baby. Amides like lidocaine, prilocaine, and mepivacaine penetrate the maternal tissues better, act faster and longer, and provide better anesthetic for the mother, but they remain in the infant for a longer time whether given by epidural or paracervical route. If given as a spinal, there is a greater chance of maternal hypotension. They are extremely useful as a substitute for a general anesthetic in C sections.

Prolonged Labor Prolonged labor is also a threat to the health of the infant. By definition a prolonged labor consists of a first and second state of more than 20 hours in either a primiparous or multiparous woman (first and second stage combined equal the time from the first contraction to a dilatation of 10 cm), over 2 hours of second stage (the stage from complete dilatation to birth) for the primiparous mother or over 1 hour of second stage for the multiparous mother. In such situations separation of the placenta may cause hypoxia, cord compression is more likely, and infection (particularly if the membranes have been ruptured) is more common. The two most common causes of prolonged labor are pelvic contractures (present in about 5 percent of the white population and 15 percent of United States Blacks), which cause pressure on the head, and abnormal presentations. Breech presentations do not generally prolong labor unless they are accompanied by a small pelvis. There are three basic types of breech deliveries; frank breech, in which the buttocks come first; a complete breech, in which both the buttocks and feet appear first; and an incomplete or footling breech, in which one or both feet constitute the presenting part. Breech deliveries have a mortality rate three to four times higher than that of cephalic presentations as well as a higher morbidity. Frequently this morbidity is caused by trauma from the increased cephalic pressure, which can result in intracranial damage, spinal cord injuries from stretching of the back, abdominal hemorrhages, dislocated hips, brachial plexus palsy, broken humerus and femur, and prolapsed cords. In addition, breech presentations are often associated with placenta previa, which also presents problems for the infants. The early separation of the placenta in placenta previa can result in hypoxia. This is more likely in a total previa, slightly less likely in a partial previa, and least likely, but still possible, in a low-lying previa.

Abruptions Abruptions are another placental cause of difficulty for the fetus. Eighty percent of placental abruptions are marginal; that is, the separation occurs along the outer margin of the placenta. These usually present the symptom of frank vaginal bleeding. The other 20 percent of abruptions are central, and since the bleeding is not allowed to escape through the margin of the placenta, this type is more likely to go unrecognized. Either type, however, presents problems for the baby. Since less surface area of the placenta is in contact with the mother's circulatory system, hypoxia from lowered oxygen transfer may result. The problem of prematurity may result from early stimulation of labor, causing further problems for the infant, and finally, the hemorrhage and blood loss can result in fetal shock and lack of sufficient oxygen to the infant's brain.

Cord Prolapse Cord prolapse is another complication of the labor and delivery process which may compromise the infant. It is most common in breech or multiple births, premature rupture of the membranes, and transverse lies. It is sometimes first detected while the nurse is doing a pelvic and can actually feel the cord, or it may be initially suspected by a monitor pattern of variable deceleration. Cords wrapped around the neck are not often a problem unless the cord is abnormally short, and they can usually be slipped over the infant's head rather easily at the time of delivery. True knots in the cord are a problem causing possible hypoxia to the infant, although they are much more rare than is usually thought.

Mechanical Injuries Mechanical injuries to the fetus are another hazard of the delivery itself. Sometimes these are limited to the skin and subcutaneous tissue. Usually these are less important, but they may be a clue that more serious damage coexists in the deeper anatomy. Common examples of these problems are caput succedaneum, cyanosis, edema of the buttocks and upper or lower extremities, diffuse scalp hemorrhage, subcutaneous fat necrosis (pressure necrosis), abrasion of the skin, petechiae, and ecchymosis. Trauma to the skull is also a possibility, but, like skin trauma, is usually not terribly serious unless it is associated with underlying brain damage. Molding, cephalhematoma, and fractures (either linear or depressed) are examples of trauma in this area. Long bones such as the clavicle, humerus, and femur may also be fractured in the delivery process and should be carefully checked in the nursery physical. Ocular signs of trauma such as subconjunctival (scleral) hemorrhage and retinal hemorrhage are common and generally innocuous. Abrasion of the cornea is also found in some babies. Damage to the central nervous system, such as hemorrhage into the brain substance, subdural hematoma, and spinal cord injury, is usually a matter of great concern, and the initial physical should include careful attention to these possibilities. Peripheral nerves may also be damaged, and this damage may be either permanent or caused temporarily by such things as pressure from nearby edema. Facial paralysis, brachial plexus injury, and phrenic nerve injury should be considered in this category. Hemorrhage into the abdominal organs, such as the liver, spleen, kidney, or adrenals, is another possibility.

Detecting Fetal Diffculties

Modern technology has greatly increased our ability to detect fetal difficulties before delivery and to be able to judge more accurately when it is appropriate to intervene in a labor and delivery process. Fetal monitors, both internal and external, are gathering more and more support and may well prove the most useful advance in perinatology to date.

There are three basic deceleration patterns of the fetal heart tones which monitors are capable of detecting and which we know are of significance. Early deceleration in which a slowing of the heart rate is shown beginning early in the contraction, lasting not longer than 90 seconds (usually not longer than 30 seconds), and not falling below a rate of 100 per minute is a normal pattern of deceleration which results from the normal compression of the head during contractions. Blood gases pH of the blood remain normal. A second pattern of late deceleration occurs later in the contractions. Such deceleration still usually lasts not longer than 90 seconds, and the rate does not often fall below 120 per minute, although it will sometimes reach as low as 60. This pattern may be accompanied by a low PO_2 and PCO_2 and is an indication of fetal distress. The third pattern is called variable deceleration. This is the situation when the deceleration seems to bear no relation to the contractions, the rate is below 100 per minute, and the length may vary from 10 seconds to several minutes. This can be accompanied by acidosis although it is not usually. This ability to monitor the fetus for dangerous deceleration patterns should enable us to improve significantly our care of the unborn child. It is probable, although not certain, that these fetal heart rate changes precede the dangerous biochemical changes so that intervention may enable us to lessen or prevent completely the damage done by such biochemical changes.

The monitoring of blood gases is another useful tool in detecting prenatally an infant's difficulty. This is done by testing capillary blood from the scalp during the actual labor. The pH of this blood correlates best with the fetal well-being. The normal range is 7.25 to 7.35; anything below 7.20 indicates distress. Serial readings are much more accurate, and two consecutive readings below 7.15 are considered indication for a C section. Although it is estimated that in about 10 percent of cases the mother's pH will be unusual, resulting in misleading readings for the baby, readings of the pH remain an excellent tool for assessing the status of the child. Another danger sign detectable in the analysis of blood from the fetal scalp is a decrease in PO_2 and an increase in PCO_2 because of lactic acid and carbon dioxide accumulation.

CARE OF THE NEWBORN IN THE DELIVERY ROOM

Although at the present time very few nurses are actually in charge of delivering babies, the nurse's role in the delivery room is quite important from the point of view of both the baby and the mother. It is important that the nurse be aware of any circumstances during the delivery which will affect the health of the infant. The position of the delivery, any difficulty encountered during delivery, and the condition of the amniotic fluid are all early important observations. Meconium-stained amniotic fluid should alert the nurse to the fact that the infant is in distress; odor from the amniotic fluid may be a clue to infection. Immediately after the baby is delivered, the physician will usually hold the infant in a head-down position and suction the nose and oropharynx with a bulb syringe. Usually both the baby and the bulb syringe are then handed to the nurse. If respirations are obstructed, continued suctioning is necessary; if not, the infant is then placed on a table which has been positioned in a 15° Trendelenberg position to help drainage of blood and mucous from the upper airways. The infant is then dried with a towel and exposed to radiant heat. A neonate has very poor thermal regulation, and it is essential that chilling be avoided, since this may cause many problems, the most common of which is a lowered blood sugar with resultant decrease of glucose available for the brain.

Assessing the Newborn

At 1 minute after delivery the nurse or physician performs the Apgar (see Table 2-5). About 90 percent of the infants born in this country receive

Table 2-5 Infant Evaluation at Birth

	0	1	2
Heart rate	Absent	Slow (below 100)	Over 100
Respiratory effort	Absent	Slow or irregular	Good crying
Muscle tone	Limp	Some flexion of extremities	Active motion
Response to catheter in nostril (tested after oropharynx is clear)	No response	Grimace	Cough or sneeze
Color	Blue or pale	Body pink, extremities blue	Completely pink

Source: V. Apgar, *Journal of the American Medical Association,* vol. 168, 1958, p. 1985.

scores of 7 or above at the 1-minute Apgar. The score is based on five characteristics of the newborn:

*A*ppearance
*P*ulse
*G*rimace
*A*ctivity
*R*espirations

Appearance refers to color. Although all infants are slightly cyanotic at birth, the color should change to pink within about 1 to 3 minutes. Extreme pallor is abnormal and probably indicates shock and the need for immediate attention. Pulse should not fall below 100. Grimace refers to the production of a cough or sneeze when a catheter is placed just inside the nose. Activity is a measure of muscle tone. Active movement rates a score of 2; some flexion of extremities rates a score of 1; a flaccid baby rates a score of 0 and is in danger and needs immediate attention. Respiration should be present by 1 minute and should be proceeded by a lusty cry.

After the 1-minute Apgar score is determined, a general assessment of the infant is performed. During this assessment, the nurse checks general appearance, auscultates the heart and lungs, palpates the abdomen (the kidney will be most easily palpated at this examination), and checks for adequate air exchange by holding a cotton wisp or stethoscope in front of the nares. If aeration is inadequate, further suctioning will be necessary.

The umbilical cord has usually been cut at birth, but at this time, the nurse will want to cut it shorter. It is important to continue observations at this time. Pulsations of the cord vessels which persist after the first few minutes indicate a distressed infant. The vessels should also be counted. If only two vessels (rather than the usual three) are present, there is a high likelihood that some type of internal anomalies, usually renal, exist.

After these procedures it will usually be time for the 5-minute Apgar, which is carried out in a similar manner to the 1-minute Apgar. This one has a greater predictive power for future problems the infant may encounter. Low 5-minute Apgars are highly correlated with later neurological problems of various types. There is a 50 percent mortality rate for infants with a 5-minute Apgar of 1 or 0.

Care of the Eyes

Next the eyes are creded. Although some hospitals use various antibiotic solutions because of their decreased irritating qualities, silver nitrate continues to be the most effective against gonorrhea. The eyes should be carefully rinsed with saline or sterile water after the silver nitrate has been in contact with the eyes for a period of 2 minutes.

Infant Respiration

For infants with depressed respiration, it is imperative that measures be taken to facilitate air exchange. A complete suctioning of the naso- and oropharynx with a DeLee trap or similar apparatus should be the first approach. The posterior pharyngeal wall should also be carefully checked since the tongue of a flaccid baby can easily fall back obstructing his passageway. A small pharyngeal airway will correct this problem. If the baby has been suctioned and an airway inserted and is still in difficulty, inflation of the lungs through an Ambu bag or similar apparatus is necessary. Oxygen should be administered in this manner under intermittent pressure. Alternating positive- and negative-pressure machines should not be used since they can do damage. Pressure of 15 to 20 cm of water is all that is usually required and is safe. There are times when the pressure must be increased over this amount, but there is always danger of bursting a lung if the pressure is too high. Whenever this procedure is employed, it is essential to auscultate the chest with a stethoscope to make sure that the oxygen is actually entering the lungs. If all the preceding measures fail, it may be necessary to proceed with direct laryngoscopy and possibly with intubation. Whether this is the responsibility of the nurse or not is a matter of controversy. It is clear that this is a dangerous procedure, since if it is incorrectly done, permanent brain damage as well as local laryngeal damage may result. On the other hand, it is a lifesaving measure, and in many hospitals there may be no one but the nurse to institute it. One thing is very clear, however; if the nurse is to be the one responsible for the procedure, it is essential that she insist on proper and adequate training. There are models available with which to practice. After dexterity with the model is perfected, it is wise to practice on something more nearly like a newborn infant. Some people choose dead newborns for this purpose; some choose live kittens. First inspection is done under direct laryngoscopy, and any visualized foreign matter such as vernix or blood must be removed by suction with a #12 French catheter. If there are still no results, a few short puffs of pressure (at about 40 or 50 cm of water) may be tried. If no machine is available, mouth-to-mouth resuscitation can be attempted. In this procedure, the mouth of the nurse should cover both the mouth and nose of the infant and she should proceed with short puffs of air. External cardiac massage is indicated if the heart does not begin beating with the insufflation. It should be done with the fingers at a rate of 120 beats per minute (i.e., about 3 beats to every respiration). IV sodium bicarbonate will probably be indicated to correct the acidosis from hypoxia as will dextrose to correct the hypoglycemia resulting from the loss of glycogen.

Newborn Behavior

The new baby normally exhibits behavior which would be worrisome at any other time. There is a definite sequence through which the infant progresses. Although distressed infants may be slower, they progress through the same stages. For the first 6 to 8 hours after birth the newborn is in a period of instability. Stage I of this instability is a condition of reactivity normally from birth to about 30 minutes. During this time, the infant is alert and active, displaying tachycardia, tachypnea, active bowel sounds, rales in his lungs, irregular respirations, and a drop in temperature. His eyes are wide open and alert (see Fig. 2-1). It is interesting to note that generally this is the same time period in which the mother is quite alert and awake, and one might wonder whether this is not the ideal time intended by nature for mother and infant to become acquainted. Usually the mother will want to see and feel her baby as soon as possible, and as long as the baby is prevented from chilling, during this period would seem an ideal time. After about 30 minutes, in Stage II, the infant's responsiveness diminishes and he sleeps. The infant's heartbeat and respirations are much more regular and somewhat slower, and the body temperature may be slightly more stable. This lasts from about the time the baby is 30 minutes old to about 4 to 6 hours old. Finally in Stage III, from about 4 or 6 hours old to about 8 hours old, the baby again becomes more alert and responsive. The gagging reflex is now active, the pulse and respirations increase, and meconium passage will commonly occur at this time. It is important in the newborn nursery to be aware of the normality of this sequence since otherwise these seemingly erratic behaviors might be a matter of concern.

Inspecting the Placenta

The nurse should inspect the placenta in the delivery room. Its size and any areas of fibrosis or calcification or infarcts are all important. Very small placentas may be an accompaniment of intrauterine growth retardation,

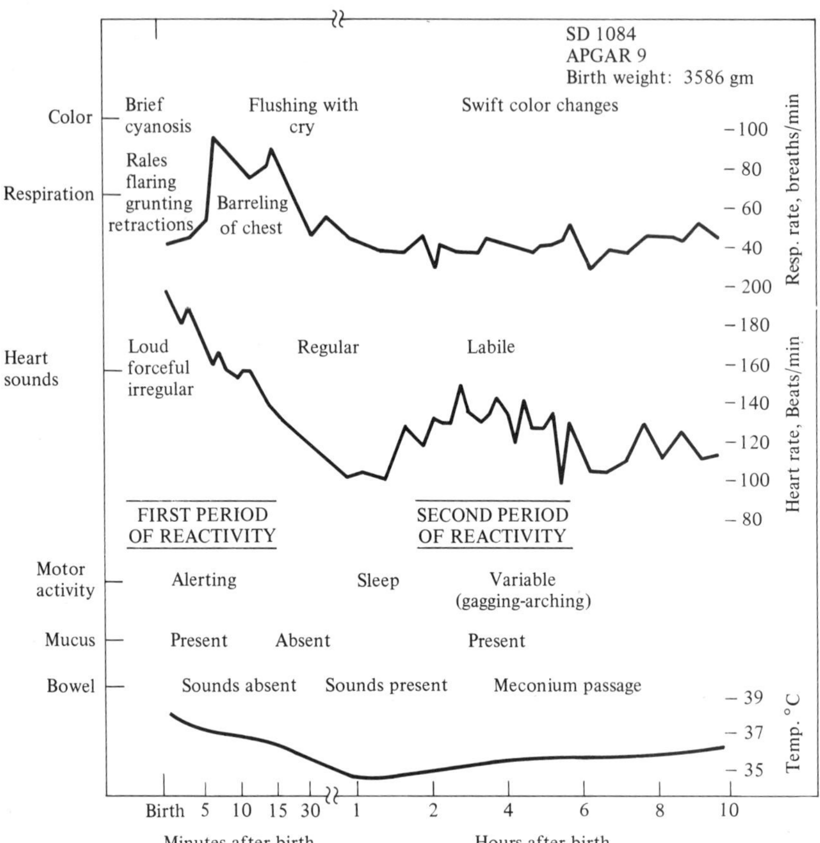

Figure 2-1 Stages of birth recovery. *(Source: Murdina M. Desmond et al., Pediatric Clinics of North America, vol. 13, 1966, p. 656.)*

while infants of diabetic mothers may have very large placentas. The angle of insertion of the cord should also be noted. The battledore type of insertion occurs when the vessels insert into the edge of the disc (see Fig. 2-2). This has been associated with small-for-gestational-age infants. Velamentous insertions, which enter into the chorioamnion rather than directly onto the placental disc (see Fig. 2-3), are also associated with small-for-gestational-age infants. Other types of insertions although commonly noted have not yet been found to be indicative of any other conditions in the baby.

THE PHYSICAL EXAMINATION OF THE NEWBORN

An important part of the nurse's responsibility to the newborn is a careful and thorough physical examination. Although all physical examinations are important, the first is perhaps more so since there are so many possibilities

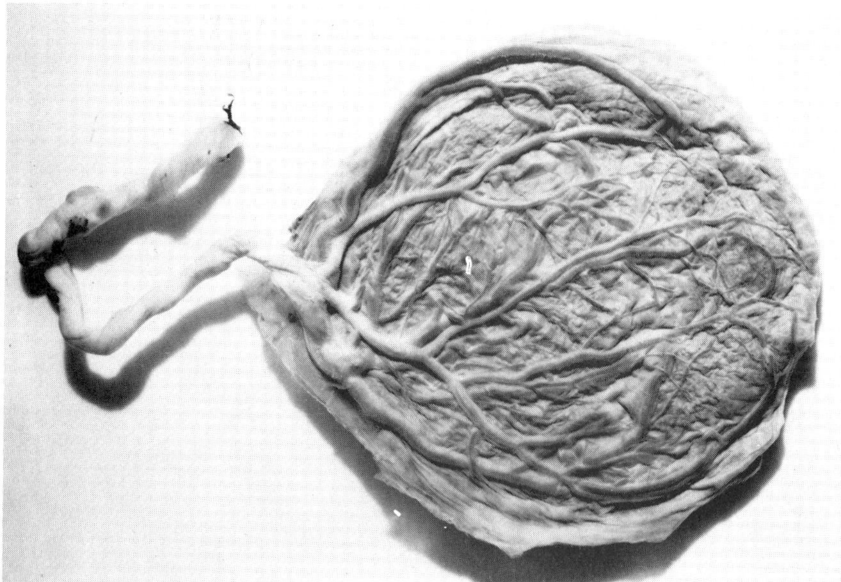

Figure 2-2 Placenta with battledore insertion. The cord inserts on the side or angle of the edge in a fashion resembling the handle of a frying pan. The ramification of surface vessels shown here is typical; occasionally the outermost passes onto the loose membrane and returns further along the circumference. *(Source: D. R. Shanklin, "The Influence of Placental Lesions on the Newborn Infant," Pediatric Clinics of North America, vol. 17, no. 1, February, 1970, p. 31.)*

for preventive health at this time. Basically, this examination is similar to other physical examinations the nurse will do and is explained more fully in the companion volume, *Pediatric Physical Diagnosis for Nurses.* There are, however, some special aspects to the physical examination of the newborn which will be discussed briefly in this section. Basically, these relate to three general areas: evaluating morbidity and mortality, evaluating minor malformations and minor deviations, and assessing gestational age. In evaluating the infant's general health, there are some important pieces of information which must be considered. Some of these are obtained from a knowledge of the history of the pregnancy and delivery and some from the physical examination. Instances such as toxemia in pregnancy, mother's age at delivery, her previous pregnancy history, and the possibility of multiple birth are all statistically related to the prognosis for the infant. Birth weight, Apgar score, and gestational age are also correlated with the newborn's health.

Minor Abnormalities

The area of evaluating minor malformations and minor deviations is also being analyzed more and more carefully. Minor abnormalities are certain unusual physical findings which may be used to predict other more serious

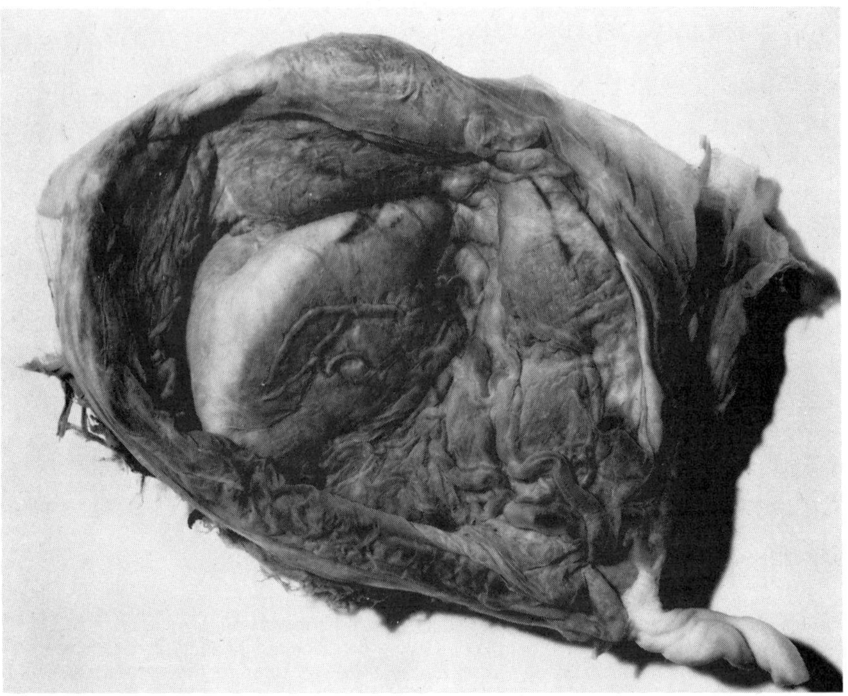

Figure 2-3 Placenta with velamentous insertion. The cord inserts onto the membranes at a variable distance from the edge of the cotyledonary placenta. The vessels often wander rather extensively across the membranes and may come to the placenta at a variety of points. *(Source: D. R. Shanklin, "The Influence of Placental Lesions on the Newborn Infant," Pediatric Clinics of North America, vol. 17, no. 1, February 1970, p. 31.)*

abnormalities. In general, 14 percent of normal infants have one so-called minor malformation. Their chances of having a major abnormality are not statistically any greater than those of a baby with no such minor malformations. There are 0.8 percent of newborns who have two such "minor malformations"; their chances of having an associated major anomaly is increased to five times that of the baby with one or none. An infant who displays three or more such anomalies (this occurs in only 0.5 percent of the population) has about a 90 percent chance of having an associated major anomaly which is or is not readily visible. Needless to say, any such baby deserves a thorough work-up. Smith (1970) has done the most work on this subject and classifies certain characteristics which should be considered minor malformations and those which should be considered normal variants. The minor malformations occur primarily in the complex areas of the body such as the face, ears, hands, and feet. Probably they should be counted only if they do not occur in normal family members. In the area of the head, Smith cites five minor abnormalities which should be considered minor malformations: a third fontanelle which is sometimes associated with mental retardation or other problems but which also can be normal, a flat occiput, a bony occipital spur, small nares, and a borderline small mandible. When examining the eye, epicanthal folds [Fig. 2-4(*a*)], Mongolian slant [Fig. 2-4(*b*)], Antimongolian slant [Fig. 2-4(*c*)], Brushfield's spots [Fig. 2-4(*d*)], and hypertelorism [Fig. 2-4(*e*)] should be considered minor malformations. Preauricular tags [Fig. 2-5(*a*)], preauricular pits [Fig. 2-5(*b*)], and different-sized auricles should also be considered in this category, as should low-set ears, i.e., those in which no part of the ear touches an imaginary line drawn from the outer canthus of the eye to the most prominent part of the occiput [Fig. 2-5(*c*)],

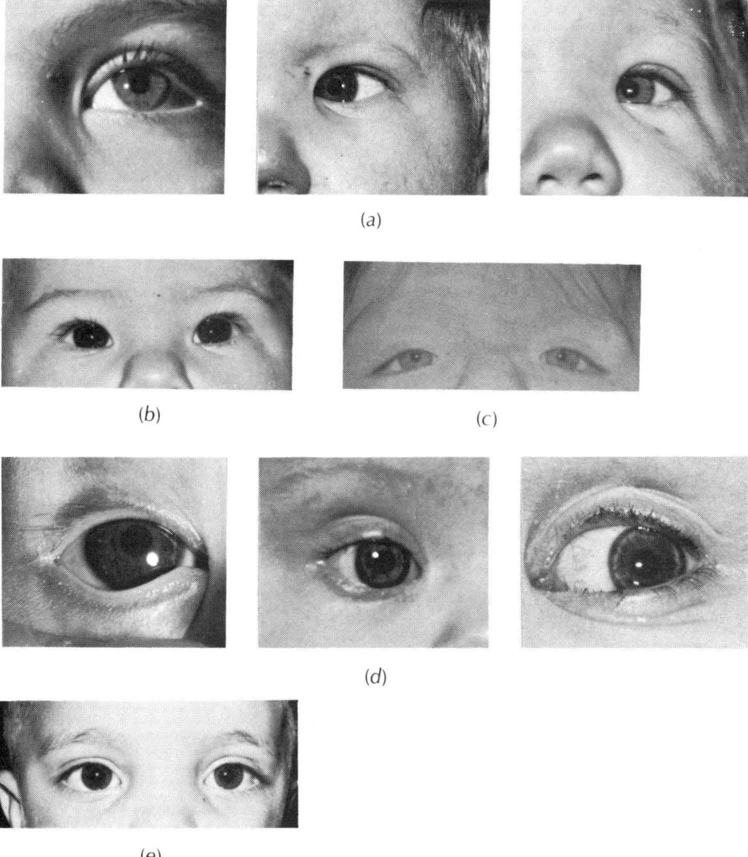

Figure 2-4 Minor abnormalities: the eye. (*a*) Varying degrees of inner epicanthic folds. (*b*) Mild lateral (Mongolian slant) displacement of inner canthi and up-slanting palpebral fissures. (*c*) Lateral displacement of inner canthi and down-slanting palpebral fissures. (*d*) Brushfield's spots: speckled ring about two-thirds of distance to periphery of iris with relative lack of patterning beyond it; found in about 20 percent of individuals versus 80 percent and more striking in Down's syndrome. (*e*) True ocular hypertelorism. *(Source: David W. Smith, Recognizable Patterns of Human Malformation, Philadelphia: Saunders, 1970, p. 338.)*

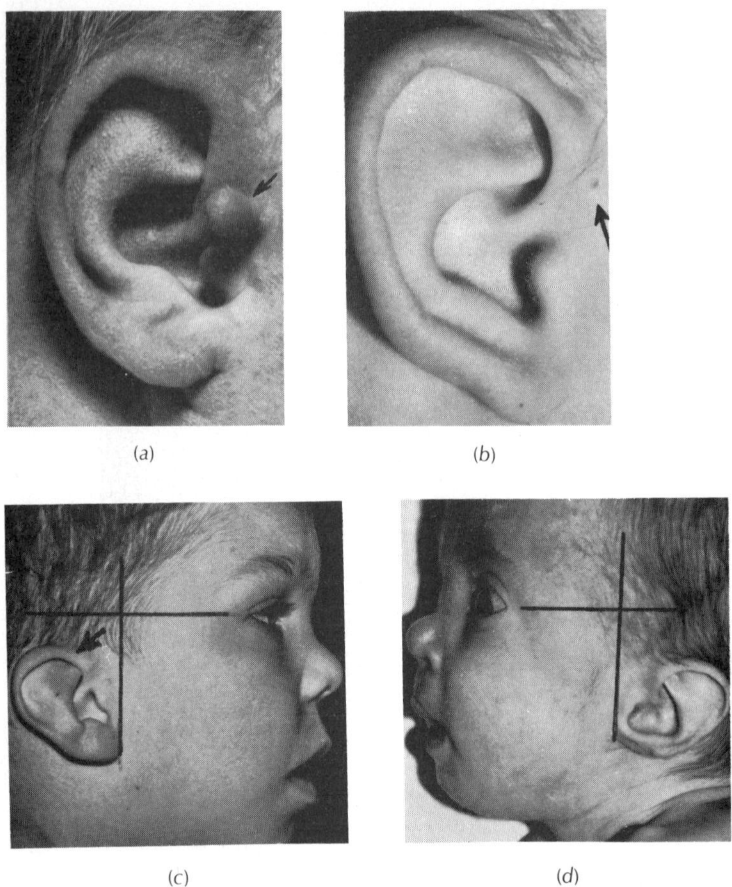

(a) (b)

(c) (d)

Figure 2-5 Minor abnormalities: the ear. (*a*) and (*b*) Cutaneous tags or pits. (*c*) Ears low set: when the lelix meets the cranium (arrow) at a level below that of a horizontal plane with the corner of the orbit. (*d*) Ears slanted. when the angle of slope of the auricle exceeds 10° from the perpendicular, a value which may be too low for prematures. *(Source: David W. Smith, Recognizable Patterns of Human Malformation, Philadelphia: Saunders, 1970, p. 339.)*

and backward-slanting ears; i.e., when the canthus-occiput line is drawn, the ear should not form more than a 10° angle with that line, as in Fig. 2-5(*d*). The skin should be examined for further minor malformations, such as deep dimples [Fig. 2-6(*a*)] excepting those naturally occurring at bony prominences, a low hairline in back [Fig. 2-6(*b*)], café-au-lait spots (i.e., light, cream-colored irregular spots on a darker background), punched-out scalp ulceration [Fig. 2-6(*c*)], capillary hemangiomata anywhere except the head and neck, two or more hair whorls, and abnormally bushy eyebrows or eyebrows which meet in the midline. The hands should be inspected to determine the presence of long, narrow fingers, syndactyly (i.e., the fusion of two digits), polydactyly (extra digits—usually very small), clinodactyly (i.e., abnormal slanting of the digits), especially in the little finger, which should not slant inward any more than 8°. These as well as unusual dermatoglyphics should also be considered minor malformations. Unusual dermatoglyphics may be in the form of palm creases, such as a simian crease (Fig. 2-7), or in the actual fingertips. Fingertip patterns are difficult to see in newborns even with magnification from the otoscope glass, and it is usually unnecessary to ascertain them. If it is necessary, fingerprints can be made in the same way that footprints are obtained in the delivery room. Dermal

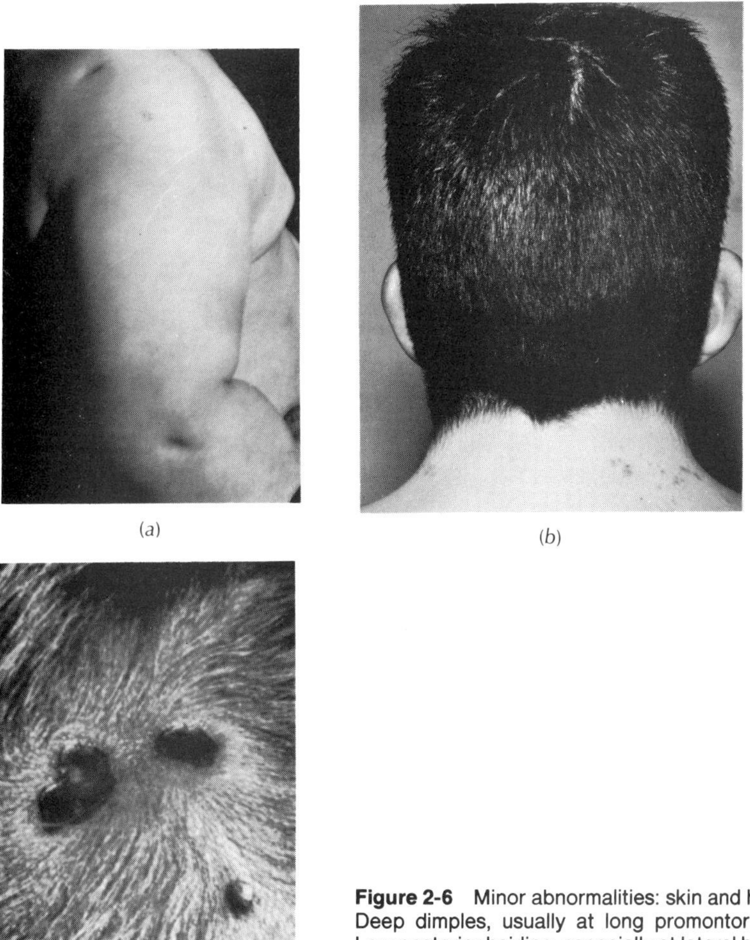

Figure 2-6 Minor abnormalities: skin and hair. *(a)* Deep dimples, usually at long promontories. *(b)* Low posterior hairline, especially at lateral borders. *(c)* "Punched-out" ulceration, posterior scalp. *(Source: David W. Smith, Recognizable Patterns of Human Malformation, Philadelphia: Saunders, 1970, p. 345.)*

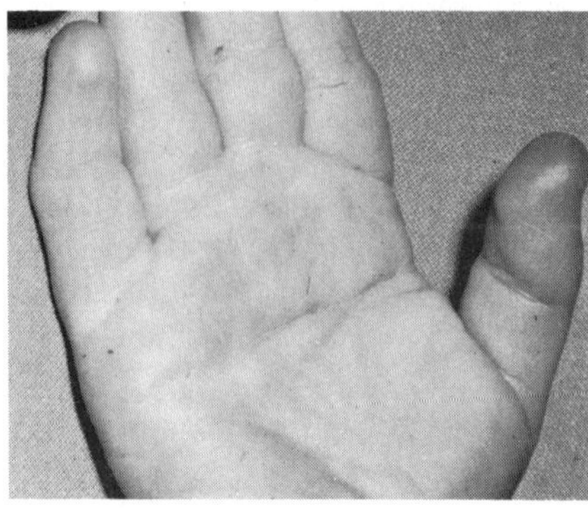

Figure 2-7 Minor abnormalities: simian crease. *(Source: David W. Smith, Recognizable Patterns of Human Malformation, Philadelphia: Saunders, 1970, p. 340.)*

patterns on the fingertips are of three types: whorls, arches, and loops (Fig. 2-8). Loops are ulnar if they open toward the ulnar side of the hand (i.e., toward the little finger) and radial if they open toward the thumb side of the hand. There is some controversy about exactly how to evaluate these patterns. Smith (1970, p. 341) says that three types of abnormalities can exist. The first of these is a high frequency of low-arch configurations, i.e., more than 6 of 10 fingers exhibiting this feature. This exists in 0.9 percent of normal babies, but in higher percentages of infants with the trisomy 18 syndrome, the XXXXY syndrome, and certain other abnormal syndromes. The second abnormal distribution is a high frequency of whorl patterns (i.e., nine or more fingers display whorls). This exists in 3.1 percent of normal infants, but in higher percentages of children with the XO syndrome, the Smith-Lemli-Opitz syndrome, and several other disease entities. Finally, Smith cites an unusual distribution of radial loop patterns. Loop patterns are not usually found on the fourth and fifth fingers of normal children but are often found there in children with Down's syndrome. It must be noted here that other investigators cite other figures for these distributions (e.g., Barness, 1971), and probably the most that can be said at this point is that unusual dermal ridges can be clues to other problems, but more research is needed before we can tell exactly how to use these clues clinically.

Hypoplasia of the fingernails (or toenails after the immediate newborn period) [Fig. 2-9(*a*)], narrow hyperconvex nails, especially of the fifth finger [Fig. 2-9(*b*)], and short broad nails [Fig. 2-9(*c*)] are further considered to be minor abnormalities. Inspection of the feet is somewhat similar to inspection of the hands. Clinodactyly of the second toe with overlapping onto the other toes [Fig. 2-10(*a*)], unusually short second toes [Fig. 2-10(*b*)], syndactyly, usually of toes two and three [Fig. 2-10(*c*)], prominent heels, prominent calcaneous, deep creases between the hallux and second toe [Fig. 2-10(*d*)], a wide space between the big toe and the adjacent toe [Fig. 2-10(*e*)], and short first metatarsal with dorsiflexion of the hallux [Fig. 2-10(*f*)] are all listed by

Smith as minor abnormalities. Two other minor abnormalities have been recognized: cubitus valgus (i.e., increased carrying angle of the elbow) and genu recurvature (i.e., hyperextension of the knee).

Minor abnormalities can also be found in the region of the thorax and other areas. A short, prominent, or depressed sternum is considered a minor abnormality. An aberrant frenulum is similarly considered in this class (Fig. 2-11), as is diastasis recti of the abdomen. A scrotum which attaches directly to the penis [Fig. 2-12(*a*)] or hypoplasia of the labia majora which makes the

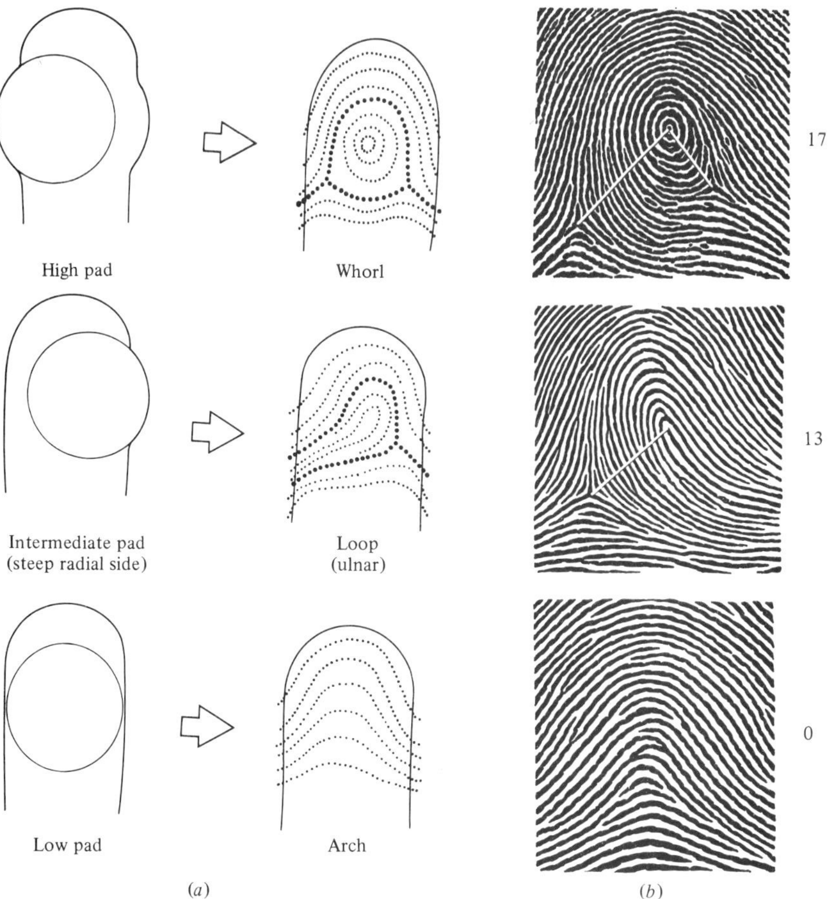

Figure 2-8 Minor abnormalities: dermal patterns on the fingertips. (*a*) Presumed relationship between fetal fingertip pads at 16 to 19 weeks of fetal life and the fingertip dermal ridge pattern, which develops at that time. *(Source: David W. Smith, Recognizable Patterns of Human Malformation, Philadelphia: Saunders, 1970, p. 343.)* (*b*) Technique for dermal ridge counting. A line is drawn between the center of the pattern and the more distal triradius, and the number of ridges which touch this line is the fingertip ridge count. The sum of the 10 fingertip ridge counts is the total ridge count; this averages 144 in the male and 127 in the female. *(Source: Sarah B. Holt, "Quantitative Genetics of Finger-Print Patterns," British Medical Bulletin, vol. 17, no. 3, 1961, p. 247.)*

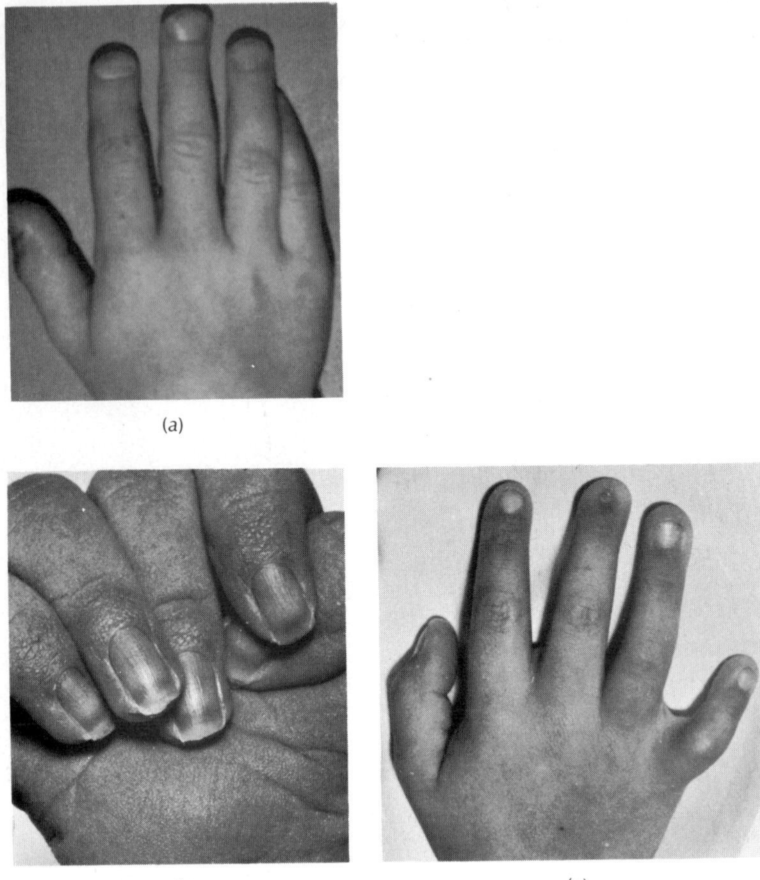

(a)

(b)

(c)

Figure 2-9 Minor abnormalities: nails. (*a*) Hypoplasia of nail and camptodactyly of fifth finger; asymmetry of short third finger. (*b*) Narrow, hyperconvex nails, especially fifth. (*c*) Short and broad nails. *(Source: David W. Smith, Recognizable Patterns of Human Malformation, Philadelphia: Saunders, 1970, p. 344.)*

clitoris appear abnormally large [Fig. 2-12(*b*)] conclude the list of minor abnormalities.

Normal Variations

There are also many minor variations which should be considered totally normal. On the skin, milia, accessory nipples, erythema toxicum, or venus spilus (a hairless mole) are all considered normal, as are the flat capillary hemangiomata which appear so frequently over the nape of the neck, eyelids, glabella, or lumbosacral areas. Other normal variations which may be found in the region of the head are cephalhematoma, caput succedaneum, facial asymmetry, and asymmetry of the scalp. Transient horizontal nystag-

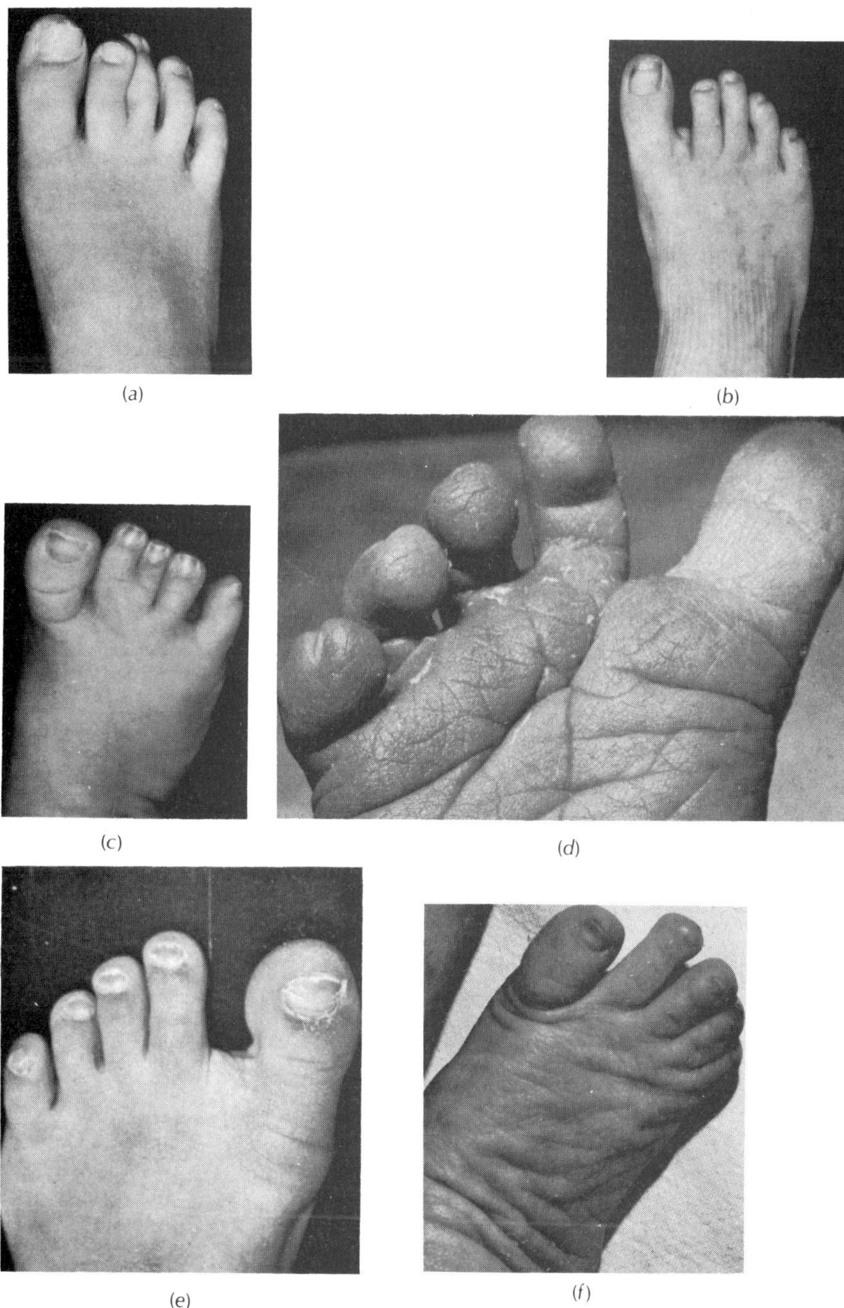

(a) (b) (c) (d) (e) (f)

Figure 2-10 Minor abnormalities: the toes. (*a*) Clinodactyly of second toe with overlapping. (*b*) Asymmetrical length of toes. (*c*) Syndactyly, most common of the second and third toes. (*d*) Deep crease between hallux and second toe. (*e*) Wide gap between hallux and second toe. (*f*) Short first metatarsal with dorsiflexion of hallux. *(Source: David W. Smith, Recognizable Patterns of Human Malformation, Philadelphia: Saunders, 1970, p. 344.)*

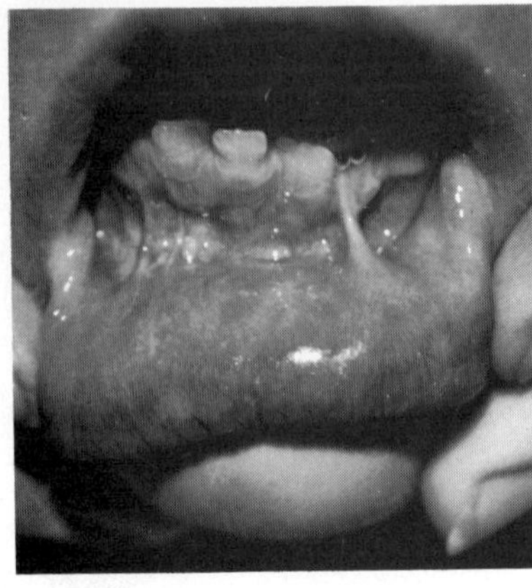

Figure 2-11 Minor abnormality: an aberrant frenulum. *(Source: David W. Smith, Recognizable Patterns of Human Malformation, Philadelphia: Saunders, 1970, p. 346.)*

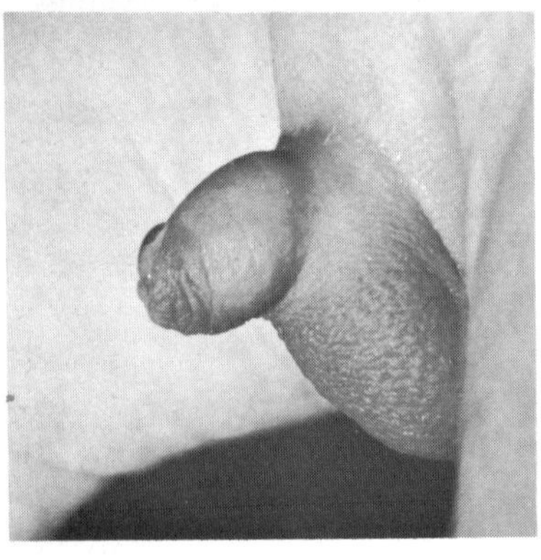

(a)

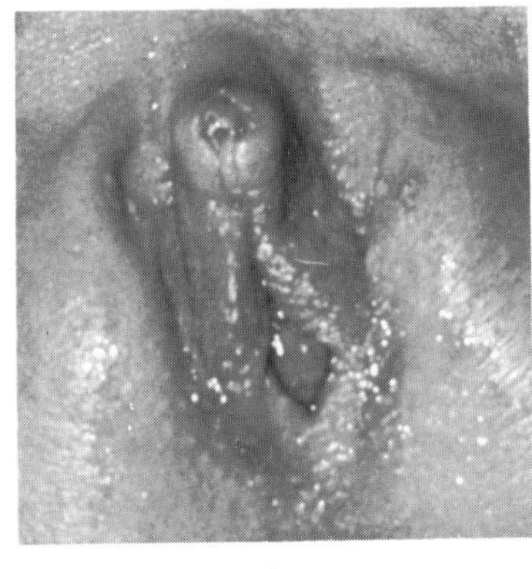

(b)

Figure 2-12 Minor abnormality: the genitalia. (*a*) Scrotum extends distally on phallus. (*b*) Hypoplasia of labia majora such that clitoris appears prominent. *(Source: David W. Smith, Recognizable Patterns of Human Malformation, Philadelphia: Saunders, 1970, p. 346.)*

mus, subconjunctival hemorrhages, and setting-sun sign are also usually normal, although the setting-sun sign can be associated with hydrocephalus. Darwinian tubercles on the ears or a mildly bent helix on the ear are also considered within normal range. In examining the mouth, Epstein's pearls on the gums, Bohn's nodules on the medial raphe of the palate, Bednar's apthae, and a high palatal arch are also considered within the range of normal. Minor variations which should *not* be considered as minor abnormalities also include the very mild syndactyly commonly seen in the second and third toes, hypoplasia of the toenails in newborns, and the normal flat foot of the neonate.

Assessing Gestational Age

The third aspect of the physical examination of the newborn which is peculiar to this age group is the assessment of the gestational age. There has been much justifiable concern about prematurity for many years, but it was not until fairly recently that we have begun to really understand how to assess prematurity. In 1961 the World Health Organization defined low birth-weight as synonymous with prematurity, any baby under 2,500 grams being considered premature. We now realize that this is not true for all babies and that one-third of what we now term small-for-gestational-age babies are actually quite near term even though they would have been considered prematures by the 1961 standards. Actually their behavior and needs are quite different from those of truly premature infants. For any given gestational age, infants who fall under the 10th percentile are considered small for gestational age, while those falling over the 90th percentile are termed large for gestational age. Prematurity is now considered strictly by the amount of time the infant has spent in the womb, not by weight. Babies who are born before the end of the 37th week are officially considered premature; those born between the beginning of the 38th and end of the 41st week are considered term, and those born after the 41st week are postterm.

Prenatal Indications of Gestational Age Much progress has been made in learning how to determine exactly how much time a specific infant has been in utero. Although the mother's history has often been considered a poor source of information, some recent studies have shown that this is accurate about 75 to 85 percent of the time. There are some problems with this method of ascertaining the exact date of conception, however. Some women have postconceptual bleeding at about the time they would normally have their period. If this occurs, they may report an episode of postconceptual bleeding as their last menstrual period. This would mean that the baby is actually a month older than would be thought by following these dates. Irregular menstrual cycles can also obscure the accurate dates, as can faulty memory of the last menstrual period.

There are other occurrences during the pregnancy which can be used to substantiate or throw suspicion on the dates obtained by calculating from the mother's last menstrual period. Fundal growth is one of these. In a normal pregnancy with only one infant, it is expected that the uterus will reach the pelvic brim by about 12 weeks and the umbilicus by 20 weeks. Thereafter, it will grow about 1 cm per week until about 35 weeks, when its growth will be restricted by the thoracic cage. This is not 100 percent reliable, however, since the exact position of the umbilicus may vary slightly in women, and individual examiners may measure slightly differently. Fetal heart tones are also used to date a pregnancy, and should be heard with the fetoscope at 18 to 20 weeks of gestation; in fact, this is such a helpful method of ascertaining dates that a woman who is seen at 17 weeks gestation when no fetal heart tones can be heard should be reappointed weekly until the heart is heard so that the examiner will know when they first become audible. If she were not seen for another month and the heart tones were then heard, it would not be known when they first became audible, and it is when they first become audible that the pregnancy is dated at 20 weeks. They can be heard earlier, of course, with the doptone; by the 12th week the nurse should expect 50 percent of the pregnancies to have the heartbeat transmitted. Some will be heard as early as the 8th week. This is not a very accurate method of ascertaining dates, however. The date when the mother first perceives movement can also be helpful, although it is less accurate. In a primipara this is approximately 18 to 19 weeks. In a multipara this is about 16 to 17 weeks. The first time the examincr should be able to ballotte the uterus should be about 24 weeks although again, this is not entirely accurate.

Certain laboratory studies can also be used to help ascertain length of gestation, particularly if there is clinical confusion concerning the dates. Many of these tests are fairly recent and are not available in all hospitals, but there is generally a regional laboratory which can be used if needed. Most of these examinations are done on amniotic fluid, and this, of course, necessitates an amniocentesis procedure. The creatinine analysis is based on the fact that the amount of creatinine increases with increasing gestation. A level over 1.8 to 2.0 mg/100 ml indicates that the fetus is at least at 36 weeks of gestation, assuming that the mother's level of creatinine is normal. The bilirubin level is sometimes used for the same purpose but is less reliable. Generally, levels should decline with increasing maturity. A lecithin/sphingomyelin (L/S) ratio is an extremely useful measure of maturity. If the ratio is over 2.0, the baby is at least at 35 to 36 weeks gestation. Not all laboratories are equipped to perform this examination, however. Ultrasound can be used to outline the size of the baby and study certain aspects of the skeletal structure for signs of increasing maturity, but a highly skilled reader is necessary for this. EKG's can also be useful, but again, special expertise is required. Amniotic cell types can also be studied. There are 12 types of amniotic cells, but the polygonal type which is shed from the skin increases sharply at 38 to 40 weeks and is a fairly good sign of maturity. X-rays can give certain radiologic information that may prove useful. For instance, the reader should be able to see the distal end of the femur at 36 weeks and the proximal end of the tibia at 38 weeks. A small-for-gestational-age infant, however, may violate these norms, and one should always keep in mind the hazards of x-rays at this time. Some clinics study the various types of vaginal cells, but this is usually thought to be unreliable. Other minor types of assessment are sometimes used, but most others are less practical.

Postnatal Indications of Gestational Age Gestational age can also be calculated postnatally and in general is quite accurate within a range of about 2 weeks. This assessment can be done accurately up until about 5 days of age, but the information is usually needed before that time. The neurological part of the examination is often not accurate during the first 48 hours, but the physical characteristics can be assessed at any time. The complete examination should not take more than 10 minutes and can be done as part of the physical. Certain physical characteristics of the skin and hair, ears, breasts, and genitalia progress in a known and orderly sequence during the last part of pregnancy, and it is knowledge of this sequence that allows us to assess gestational age. For instance, it is known that the amount of pitting edema over the tibia decreases with increasing gestational age. Skin becomes thicker and turns from dark red to pink to pale with increased age. The opacity of the skin deepens, allowing fewer vessels to be visible, while the area covered by lanugo decreases. There are only one or two creases across the soles of the feet in a 36-week-old infant, while a 37 to 38-week-old will have creases down about three-fourths of the foot, leaving the heel smooth. Past 38 weeks, the examiner will expect the entire foot, including the heel, to be covered with creases. Scalp hair also changes with increasing gestational age. Until about 38 weeks it is fuzzy and tends to lie in clumps, but after that time will appear as silky, single strands. The ear also changes with increasing gestation. The cartilage becomes firmer, allowing the folded pinna to spring back faster as the child becomes more mature. Similarly the incurving of the pinna increases with age. Certain characteristics of the breasts also display an orderly developmental sequence. The nipples gradually become more and more clearly defined and the areola begins to rise above the contour of the breast. Breast tissue itself is not palpable before 33 weeks but by 35 weeks should be about 3 mm; by 37 to 38 weeks it should be about 4 mm; and by 38 weeks it should be about 7 mm. This may not be reliable in infants who are small for gestational age. Genitalia also shows signs of change as gestation progresses. The little girl will show larger and larger labia majora until at term they finally completely cover the labia minor. In the male of about 36 weeks gestation, testes will be found at the junction of the sac and the abdomen, while rugae will be found only on a small area of the inferior scrotum. Gradually the testes descend further into the scrotum and the number of rugae increase until at term the testes are completely descended and rugae cover the entire scrotum.

Certain neurological findings can also be used to estimate gestational age although they may be unreliable for the first 48 hours and can be obscured by any trauma or neurological difficulties which may or may not be connected with the gestational age. They are very useful since their sequence seems to be the same whether the child reaches a certain age in utero or outside. In other words, an infant who is born at 36 weeks gestation will 4 weeks later show the typical neurological findings of a full-term infant. Many neurological findings have been used and found relevant to gestational age. Among these are the heel-ear maneuver, the scarf maneuver, head lag, ventral suspension, horizontal suspension, and trunk righting. Exact ratings of these maneuvers are shown on the accompanying charts. Resting position is also important, being primarily extension until about 32 weeks. From 32 to 36 weeks it consists of extension when supine but flexion when prone. After that time flexion predominates in all positions. Along with flexion, increased tone results in increased recoil, and this is also seen in the accompanying charts. Flexion angles such as the wrist, popliteal, and ankle are also shown in their relation to gestational age on the charts. Certain reflexes such as the sucking, rooting, grasp, Moro, tonic neck, crawling, neck righting, knee jerks, and the cremasteric reflex also progress with increasing maturity but not all are useful, either because they are unpredictable or because they mature so early (e.g., the grasp is mature at 26 weeks) that they are of little clinical value in most situations. Those which are most reliable for gestational age are the pupillary reflex, which begins from 29 to 31 weeks; the glabellar, which matures at 32 to 34 weeks; the head righting in prone position, which does not appear until after 40 weeks; traction (when the examiner pulls the infant up by the hands only), which appears at 33 to 36 weeks; and the turning of the head to light, which begins at 32 to 36 weeks. All these known gestational changes have been studied and certain of them chosen for consistency, ease of assessment, and simplicity; methods of scoring them were evolved. Two such examples are the chart evolved by Lubchenko (Fig. 2-13) and that evolved by Dubowitz (Table 2-6). These give more precise details on how to evaluate each specific characteristic and assign it to a gestational age in weeks.

Some postnatal laboratory tests can also be useful, but they are less useful than a careful gestational assessment of physical and neurological characteristics. Fetal hemoglobin should be about 80 percent in a full-term infant. A higher percentage indicates some degree of prematurity. Alkaline phosphatase in meconium can also be measured, but this test is generally available only in research laboratories. Immunoglobulins can also give important gestational information. It is known that the fetal IgG is equal to the maternal level at about 33 weeks. IgA and IgD are not useful for this kind of dating, and IgM is still controversial.

Reduced Intrauterine Growth We do not yet know all the causes of decreased intrauterine growth, but there are some specifics that are known. It is suspected that high altitudes and malnutrition are two causes, although there is still some controversy over these. It seems to be agreed that cigarette smoking in excess of 20 cigarettes per day increases the chances that an infant will be small for gestational age, although it is not clear whether this is due only to the smoking during the pregnancy or may be partially attributed to the fact that the woman was a heavy smoker even before the pregnancy. Noninfectious diseases of the mother such as cardiorenal disease, toxemia (which presumably decreases the blood flow through the placenta), chronic hypertension, sickle cell C, narcotic addiction, and diabetes of class D or F (i.e., the most severe types of diabetes) all seem to be influential in retarding the intrauterine growth of an infant as do infectious diseases such

PHYSICAL FINDINGS	EST GA	WEEKS GESTATION																				
		24	25	26	27	28	29	30	31	32	33	34	35	36	37	38	39	40	41	42	43	44
EXAMINATION FIRST HOURS																						
VERNIX		APPEARS	COVERS BODY														DECREASE IN AMOUNT		NO VERNIX			
BREAST TISSUE		NONE											1 - 2 MM		4 MM		7 MM OR MORE					
NIPPLES		BARELY VISIBLE								WELL DEFINED FLAT AREOLA					WELL DEFINED, RAISED AREOLA							
SOLE CREASES		NONE								1, ANTERIOR TRANSVERSE		2, ANTERIOR TRANSVERSE			ANTERIOR 2/3 SOLE		CREASES INVOLVING HEEL					
EAR CARTILAGE		PINNA SOFT, STAYS FOLDED										RETURNS SLOWLY FROM FOLDING			THIN CARTILAGE, SPRINGS BACK		FIRM, REMAINS ERECT FROM HEAD					
EAR FORM		FLAT, SHAPELESS										BEGINNING INCURVING OF PERIPHERY			PARTIAL INCURVING UPPER PINNA			WELL DEFINED INCURVING ALL OF UPPER PINNA				
GENITALIA - TESTES & SCROTUM		UNDESCENDED						TESTES HIGH IN CANAL, FEW RUGAE						TESTES LOWER MORE RUGAE			TESTES DESCENDED, PENDULOUS SCROTUM, RUGAE COMPLETE					
LABIA & CLITORIS		LABIA MAJORA WIDELY SEPARATED, PROMINENT CLITORIS												LABIA MAJORA NEARLY COVER LABIA MINORA			LABIA MINORA & CLITORIS COVERED					
HAIR (APPEARS ON HEAD @ 20 WKS)		EYEBROWS & LASHES						FINE, WOOLLY HAIR								HAIR SILKY, SINGLE STRANDS						
LANUGO (APPEARS @ 20 WKS)		LANUGO OVER ENTIRE BODY				VANISHES FROM FACE					SLIGHT LANUGO OVER SHOULDERS					NO LANUGO						
SKIN TEXTURE		THIN										SMOOTH, MEDIUM THICKNESS							DESQUAMATION			
SKIN COLOR & OPACITY		TRANSLUCENT, PLETHORIC, NUMEROUS VENULES (ABDOMEN)													PINK, FEW LARGE VESSELS OVERALL			PALE PINK, NO VESSELS SEEN				
SKULL FIRMNESS		SOFT TO 1 INCH FROM ANTERIOR FONTANELLE											SPRINGY AT EDGES OF FONTANELLE CENTER FIRM			BONES HARD SUTURES EASILY DISPLACED			BONES HARD, CANNOT BE DISPLACED			
POSTURE - RESTING		LATERAL DECUBITUS				HYPOTONIA		SLIGHT INCREASE IN TONE, LOWER EXTREMITY				FROG-LIKE		TOTAL FLEXION								
RECOIL		ABSENT						SLIGHT, LOWER EXTREMITIES				NONE UPPER EXTREMITIES GOOD LOWER EXTREMITIES		SLOW UPPER EXTREMITIES			GOOD UPPER EXTREMITIES					
LATER EXAMINATION																						
TONE - HEEL TO EAR		NO RESISTANCE						SLIGHT RESISTANCE				DIFFICULT		ALMOST IMPOSSIBLE		IMPOSSIBLE						
SCARF MANEUVER		NO RESISTANCE										MINIMAL RESISTANCE		FAIR RESISTANCE		DIFFICULT						
NECK EXTENSORS		ABSENT						SLIGHT				FAIR		GOOD								
NECK FLEXORS		ABSENT										MINIMAL				FAIR						
REFLEXES - MORO		BARELY APPARENT			COMPLETE, EXHAUSTIBLE				GOOD, COMPLETE			NO ADDUCTION				COMPLETE WITH ADDUCTION						
PUPILS TO LIGHT					REACT																	
GRASP		FEEBLE			FAIR				SOLID, INVOLVES ARMS						MAY PICK INFANT UP							
ROOTING		MINIMAL c̄ REINFORCEMENT			GOOD c̄ REINFORCEMENT				GOOD													
CROSSED EXTENSION		SLIGHT WITHDRAWAL						WITHDRAWAL				WITHDRAWAL & EXTENSION				WITHDRAWAL, EXTENSION, ADDUCTION						
AUTOMATIC WALK		ABSENT										MINIMAL				FAIR, TOES		GOOD, HEELS				
TRUNK ELEVATION		ABSENT										SLIGHT			GOOD							
GLABELLAR TAP		ABSENT						APPEARS					PRESENT									
HEAD TURNS TO LIGHT		ABSENT								APPEARS				PRESENT								
CLINICAL ESTIMATE, GA																						
CALCULATED GA																						
		24	25	26	27	28	29	30	31	32	33	34	35	36	37	38	39	40	41	42	43	44
		WEEKS GESTATION																				

Figure 2-13 Lubchenko's assessment of gestational age. *(Source: Lulu Lubchenko, "Assessment of Gestational Age and Development at Birth," Pediatric Clinics of North America, vol. 17, no. 1, February 1970, p. 127.)*

Table 2-6 Dubowitz Gestational Scoring Chart

External sign	Score*				
	0	1	2	3	4
Edema	Obvious edema of hands and feet; pitting over tibia	No obvious edema of hands and feet; pitting over tibia	No edema		
Skin texture	Very thin, gelatinous	Thin and smooth	Smooth; medium thickness. Rash or superficial peeling	Slight thickening. Superficial cracking and peeling especially of hands and feet	Thick and parchment-like; superficial or deep cracking
Skin color	Dark red	Uniformly pink	Pale pink; variable over body	Pale; only pink over ears, lips, palms, or soles	
Skin opacity (trunk)	Numerous veins and venules clearly seen, especially over abdomen	Veins and tributaries seen	A few large vessels clearly seen over abdomen	A few large vessels seen indistinctly over abdomen	No blood vessels seen
Lanugo (over back)	No lanugo	Abundant; long and thick over whole back	Hair thinning especially over lower back	Small amount of lanugo and bald areas	At least $\frac{1}{2}$ of back devoid of lanugo
Plantar creases	No skin creases	Faint red marks over anterior half of sole	Definite red marks over > anterior $\frac{1}{2}$; indentations over < anterior $\frac{1}{3}$	Indentations over > anterior $\frac{1}{3}$	Definite deep indentations over > anterior $\frac{1}{3}$

Nipple formation	Nipple barely visible; no areola	Nipple well defined; areola smooth and flat, diameter < 0.75 cm	Areola stippled, edge not raised, diameter N 0.75 cm	Areola stippled, edge raised, diameter > 0.75 cm
Breast size	No breast tissue palpable	Breast tissue on one or both sides, < 0.5 cm diameter	Breast tissue both sides; one or both 0.5–1.0 cm	Breast tissue both sides; one or both n 1 cm
Ear form	Pinna flat and shapeless, little or no incurving of edge	Incurving of part of edge of pinna	Partial incurving whole of upper pinna	Well-defined incurving whole of upper pinna
Ear firmness	Pinna soft, easily folded, no recoil	Pinna soft, easily folded, slow recoil	Cartilage to edge of pinna, but soft in places; ready recoil	Pinna firm, cartilage to edge; instant recoil
Genitals				
Male	Neither testis in scrotum	At least one testis high in scrotum	At least one testis right down	
Female (with hips 1/2 abducted)	Labia majora widely separated, labia minora protruding	Labia majora almost cover labia minora	Labia majora completely cover labia minora	

* If score differs on two sides, take the mean.

Source: L. M. S. Dubowitz, V. Dubowitz, and C. Goldberg, "Clinical Assessment of Gestational Age in the Newborn Infant," *Journal of Pediatrics,* vol. 77, 1970, p. 1; adapted from V. Farr et al., *Developmental Medicine and Child Neurology,* vol. 8, 1966, p. 507.

as rubella, herpes simplex, cytomegalus infectious disease, toxoplasmosis, syphilis, malaria, and certain bacterial infections. Rubella and hepatitis are likely to precipitate premature labor but do not seem to result in small-for-gestational-age babies. The placenta has been implicated in certain research studies as a possible cause of small-for-gestational-age infants. Structural defects such as infarcts, fibrosis, or early separation as may happen in placenta abruptio or placenta previa have been suggested as possible causes, as has a single umbilical artery and the battledore and velamentous insertion of the cords (see Figs. 2-2 and 2-3).

Certain characteristics of the fetus itself may be causal in reducing intrauterine growth. Multiple gestations almost always affect intrauterine growth rate, usually more severely in one fetus than the others. With twins, a decrease in the rate of growth usually begins at about 30 weeks. Congenital anomalies such as anencephaly, heart disease, or chromosomal and genetic problems such as trisomy 16 (which results in small and often postterm infants), trisomy 18 (which also results in small, postterm infants as well as a small placenta with a single umbilical artery), trisomy D (which results in infants which are smaller than normal but not as small as those with trisomy 18), cri-du-chat syndrome, Down's syndrome, Turner's syndrome, and Noonan's syndrome (though this is not true for Klinefelter's syndrome and the various Poly X syndromes). Intrauterine infections such as rubella, cytomegalovirus disease, toxoplasmosis, and syphilis may also be causal. Teratogenic drugs or radiation end this list of possible causes for decreased intrauterine growth.

Increased Intrauterine Growth The etiology of infants who are large for gestational age is also somewhat unclear, but again causes for specific cases are known. Some of these include renal or cardiac difficulties in the infant which are accompanied by edema as well as diabetes in the mother. The larger of two discordant twins is also often large for gestational age because of a twin-to-twin transfusion in which the one twin receives much too much fluid.

Effects of Size Prognosis of infants who are either small or large for gestational age has been investigated to some extent. Small babies are more likely to be hypoxic before labor, and therefore birth recovery is usually slower and the infant often receives a lower Apgar score. Similarly, the infant is more likely to aspirate meconium during delivery and suffer from problems arising from this. The small infant is much more likely to be hypoglycemic soon after birth, and if this is untreated and the brain receives decreased amount of nourishment, the child is likely to show a lower IQ and an increased number of neurological problems later. For this reason it is extremely important to monitor the blood glucose of all small-for-gestational-age infants closely. Usually this hypoglycemia begins 12 to 24 hours after birth but sometimes before. Monitoring should be continued for 3 to 4 days. Symptoms of hypoglycemia include cyanosis and a weak, high-pitched cry (much like hypocalcemia), but it can also be completely asymptomatic.

These babies are much more likely to lose heat rapidly, thus increasing the problem of hypoglycemia. They also have a greater chance of suffering from intrapulmonary hemorrhage as well as cerebral edema. Although this latter is uncommon, it is important when it occurs and will usually be heralded by widened sutures and bulging fontanelle, most often within the first 24 to 48 hours. These babies have 30 times as many anomalies as infants who are average for gestational age, but it is probably the anomaly which causes the decreased size rather than the other way around. These children will probably always remain small. On autopsy, the cerebellum appears to be the part of the brain most affected.

Less is known about the prognosis of infants who are large for gestational age. They are also quite likely to be hypoglycemic and should be monitored carefully. They are more likely to encounter birth trauma because of their size. Finally, they are more likely to suffer from transposition of the aorta. Figure 2-14 summarizes findings associated with various combinations of weights and gestational ages.

Prematurity Although we are now able to distinguish premature infants from infants who are small for gestational age, the causes for both are uncertain. Certain statistical associations have been made. For instance, we know that increased blood pressure in the mother, toxemia, cervical incompetence, placenta abruptio, placenta previa, decreased maternal stature, lack of prenatal care, lower socioeconomic status, history of previous premature births, and poor maternal nutrition are all correlated highly with premature delivery, although we are not certain whether they are all causal and if they are, exactly what the causal mechanism entails. The prognosis for the premature is generally much worse than that for the small- or large-for-gestational-age infant. The most serious problem is the well-known hyaline membrane disease, but such an infant is also at increased risk from infection, anemia, and asphyxia. The infant's chances of suffering from neurological problems and a decreased intelligence quotient later in life are also increased.

Postmaturity Less is known about postmaturity although it is estimated to occur in 12 percent of all pregnancies and is defined as a pregnancy which is prolonged past the end of the 41st week. These babies are often small for gestational age although occasionally one is found to be average for gestational age. Usually they appear wasted, probably because of intrauterine malnourishment secondary to placental dysfunction. The mortality of postmature infants is two to three times that of term babies, and 75 to 85 percent of these deaths occur during labor, apparently because the child has

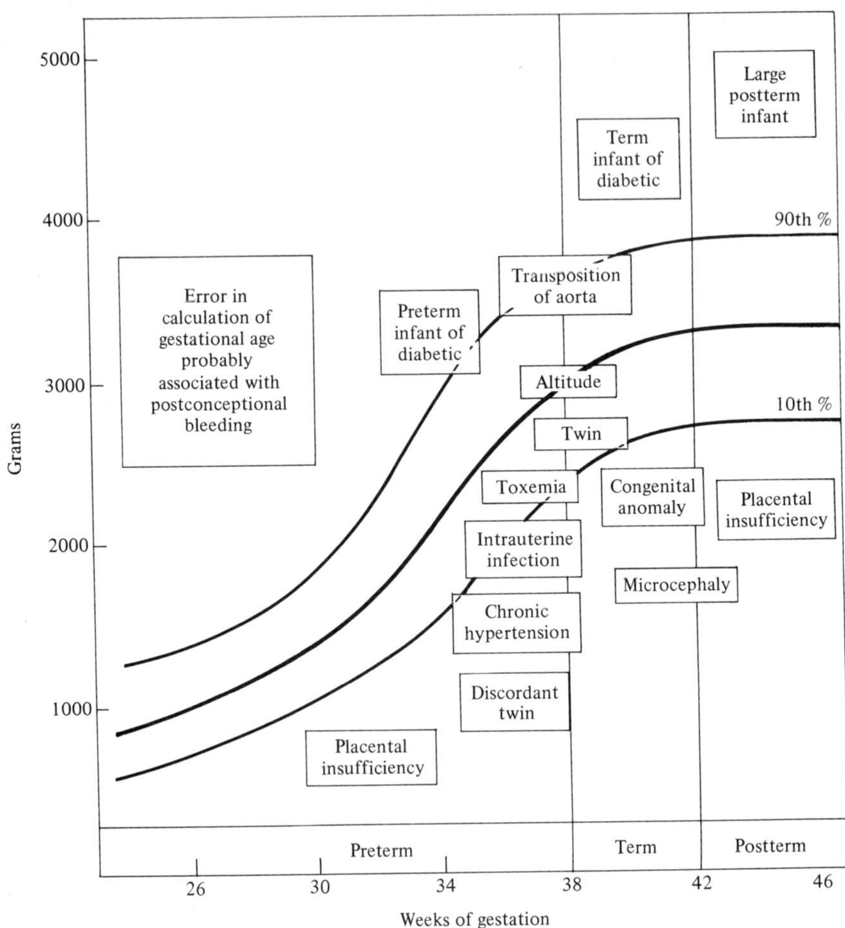

Figure 2-14 Conditions associated with deviations of intrauterine growth and weight. *(Source: Nutricia Symposium. Leiden, Holland, H. E., Stenfert Kroese, N. V., 1968.)*

been subjected to a marginally low supply of oxygen even before labor because of the malfunctioning placenta and is unable to stand the additional strain of labor.

Not only are the weight, length, and head circumference important in their relation to the gestational age, but they are important in relation to each other, and certain specific types of relationships are characteristic of certain problems (see Fig. 2-15). Down's syndrome, for instance, is often associated with an infant in which the head and weight are both significantly less than usual, but the length, although it may be slightly less than normal, is not as deviant as the other two measurements. Infants suffering from rubella often are of normal length although the head circumference and weight are generally less than that of a normal infant. In intrauterine growth retardation (i.e., infants small for gestational age) the weight seems to be most affected, the length somewhat less affected, and the head circumference least affected.

POSSIBLE NEONATAL PROBLEMS

The neonatal period is certainly one of the most physiologically unstable periods an individual ever goes through. There are many potential dangers, some of them more common than others. The nurse involved in ambulatory pediatrics will not be treating these problems, but does need to be alert to them so that help can be given immediately.

Jaundice

Certainly the most common of these neonatal dangers is jaundice. The word *jaundice* refers to the yellow coloration seen in the skin, mucous membranes

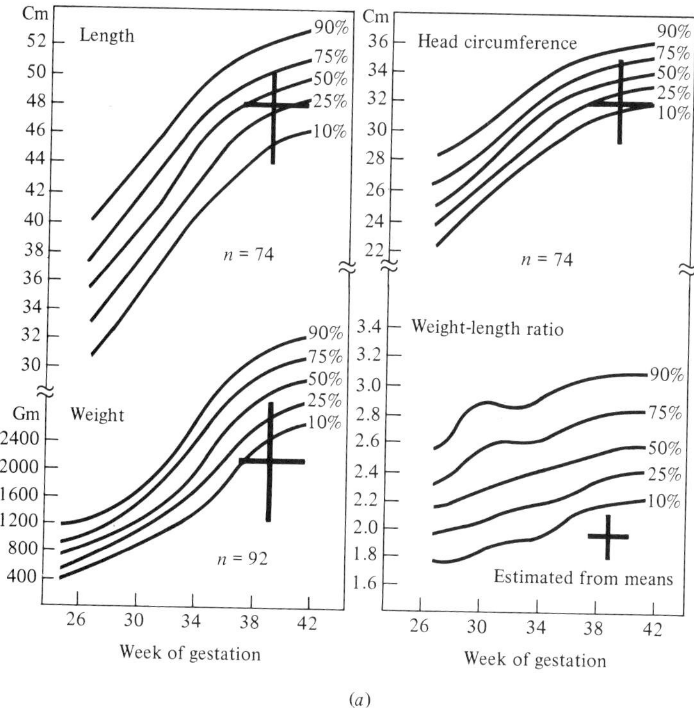

Figure 2-15 Height, weight, and head circumference relationships of the newborn. (*a*) Normal values. (*b*) The median birthweight and gestational age of infants with osteogenesis imperfecta markedly deviant, being 1,500 gm and 37 weeks. (*c*) In newborns with Down's syndrome the weight, length, and head circumference are affected. The parameter least affected is length. *(Source: Lulu Lubchenko, "Assessment of Gestational Age and Development at Birth," Pediatric Clinics of North America, vol. 17, no. 1, February 1970, p. 137.)*

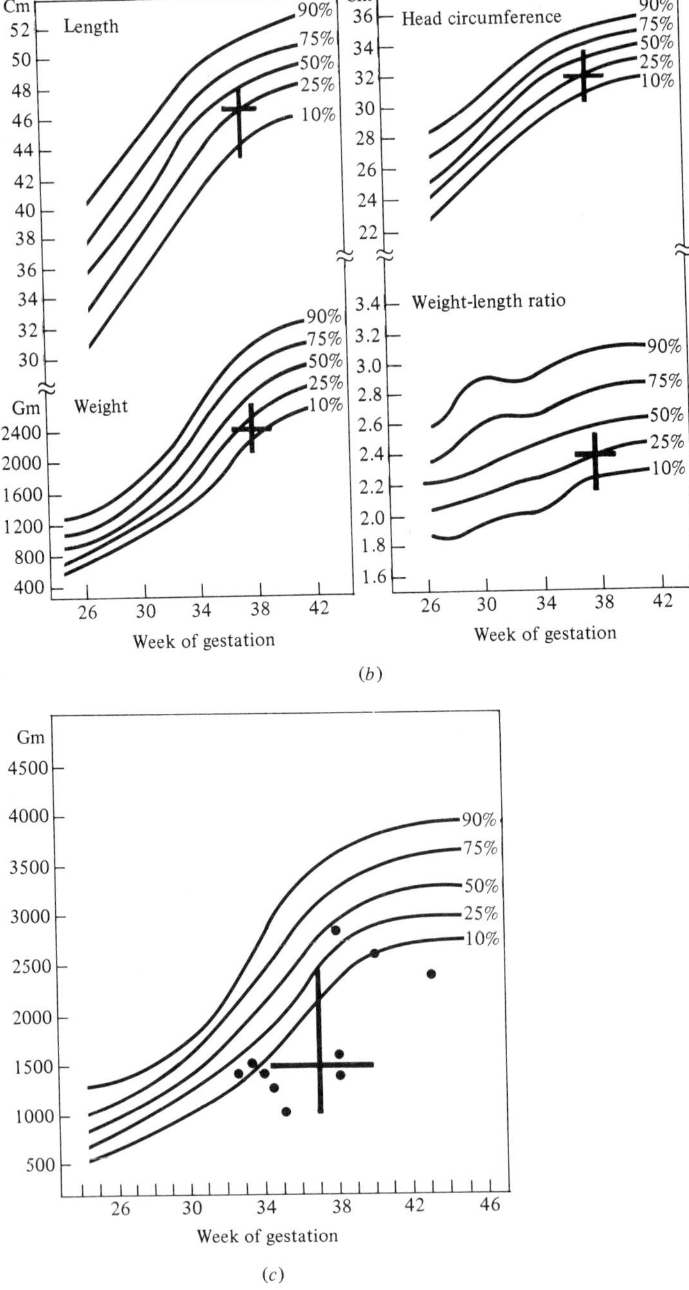

Figure 2-15 ***(Cont'd)***

and sclera as a result of high levels of bilirubin in the blood. There are two types of bilirubin, direct or conjugated and indirect or unconjugated. Direct bilirubin has been conjugated with a glucuronide molecule in the liver, resulting in a water-soluble compound which can be excreted through the urine and is generally not potentially harmful to the body. Indirect bilirubin has not yet been conjugated in the liver and is potentially more damaging to the body. It is only fat soluble and can thus not be excreted through the kidney. It is, however, attracted to certain body and brain tissues which contain fat, and it is here that the possible damage may result. This is particularly true in the brain, where it is called *kernicterus* and leaves permanent impairment. Indirect or unconjugated bilirubin can be either bound or unbound. The bound type is that which has become attached to albumin molecules in the blood. When this attachment occurs, the molecule can no longer pass out through the vessel walls into the body and nervous tissue and is thus rendered safe. It is the unconjugated, unbound bilirubin which is most likely to leave the cardiovascular spaces and enter the susceptible tissues. The unbound type results from situations in which there is a lack of albumin to attach to or where the albumin is replaced in its attachment with the bilirubin by such chemical entities as free fatty acids, sulfonomides, salicylates, and sodium benzoates. This is one reason why one must be so careful of certain medications in very young infants. An acid pH in the blood will also cause the displacement of albumin and will free more bilirubin to pass into the body proper. Most laboratory tests do not differentiate these two types of indirect bilirubin, but in certain circumstances it is important to do so since it is the unbound type that is most dangerous. This can be discovered by a laboratory determination of the albumin-binding capacity of the blood.

Clinically, jaundice does not usually appear until the bilirubin level exceeds 4 to 6 ml. Since most newborns have immature hepatic systems, most will display some amount of jaundice. The term *physiological jaundice* has been used to refer to such a normal, nondamaging type of jaundice. It is expected to reach its peak in full-term infants by about 3 to 4 days and in premature infants in about 5 to 6 days. It is important to remember, however, that even physiological jaundice can cause damage if it reaches excessive levels. To be considered normal, the infant must be otherwise well and the jaundice must not begin before 24 hours in a full-term infant or 48 hours in a premature child. It must be gone before 1 week in a full-term child and before 9 to 10 days in a premature child. It must never exceed 12 mg/100 ml in the serum, and almost all this must be of the unconjugated type. Clinically one can judge the extent of jaundice partly by the depth of color and partly by how far down the trunk it has extended. Jaundice proceeds in a cephalocaudal direction, and early mild jaundice will usually not extend beyond the chin or neck. Moderate jaundice will not extend beyond the trunk, and severe jaundice will usually cover the infant from head to toes. If there is any question, however, laboratory studies are imperative since there is a certain element of subjectivity to the clinical interpretation.

Certain pathological conditions are also manifested in jaundice. Generally, these conditions are those which cause breakdown of the red blood cells at an excessive rate of speed either within or outside of the vessels or which interfere with the ability of the liver to excrete these breakdown products.

The most dangerous result of jaundice is kernicterus, in which the bilirubin is deposited in the brain and central nervous system tissue. Common symptoms associated with this are either those of central nervous system depression, such as coma, lethargy, decreased Moro reflex, hypotonia, and decreased sucking and rooting, or those of excitation of the central nervous system, such as twitching, opisthotonis, high-pitched cry, and seizures. Kernicterus occurs at approximate levels of 20 mg/100 ml in a full-term infant and 15 mg/100 ml in a premature infant. However, even more important than the level of bilirubin is the knowledge of how much of that bilirubin is bound. In laboratories which can determine albumin-binding capacities, this test is an extremely useful tool. Albumin can, in fact, be given to the infant in order to bind more bilirubin, thus trapping it inside the vascular walls and protecting the extravascular organs such as the brain. Kernicterus is an extremely dangerous situation not only because of the immediate central nervous system problems but because of the poor long-term prognosis in terms of intelligence and various motor problems. As discussed before, several types of treatment are available, including exposure to fluorescent lights, exchange transfusion, and in some places experimental administration of phenobarbital to the mother prenatally or to the baby postnatally.

Respiratory Distress

Respiratory distress syndrome is another rather common problem during the neonatal period restricted primarily, but not exclusively, to premature infants. Again, the nurse will not usually be involved in treatment, but must be alert to the symptoms which occur rather soon after birth. Sternal retractions, tachypnea, grunting respirations, flaring nostrils, barrel chest, and decreased breath sounds are all danger signs in this regard.

Anemia

A third problem which is relatively common during this period is anemia. Certain infants are more "at risk" for this complication than others. Infants of low birth weight, infants with sepsis, premature infants, twins, and infants born after any obstetric problem, particularly placenta previa or placenta abruptio, are much more likely than other babies to be anemic. A full-term baby has 70 to 80 percent fetal hemoglobin, while a preterm infant has about 80 to 90 percent fetal hemoglobin. During the first few months this is gradually lost, to be replaced by mature hemoglobin. By about 3 months, this transition should be almost complete. This time period often coincides with a *physiologic anemia.* This occurs in term infants about 2 to 3 months, but usually is seen earlier in prematures. In the past this physiological anemia was not treated. Within the last few years, however, a good deal of controversy has arisen over whether iron should be given to all infants prophylactically because of this drop in iron. The American Academy of Pediatrics has issued a statement saying that it does indeed feel this prophylactic use of iron is useful, given either in iron-fortified milks or medicinally. A term infant, the academy says, should receive a prophylactic dose of 0.8 to 1.0 mg/kg/day (up to 15 mg/day) while a premature infant should receive 2.0 mg/kg/day (up to 15.0 mg/day). Therapeutic doses should be given only if real anemia is present, and this should consist of elemental iron in the amounts of 6.0 mg/kg/day. It is sometimes useful to know that iron absorption can be increased by the addition of vitamin C or by giving the iron only between regular feedings since the phosphates and phytates of food interfere with iron absorption.

Hypoglycemia

A fourth important and reasonably common problem of the neonate is hypoglycemia. Normal full-term infants whose weight is average for gestational age should be born with glycogen stores which are about 90 percent used up by the third postdelivery hour. From then on for the first 2 to 3 days, carbohydrate is the primary energy source. After that infants will rely much more heavily on fat for their metabolic needs. The normal range of blood sugar in the newborn is about 30 to 125 mg/100 ml in full-term infants of 2,500 gm. In babies who are large for their gestational age, this range is lower, about 20 to 100 mg/100 ml. Blood sugar levels below these are a matter of concern since the brain is being deprived of essential nourishment when the blood sugar is low. Sometimes the resultant hypoglycemia will be asymptomatic, and all suspect infants should have their blood sugar monitored carefully with or without symptoms. Symptoms, when they do appear, may be vague and often mimic a wide variety of other diseases. Cyanosis, irregular and rapid respirations, tremors, pallor, apnea, sweating, poor feeding, and convulsions may all be results of low blood sugar.

Certain groups of babies are more likely to have problems with hypoglycemia, and these groups should be considered high risk and should be carefully monitored. Included in these groups are babies who are small for their gestational age. Presumably, these infants suffered some degree of intrauterine malnutrition and are more likely to use up their blood sugar quickly after birth. About 20 percent of such babies have been shown to have hypoglycemia, and of these 50 to 90 percent manifest symptoms. About twice as many males as females seem to be affected. Infants that do manifest symptoms generally will do so within 24 to 72 hours after birth, but some may show symptoms as early as 3 hours after birth or as late as 7 days after birth. Generally, it is recommended that the dextrostix test for blood sugar should be done about twice during the first 24 hours and then three times daily for 4 days in babies who are small for their gestational age. Infants of diabetic mothers form another group which is at high risk for developing hypoglycemia. These babies are usually large for gestational age and most often develop the hypoglycemia within 2 to 4 hours after delivery. Dextrostix tests are recommended at 1, 2, 4, and 6 hours after birth. Also to be watched closely for this problem are erythroblastotic infants, who should be checked every 4 to 6 hours the first day and then daily for the succeeding 4 days. Premature infants are also prone to develop low blood sugar and are generally given IV glucose routinely if they are under 1,250 gm since almost all of them have decreased glycogen and glucagon storage. They, like any infant who is suspected of having hypoglycemia, should be assiduously protected against loss of body heat since this expends energy in the form of blood sugar and further depletes the brain.

Treatment of hypoglycemia is sugar. When possible, this is given orally but can be given as IV glucose if necessary. Sometimes glucagon is given to infants of diabetic mothers for the purpose of releasing their glycogen stores. This would be useless in small-for-gestational-age infants, however, since they have no glycogen stores. The prognosis of untreated hypoglycemia is very poor. If it is symptomatic, most will die without treatment and 30 to 60 percent will have long-range central nervous system problems even with treatment. The forecast for hypoglycemia without symptoms is not clear since as yet no good long-term studies are available.

Hypocalcemia

Another fairly common neonatal problem is hypocalcemia. In general, the newborn's range of blood calcium should be between 8 and 10 mg/100 ml. Anything below a level of 7 is certainly a reason for concern. Infants with hypocalcemia may be asymptomatic; if they do display symptoms, however, the specific symptoms will depend on how long after delivery they develop. There are two peak times for hypocalcemia; the first occurs during the first 48 hours, the second appears later, usually between 5 and 10 days. If symptoms occur during the first 48 hours, they will most often consist of apnea, high-pitched cry, cyanosis, edema, and abdominal distention. Symptoms developing during the later time period are more likely to consist of tremors, twitching, convulsions, or tetany. This form of neonatal tetany may result from a type of milk with a low calcium phosphorus ratio (like evaporated milk), causing hyperphosphatemia which depresses the parathyroid, which in turn depresses the level of serum calcium. A full half of all prematures will suffer from some degree of hypocalcemia. Other infants who should be considered at risk for hypocalcemia are those who suffer from any type of perinatal asphyxia; those who are small for gestational age; those born of diabetic mothers (25 percent of this group have hypocalcemia); those whose mothers are hypocalcemic or who suffered from toxemia, abruptio placenta, or placenta previa during pregnancy; and those who do not receive oral feedings for 24 to 48 hours. Treatment for hypocalcemia consists of IV calcium gluconate administered very slowly (this can be a dangerous procedure and the infant must be carefully monitored for bradycardia). This cannot be given intramuscularly since it causes necroses of the muscle. After the acute emergency is over, it may be given orally.

Hypomagnesemia

Hypomagnesemia is less common, and some investigators do not feel that it even presents a problem. Others, however, feel that it does and point to such symptoms as a weak cry, apnea, hypotonia, and cyanosis and say that it is much more likely if the mother has been given magnesium sulfate.

Narcotic Addiction

Narcotic addiction can be a very serious neonatal problem for certain newborns. Generally it occurs in infants whose mothers were taking 6 to 12 mg of heroin a day during pregnancy. This is often difficult to estimate, however, since street dosages are frequently inaccurate. Symptoms in the newborn usually occur within 24 hours although it is possible for them to develop any time up until 5 days of age. Excitability of the autonomic system is responsible for the majority of symptoms, such as tremors, high-pitched cry, hyperactivity, yawning, sneezing, increase of mucus, poor feeding, vomiting, and diarrhea. This is a very serious condition with mortality estimates that range from 9 to 94 percent. Treatment consists of either phenobarbital or chlorpromazine. Women who are on methadone may also have infants who suffer from withdrawal symptoms, but this is usually much less severe.

Infection

Certainly one of the most dangerous of newborn ailments is infection. Infection in the neonate seems to be quite different from infection in older children or adults. Different organisms are usually responsible (most often Gram-negative organisms), and the symptoms may be quite unfamiliar to the clinician not accustomed to newborns. Fever is seldom evident, and in general the symptoms are quite vague and diffuse. Often lethargy and feeding difficulties are the only manifestations of infections. Because of the newborn's small size, local infection is quite likely to become systematic rather quickly, and 20 percent of these cases result in sepsis. Sepsis may in turn result in other problems such as hyperbilirubinemia with associated kernicterus and later neurological complications. Infants who should be considered as high risk for infections include all prematures, any infant whose labor and delivery have been excessively long, and any infant who suffered from premature rupture of the membrane (i.e., more than 24 hours before delivery).

Knowledge of the etiology of newborn infections is important to the nurse concerned with ambulatory pediatrics. Etiological agents can be bacteria, viruses, protozoa, or fungi. The most commonly cited bacteria are

Gram negative, usually E. coli and Pseudomonas aeruginosa. A few Gram-positive organisms like streptococcus, Group B and Listeria monocytogenes have also been implicated. Viral causes are less common although still important; several viruses known to be capable of infecting the infant through the mother during pregnancy are listed in Table 2-7. The one important protozoan known to infect the newborn is the toxoplasmosis protozoan discussed previously; the one fungus known to be important in this situation is Candida albicans, which is frequently present in the vagina of pregnant women and causes monilia infections that are usually quite resistant to treat-

Table 2-7 Viruses Affecting the Fetus

Virus	Fetal/neonatal disorders
Rubella	Microcephaly, meningoencephalitis (chronic), cataracts, microphthalmia, glaucoma, deafness, hepatitis, jaundice, hepatosplenomegaly, pneumonitis, cardiovascular anomalies, myocardial necrosis, thrombocytopenia, anemia, purpura, inguinal hernia
Cytomegalovirus	Microcephaly, cerebral calcification, hydrocephalus, encephalitis, chorioretinitis, hepatitis, jaundice, hepatosplenomegaly, pneumonitis, cardiac anomalies, thrombocytopenia, purpura, anemia, inguinal hernia
Herpesvirus hominis	Meningoencephalitis, microcephaly, cerebral calcification, herpetic rash, hepatitis, jaundice, pneumonitis, thrombocytopenia, anemia, coagulopathy, keratoconjunctivitis, chorioretinitis
Coxsackie group B	Meningoencephalitis, myocarditis, hepatitis, jaundice, thrombocytopenia
Varicella-zoster	Chicken pox rash, pneumonitis, hepatitis
Variola	Smallpox rash, pneumonitis, hepatitis, meningoencephalitis
Vaccinia	Vaccinia rash, pneumonitis, hepatitis, stillbirth
Poliomyelitis	Spinal or bulbar polio similar to adult, myocarditis, pneumonitis, stillbirth, abortion
Rubeola	Measles as in later life (usually benign), stillbirth, abortion
Western equine encephalomyelitis	Meningoencephalitis
Mumps	Congenital parotitis, ? congenital malformations
Hepatitis (B)	Neonatal hepatitis

Source: Sheldon B. Korones, *High-Risk Newborn Infants,* Mosby: St. Louis, 1972, p. 193; modified from J. L. Sever and L. R. White, "Intrauterine Viral Infections," *Annual Review of Medicine,* vol. 19, 1968, p. 471.

ment during pregnancy. If the infection is not cleared up by the time of delivery, it is possible for the infant to contract the infection during delivery. In the infant, the result is usually oral thrush.

There are three main sources of these organisms. Contaminated nursery equipment is a very important one, and all such equipment should be cultured frequently. Nursery personnel are also implicated in many epidemics, and regular cultures may be important in this area too. Transmission of the infective organism from the mother to the infant is also important. It may be transmitted through the blood stream, from the amniotic fluid, through the birth canal before delivery by the ascending route (such as occurs in herpes virus infections or in cytomegalus infectious disease), or from the birth canal by contact during delivery (such as occurs in gonorrhea, monilia, and herpes infections).

Detecting Infections Detection of infections is important, but not always easy. As stated before, the symptoms are frequently vague and nondescript, and therefore the clinician must be constantly on the alert for sepsis. Certain laboratory techniques can be of help in this detection. Gastric contents can be analyzed for neutrophils. The umbilical cord can be examined for polymorphonuclear leukocytes, and the amniotic membranes can be examined. The baby's throat, axillae, ear canals, and inguinal folds can be cultured within 1 to 2 hours after delivery. Probably the most important laboratory technique in this regard is the analysis of circulating antibodies (called humoral antibodies) in the neonate's blood stream. There are several types of such antibodies or immunoglobulins as they are called: IgG, IgM, IgA, and IgD, but these studies are generally concerned primarily with IgG and IgM. IgG is an immunoglobulin which passes freely from the mother through the placenta to the infant. It is produced by the mother and is therefore effective only against those things to which the mother is immune. It begins accumulating in the 3rd month of gestation and is equal to the mother's level by the time of delivery; premature infants, therefore, receive less of it. These immunoglobulins generally persist in the infant until about 3 months of age, at which time the infant has produced enough of his or her own IgG to afford protection. In general, IgG is reasonably protective against Gram-negative organisms, but less effective in the case of Gram-positive organisms. This is very helpful since it is usually the Gram-negative organisms which the infant has the most difficulty with.

IgM, on the other hand, is an immunoglobulin which the fetus produces, beginning at about the 20th week of gestation. It is not transmitted from the mother. In normal infants, the level of IgM is below 20 mg/100 ml at birth. An infant who has been exposed to infection during the gestational period, however, will have been stimulated to produce higher levels of IgM, and one generally assumes that a newborn with sepsis with a higher level of IgM is manifesting an infection contracted before birth from the mother rather than one found on the nursery equipment or harbored by the nursery personnel. This is often an important distinction to make. A high level of IgM does indicate that the infant is suffering from an infection contracted while in utero. It does not, however, tell which specific infective agent was responsible, and further tests are necessary for this information.

Common Sites of Infection Although newborn infection can theoretically occur in any area, there are six anatomical sites in which it is more common. The first of these is the lungs, and pneumonia during the neonatal period is generally caused by E. coli, staphylococci or Group B streptococci. It can be either congenital or acquired. The congential type is more serious and will usually show up immediately or at least within 48 hours after delivery.

Septicemia in which the infection is spread by the bloodstream throughout the body is an extremely hazardous situation in the new baby. It is more common in male infants and in premature infants. Its symptoms are primarily nonspecific and frequently consist of generalized lethargy, poor feeding, sometimes vomiting and diarrhea, abdominal distention, abnormal respiration, jaundice, skin lesions, and meningitis (with accompanying neurological signs in about one-third of the infants). It is essential to obtain cultures of blood, urine, and spinal fluid with any such symptoms, but generally treatment must be begun before such cultures are read.

Infection of the meninges also occurs in newborns, especially in premature infants. This is 60 to 75 percent fatal and is manifested by various signs. A full, sometimes bulging anterior fontanelle is frequently noticed. Coma and convulsions occur in approximately one-half of these children, and opisthotonos is seen in about one-fourth of them. Kernig's or Brudzinski's signs are unusual in the newborn, and their absence should not reassure the examiner.

Diarrhea is another type of infection occuring in neonates. Generally the causative organism in E. coli although salmonella, shigella, and staphlococci have also been implicated. The diarrhea may also be accompanied by vomiting and weight loss. Culture of the stools is imperative.

Conjunctivitis is another possible type of neonatal infection and can be caused by staphlococci and pseudomonas although the most well-known infection in this area is the gonococcus, which will cause blindness without treatment. Polymixin, bacitracin, or neomycin are most generally used for neonatal conjunctivitis.

The last common site of infection to be mentioned here is the omphalitis. The cord stump must be inspected daily, and mothers must be carefully taught how to apply good cord care before leaving the hospital. A very slight erythema around the stump is sometimes seen and may be normal, but any more than this is a serious danger and can easily lead to septicemia.

BIBLIOGRAPHY

Adamsons, K.: "The Role of Thermal Factors in Fetal and Neonatal Life," *Pediatric Clinics of North America,* vol. 13, 1966, p. 599.

———, and I. Joelsson: "The Effects of Pharmacologic Agents upon the Fetus and Newborn," *American Journal of Obstetrics and Gynecology,* vol. 96, p. 437.

———, and M. E. Towell: "Thermal Homeostasis in the Fetus and Newborn," *Anesthesiology,* vol. 26, 1965, p. 531.

———, G. M. Gandy, and L. S. James: "The Influence of Thermal Factors upon Oxygen Consumption of the Newborn Human Infant," *Journal of Pediatrics,* vol. 66, 1965, p. 495.

Amiel-Tison, C.: "Neurological Evaluation of the Maturity of Infants," *Archives of Disease in Childhood,* vol. 43, 1969, p. 89.

Annotations: "Feeding Reflexes in Infancy," *Developmental Medicine and Child Neurology,* vol. II, 1969, pp. 641-653.

Apgar, V.: "The Newborn (Apgar) Scoring System," *Pediatric Clinics of North America,* vol. 13, 1966, p. 645.

———, and L. S. James "The First Sixty Seconds of Life," in H. Abramson: (ed.), *Resuscitation of the Newborn Infant,* St. Louis: Mosby, 1966.

———, and L. S. James: "Resuscitation Procedures in the Delivery Room," in H. Abramson (ed.), *Resuscitation of the Newborn Infant,* St. Louis: Mosby, 1966.

Arias, I. M., et al.: "Prolonged Neonatal Unconjugated Hyperbilirubinemia Associated with Breast Feeding," *Journal of Clinical Investigation,* vol. 43, 1964, p. 2037.

Barnett, Clicord R., et al.: "Neonatal Separation: The Maternal Side of Interactional Deprivation," *Pediatrics,* vol. 45, 1970, p. 2.

Battaglia, F. C., and L. O. Lubchenco: "A Practical Classification of Newborn Infants by Weight and Gestational Age," *Journal of Pediatrics,* vol. 71, 1967, p. 159.

Beard, A. G., et al.: "Neonatal Hypoglycemia: A Discussion," *Journal of Pediatrics,* vol. 79, 1971, p. 314.

Behrman, R. E., et al.: "In Utero Disease and the Newborn Infant," in I. Schulman et al. (ed.), *Advances in Pediatrics,* vol. 17, Chicago: Year Book, 1970.

Benirschke, K., and S. G. Driscoll: "The Pathology of the Human Placenta," New York: Springer-Verlag, 1967.

Berendes, H., and J. S. Drage: "Apgar Scores and Outcome of the Newborn," *Pediatric Clinics of North America,* vol. 13, 1966, p. 635.

Bodegard, G. and G. H. Schwieler: "Control of Respiration in Newborn Babies," *Acta Pediatrica Scandinavica,* vol. 60, 1971, pp. 181-186.

Brown, R. J. K., and P. G. Wallis: "Hypoglycemia in Newborn Infants," *Lancet,* vol. 1, 1963, p. 1278.

Brown, W. A., T. Manning, and J. Grodin: "The Relationship of Antenatal and Perinatal Psychologic Variables to the Use of Drugs in Labor," *Psychosomatic Medicine,* vol. 34, 1972, p. 2.

Campbell, D., J. Kuyek, et al.: "Motor Activity in Early Life," *Biology of the Neonate,* vol. 18, 1971, pp. 108-120.

Cannell, D., and C. P. Vernon: "Congenital Heart Disease in Pregnancy," *American Journal of Obstetrics and Gynecology,* vol. 85, 1969, p. 744.

Casaer, P., and Y. Akiyama: "The Estimation of the Postmenstrual Age: A Comprehensive Review," *Developmental Medicine and Child Neurology,* vol. 12, 1970, pp. 697-729.

Catz, C., and S. J. Yaffe: "Pharmacological Modification of Bilirubin Conjugation in the Newborn," *Journal of Dis. Child.,* vol. 104, 1962, p. 516.

Chantler, C., J. D. Baum, and D. A. Norman: "Dextrostix in the Diagnosis of Neonatal Hypoglycemia," *Lancet,* vol. 2, 1967, p. 1395.

Chase, H. Peter, et al.: "Alterations in Human Brain Biochemistry Following Intrauterine Growth Retardation," *Pediatrics,* vol. 50, 1972, p. 3.

Chown, B.: "Anemia from Bleeding of the Fetus into the Maternal Circulation," *Lancet,* vol. 1, 1954, p. 1213.

Clarke, P. C. N., and I. J. Carre: "Hypocalcemic, Hypomagnesemic Convulsions," *Journal of Pediatrics,* vol. 70, 1967, p. 806.

Clifford, S. H.: "Postmaturity with Placental Dysfunction; Clinical Syndrome and Pathologic Findings," *Journal of Pediatrics,* vol. 44, 1954, p. 1.

Cohen, Sanford N., and W. A. Olson,: "Drugs That Depress the Newborn Infant," *Pediatrics Clinics of North America,* vol. 12, 1970, p. 4.

Colman, H. I., and J. Rienzo: "The Small, Term Baby," *Obstetrics and Gynecology,* vol. 19, 1962, p. 87.

Cornblath, M., G. Joassin, B. Weisskopf, et al.: "Hypoglycemia in the Newborn," *Pediatric Clinics of North America,* vol. 13, 1966, p. 905.

Craig, W. S., and M. F. Buchanan: "Hypocalcemic Tetany Developing within 36 Hours of Birth," *Archives of Disease in Childhood,* vol. 33, 1958, p. 505.

Dahm, L. S., and L. S. James: "Newborn Temperature and Calculated Heat Loss in the Delivery Room," *Pediatrics,* vol. 49, April 1972, p. 4.

Davies, P. A.: "Bacterial Infection in the Fetus and Newborn," *Archives of Disease in Childhood,* vol. 46, 1971, p.1.

———, and W. Aherne: "Congenital Pneumonia," *Archives of Disease in Childhood,* vol. 37, 1962, p. 598.

Davis, L. E., et al.: "Cytomegalovirus Mononucleosis in a First Trimester Pregnant Female with Transmission to the Fetus," *Pediatrics,* vol. 48, 1971, p. 200.

Day, R. L., L. Caliguiri, C. Kamenski, et al.: "Body Temperature and Survival of Premature Infants," *Pediatrics,* vol. 34, 1964, p. 171.

Desmond, Murdina M., A. J. Rudolph, and P. Phitaksphralwan: "The Transitional Care Nursery," *Pediatric Clinics of North America,* vol. 13, 1966, p. 651.

———, et al.: "Cogenital Rubella Encephalitis," *Journal of Pediatrics,* vol. 71, 1967, p. 311.

———, et al.: "The Relation of Maternal Disease to Fetal and Neonatal Disorders," *Pediatric Clinics of North America,* vol. 8, 1961, p. 421.

Drillien, C. M.: "The Small-for-Date Infant; Etiology and Prognosis," *Pediatric Clinics of North America,* vol. 17, 1970, p. 9.

Droegemueller, E., et al.: "Amniotic Fluid Examination as an Aid in the Assessment of Gestational Age," *American Journal of Obstetrics and Gynecology,* vol. 104, 1969, p. 424.

Du, J. N. H., and T. K. Oliver, Jr.: "The Baby in the Delivery Room," *Journal of the American Medical Association,* vol. 207, 1969, p. 1502.

Dubowitz, L. M. S., V. Dubowitz, and C. Goldberg: "Clinical Assessment of Gestational Age in the Newborn Infant," *Journal of Pediatrics,* vol. 77, 1970, p.1.

Eichenwald, H. F.: "Cogenital Toxoplasmosis; A Study of 150 Cases," *American Journal of Diseases of Children,* vol. 94, 1957, p. 411.

Farr, V., D. F. Kerridge, and R. G. Mitchess: "The Value of Some External Characteristics in the Assessment of Gestational Age at Birth," *Devel. Med. Child Neurol.* vol. 8, 1966, pp. 657-666.

Finnstrom, O.: "Studies on Maturity in Newborn Infants, *Acta Paediatrica Scandinavica,* vol. 60, 1971, p. 685-694.

Friend, D. G.: "Current Drug Therapy, Drugs and the Fetus," *Clinical Pharmacology and Therapy,* vol. 4, 1963, p. 141.

Fuchs, F., and L. L. Cederquist: "Recent Advances in Antenatal Diagnosis by Amniotic Fluid Analysis," *Clinical Obstetrics and Gynecology,* vol. 13, 1970, p. 178.

Gittleman, I. F., et al.: "Hypoglycemia Occurring on the First Day of Life in Mature and Premature Infants," *Pediatrics,* vol. 18, 1956, p. 721.

Glass, L., W. A. Silverman, and J. C. Sinclair: "Effect of the Thermal Environment on Cold Resistance and Growth of Small Infants after the First Week of Life," *Pediatrics,* vol. 41, 1968, p. 1033.

Goodfriend, M. L. J., I. A. Shey, and M. D. Klein: "The Effects of Maternal Narcotic Addiction on the Newborn," *American Journal of Obstetrics and Gynecology,* vol. 71, 1956, p. 26.

Gotoff, S. P., and R. E. Behrman: "Neonatal Septicemia," *Journal of Pediatrics,* vol. 76, 1970, p. 142.

Gruenwald, P.: "Chronic Fetal Distress and Placental Insufficiency," *Biology of the Neonate,* vol. 5, 1963, p. 215.

———: "The Fetus in Prolonged Pregnancy," *American Journal of Obstetrics and Gynecology,* vol. 89, 1964, p. 503.

———: "Growth of the Human Fetus. I. Normal Growth and Its Variation," *American Journal of Obstetric Gynecology,* vol. 94, 1966, p. 1112.

Haworth, J. C., et al.: "Hypoglycemia Associated with Symptoms in the Newborn Period," *Canadian Medical Association Journal,* vol. 88, 1963, p. 23.

Hildebrandt, R. J., et al.: "Cytomegalovirus in the Normal Pregnant Woman," *American Journal of Obstetrics and Gynecology,* vol. 98, 1967, p. 1125.

Hill, R. M., and M. M. Desmond: "Management of the Narcotic Withdrawal Syndrome in the Neonate," *Pediatric Clinics of North America,* vol. 10, 1963, p. 67.

Hodgeman, J. E.: "Clinical Evaluation of the Newborn Infant," *Hospital Practice,* vol. 4, 1969, p. 70.

Hogan, G. R., and J. E. Milligan: "The Plantar Reflex of the Newborn," *New England Journal of Medicine,* vol. 285, 1970, p. 9.

Holmes, G., J. Miller, and E. Smith: "The Role of Neonatal Hyperbilirubinemia in the Production of Long-Term Neurologic Deficits," *American Journal of Diseases of Children,* vol. 44, 1969, p. 356.

Hunscher, H. A., and W. T. Tompkins: "The Influence of Maternal Nutrition on the Immediate and Long-Term Outcome of Pregnancy," *Clinical Obstetrics and Gynecology,* vol. 13, 1970, p. 130.

Keen, J. H.: "Significance of Hypocalcemia in Neonatal Convulsions," *Archives of Disease in Childhood,* vol. 44, 1969, p. 356.

Kivalo, I., S. Timonen, and O. Castren: "The Influence of Anaesthesia and the Induction-Delivery Interval on the Newborn Delivered by Caesarean Section," *Journales Chirurgiae et Gynaecologiae Fenniae,* vol. 60, 1971, pp. 71-75.

Kincaid-Smith, P.: "Bacteriuria and Urinary Infection in the Kidney in Pregnancy," *Clinical Obstetrics and Gynecology,* vol. 11, 1968, p. 533.

Koenigsberger, M. R.: "Judgment of Fetal Age," *Pediatric Clinics of North America,* vol. 13, 1966, p. 823.

Knobloch, H., and B. Pasamanick: "The Developmental Behavioral Approach to the Neurologic Examination in Infancy," *Child Development,* vol. 33, 1962, pp. 181-198.

Korones, S. B., L. E. Ainger, G. R. Monif, et al.: "Congenital Rubella Syndrome; New Clinical Aspects with Recovery of Virus from Affected Infants," *Journal of Pediatrics,* vol. 67, 1965, p. 166.

———, J. A. Roane, M. R. Gilkeson, et al.: "Neonatal IgM Response to Acute Infection," *Journal of Pediatrics,* vol. 75, 1969, p. 1261.

———, J. Todaro, J. A. Roane, et al.: "Maternal Virus Infection after the First Trimester of Pregnancy and Status of Offspring to Four Years of Age in a Predominantly Negro Population," *Journal of Pediatrics,* vol. 77, 1970, p. 245.

Korner, A. F.: "Neonatal Startles, Smiles, Erections, and Reflex Sucks as Related to State, Sex, and Individuality," *Child Development,* vol. 40, 1969, pp. 1039-1053.

Lin-fu, J. S. L.: "Neonatal Narcotic Addiction," U.S. Department of Health, Education, and Welfare, Welfare Administration, Children's Bureau, 1967.

Lubchenco, L. O.: "Intrauterine Growth as Estimated from Liveborn Birthweight Data at 24 to 42 Weeks of Gestation," *Pediatrics,* vol. 32, 1963, p. 793.

———, C. Hansman, and E. Boyd: "Intrauterine Growth in Length and Head Circumference as Estimated from Live Births at Gestational Ages from 26 to 42 Weeks," *Pediatrics,* vol. 37, 1966, p. 403.

———, and H. Bard: "Incidence of Hypoglycemia in Newborn Infants Classified by Birth Weight and Gestational Age," *Pediatrics,* vol. 47, 1971, p. 831.

Milligan, J. E., et al.: "Retention of the Moro Response in the Newborn," *Developmental Medicine and Child Neurology,* vol. 12, 1970, pp. 6-15.

Mizrahi, A., R. D. London, and D. Gribetz: "Neonatal Hypocalcemia—Its Causes and Treatment," *New England Journal of Medicine,* vol. 278, 1968, p. 1163.

Moya, R., and V. Thorndike: "The Effects of Drugs Used in Labor on the Fetus and Newborn," *Clinical Pharmacology and Therapeutics,* vol. 4, 1963, p. 628.

Naeye, R. L.: "Human Intrauterine Parabiotic Syndrome and Its Complications," *New England Journal of Medicine,* vol. 768, 1963, p. 804.

———: "Abnormalities in Infants of Mothers with Toxemia of Pregnancy," *American Journal of Obstetrics and Gynecology,* vol. 95, 1966, p. 276.

———, K. Benirschke, J. W. C. Hagstrom, and C. C. Marcus: "Intrauterine Growth of Twins as Estimated from Live Born Birthweight Data," *Pediatrics,* vol. 37, 1966, p. 409.

Nahmias, A. J., C. A. Alford, and S. B. Korones: "Infection of the Newborn with Herpesvirus Hominis," *Advances in Pediatrics,* vol. 17, 1970, p. 185.

Neligan, G. A., E. Robson, and J. Watson: "Hypoglycemia in the Newborn; A Sequel of Intrauterine Malnutrition," *Lancet,* vol. 1, 1963, p. 1282.

Nelson, W. E.: "Categorization by Weight and Gestational Age of the Infant at Birth," *Journal of Pediatrics,* vol. 71, 1967, p. 309.

Niswander, K. R., and H. Berendes: "Effect of Maternal Cardiac Disease on the Infant," *Clinical Obstetrics and Gynecology,* vol. 11, 1968, p. 1026.

Oliver, T. K., Jr.: "Temperature Regulation and Heat Production in the Newborn," *Pediatric Clinics of North America,* vol. 12, 1965, p. 765.

Paine, R. S.: "Neurologic Examination of Infants and Children," *Pediatrics Clinics of North America,* vol. 7, 1960, p. 471.

Parmalee, A. H.: "Sleep Studies for the Neurological Assessment of the Newborn," *Neuropaediatrie,* vol. 1, 1970, p. 3.

———,et al.: "Neurological Evaluation of the Premature Infant," *Biology of the Neonate,* vol. 15, 1970, pp. 65-78.

Partington, M. W., E. Lang, and D. Campbell: "Motor Activity in Early Life," *Biology of the Neonate,* vol. 18, 1971, p. 94-107.

Pildes, R., et al.: "The Incidence of Neonatal Hypoglycemia—A Complete Survey," *Journal of Pediatrics,* vol. 70, 1967, p. 76.

Reisner, S. H., A. E. Forbes, and M. Cornblath: "The Smaller of Twins and Hypoglycemia," *Lancet,* vol. 1, 1965, p. 524.

Robinson, R. J.: "Assessment of Gestational Age by Neurological Examination," *Archives of Disease in Childhood,* vol. 41, 1966, p. 427.

Schlesinger, E.R., and N. C. Allaway: "The Combined Effect of Birthweight and Length of Gestation on Neonatal Mortality among Single Premature Births," *Pediatrics,* vol. 15, 1955, p. 698.

Seeds, E. A.: "Adverse Effects on the Fetus of Acute Events in Labor," *Pediatric Clinics of North America,* vol. 17, 1970, p. 811.

Sever, J., and L. R. White: "Intrauterine Viral Infections," *Annual Review of Medicine,* vol. 19, 1968, p. 471.

Shanklin, D. R.: "The Influence of Placental Lesions on the Newborn Infant," *Pediatric Clinics of North America,* vol. 17, 1970, p. 25.

Silverman, W. A., et al.: "The Oxygen Cost of Minor Changes in Heat Balance of Small Newborn Infants," *Paediatrica Scandinavica,* vol. 55, 1966, p. 294.

———, and J. C. Sinclair: "Infants of Low Birth Weight," *New England Journal of Medicine,* vol. 274, 1966, p. 448.

Sinclair, J. C.: "Heat Production and Thermoregulation in the Small-for Date Infant," *Pediatric Clinics of North America,* vol. 17, 1970, p. 147.

Sisson, T. R. C., et al.: "Retinal Changes Produced by Phototherapy," *Journal of Pediatrics,* vol. 77, 1970, p. 2.

Smith, R. T., E. S. Platou, and R. A. Good: "Septicemia of the Newborn; Current Status of the Problem," *Pediatrics,* vol. 17, 1957, p. 549.

Starr, J. G., and Gold, E.: "Screening of Newborn Infants for Cytomegalovirus Infection," *Journal of Pediatrics,* vol. 73, 1968, p. 820.

Sutherland, J. M., and I. J. Light: "The Effect of Drugs on the Developing Fetus," *Pediatric Clinics of North America,* vol. 12, 1965, p. 781.

Tahti, E., J. Lind, K. Osterlund, and E. Rylander: "Changes in Skin Temperature of the Neonate at Birth," *Acta Paediatrica Scandinavica,* vol. 61, 1972, pp. 159-164.

Towell, M. E.: "The Influence of Labor on the Fetus and the Newborn," *Pediatric Clinics of North America,* vol. 13, August 1966, pp. 575-598.

Usher, R. H.: "Clinical and Therapeutic Aspects of Fetal Malnutrition," *Pediatric Clinics of North America,* vol. 17, 1970, p. 169.

———, R. McLean, and K. E. Scott: "Judgment of Fetal Age. II Clinical Significance of Gestational Age and an Objective Method for Its Assessment," *Pediatric Clinics of North America,* vol. 17, 1970, p. 835.

Winick, M.: "Cellular Growth of Human Placenta. III Intrauterine Growth Failure," *Journal of Pediatrics,* vol. 71, 1967, p. 390.

———: "Cellular Growth in Intrauterine Malnutrition," *Pediatric Clinics of North America,* vol. 17, 1970, p. 69.

Yankauer, A.: "Evaluation of the Routine Physical Examination of Infants in the First Year of Life: Observations," *Pediatrics,* vol. 45, 1970, p. 6.

Yerushalmay, J.: "Mother's Cigarette Smoking and Survival of Infant," *American Journal of Obstetrics and Gynecology,* vol. 88, 1964, p. 505.

———: "The Classification of Newborn Infants by Birth Weight and Gestational Age," *Journal of Pediatrics,* vol. 71, 1967, p. 164.

Zabriskie, J. R.: "Effect of Cigarette Smoking during Pregnancy; Study of 2,000 Cases," *Obstetrics and Gynecology,* vol. 21, 1963, p. 405.

Zelazo, P.: "Walking in the Newborn," *Science,* vol. 176, 1972, p. 21.

Chapter 3

Well-Child Management

IMMUNIZATIONS

Certainly one of the most striking advances in pediatric health care has been the impressive decrease in infectious diseases in the past 30 years. Although this decrease is partially due to better standards of cleanliness and to antibiotics, immunizations have played a large and important role and are among the most widely accepted measures of preventive health care. The number of diseases against which we are able to immunize is daily increasing, as is our knowledge concerning the proper use of the immunizing agents which we already possess. This is a rapidly changing field, and it is important that the nurse in ambulatory pediatrics keep abreast of current developments. Although the literature in this field can be rather technical and cumbersome, there are several sources which summarize the current status and policies on the various immunization procedures. The two basic policy-forming bodies are the American Academy of Pediatrics Committee on Infectious Diseases and the Advisory Committee on Immunization Practices (ACIP) of the U.S. Public Health Service sponsored by the Center for Disease Control. The ACIP publishes its recommendations weekly in a newsletter called *Morbidity and Mortality Weekly Report,* printed by the National Communicable Disease Center, Atlanta, Georgia, a part of the U.S. Department of Health, Education, and Welfare. This report tells the prevalence and incidence of certain infectious diseases in various parts of the country, as well as any change in recommendations on immunization practices. Every nurse practicing in the field of preventive health care should ask to have her name placed on the mailing list for this newsletter. The American Academy of Pediatrics publishes its recommendations in the so-called Redbook, officially the *Report of the Committee on Infectious Diseases,* which is updated periodically. Since the ACIP is concerned primarily with public health issues and the American Academy of Pediatrics is concerned with pediatric and general practice, there are times when their specific recommendations may differ slightly, but basically, their recommendations are similar. Another helpful publication needed by the nurse in certain circumstances is government publication 384, *Immunization Information for Foreign Travel,* obtainable for 25¢ from the Superintendent of Documents, Government Printing Office, Washington, D.C. Recommendations for specific immunizations for travel or other special circumstances can also be obtained from the disease control section of the local public health agency.

Active and Passive Vaccines

There are basically two types of vaccines available: those which confer active immunization and those which confer passive immunization. In active immunization a substance is introduced into the body which will stimulate the individual's body to produce antibodies to a specific antigen (in this case, a disease organism). This substance is generally the disease organism itself, but in certain instances may be only a form of the toxin produced by that organism. Depending on the virulence and certain other characteristics of the organism, it may be used in the vaccine in a live, killed, or attenuated form; in the attenuated form the organism remains alive, but its virulence has been significantly decreased by certain laboratory procedures.

Passive immunization is also possible, although it is less reliable and produces a much shorter immunity (generally only about 1 to 6 weeks) than the active form of immunization. It consists of the injection of already formed antibodies and will usually take effect about 2 days after injection; therefore in certain circumstances when persons have been exposed to a disease which has an incubation period of longer than 2 days, they can be given passive immunization to keep them immune until the danger of contracting the disease from this exposure is over; they will have to get an active form of immunization later, however, to remain immune. Another circumstance in which passive immunization is useful is in cases of hypogammaglobulinemias where the danger of injecting the actual organism is too great, since the individual will probably not be able to produce enough antibodies even to protect himself from the small number of organisms in the injection itself. Finally, passive immunization is useful in situations in which a person has been exposed to a disease for which no active immunization has yet been developed, such as infectious hepatitis.

There are two main categories of passive immunizations: a generalized immune serum globulin (ISG) and certain specific immune serum globulins. The more generalized type (formerly called gammaglobulin) is a concentration of pooled blood serum. Its effectiveness has been proven for four specific disease entities: measles, polio, infectious hepatitis, and hypogammaglobulinemias (in this case it is used as a replacement therapy) (Krugman, 1973). It is not protective against serum hepatitis although this was previously thought to be the case; neither is it protective against chickenpox although it does seem to modify this disease if given within 1 to 3 days of exposure (it would generally not be important to modify this disease unless the child was high risk because of some preexisting pathological condition such as leukemia). Finally, although it may prevent symptoms of rubella in pregnant women, it does not prevent the viremia which causes the damage to the fetus.

Specific immune globulins for certain diseases such as mumps, rubella, tetanus, pertussis, and vaccinia are also available and will be discussed in the sections in this chapter on these diseases.

In general, passive immunization is the responsibility of the physician. Human ISG is always preferable to the serum globulin of any animal, particularly the horse; any situation in which horse or other animal serum is needed for passive immunization is definitely the responsibility of the physician. However, the nurse should be aware of the dangers of horse serum injections. A great possibility of allergic reactions exist in this situation, particularly to individuals who have had previous exposure to such serum or who have known sensitivity to horses or horse products. It is possible to develop an extreme reaction even with the first exposure, however, and any time horse serum is used, adequate equipment should be available for handling anaphylactic shock. Sensitivity tests should always be done prior to the injection of horse serum. There are two types of sensitivity tests: the skin test and the conjunctival test. Even the small amount used in a skin test has been known to be fatal; this has never been described in a conjunctival test, however. Negative sensitivity tests are not absolute guarantees against allergy, and anaphylactic shock to the injection can occur even though the sensitivity tests were negative.

Even in cases where anaphylactic shock does not occur, a delayed serum sickness consisting of fever, urticaria, joint pains, and lymphadenopathy may occur later (after the second injection this may be several hours to several days later; after the first injection it is usually between 5 and 10 days later).

Depot and Aqueous Vaccines

Vaccines come in two basic types of preparations: depot (adjuvant) and aqueous. Depot preparations contain alum, aluminum hydroxide or phosphate, or mineral or other types of oil to allow for a slower release into the body. These should always be given intramuscularly since subcutaneous injections will cause irritation. Injections should be given into muscle masses in the anterior lateral thigh in infants or the deltoid or triceps in older children; this avoids the possibility of sciatic nerve damage, which is more likely in young children than adults. Common examples of depot injections are tetanus, diphtheria, pertussis, and the combined DPT vaccines.

Aqueous solutions can be given either intramuscularly or subcutaneously or in certain circumstances, intradermally. These cause fewer local reactions and are absorbed more quickly. Theoretically they cause earlier immunity but do not last as long as the depot type; the difference, however, is insignificant in most cases. Diphtheria, pertussis, and tetanus vaccines are also available in aqueous form, as are measles and influenza vaccines.

Precautions and Contraindications

Although immunizations have been an extremely important addition to preventive health care in this country, they are not without their disadvantages. The nurse working in this area must be fully aware of these and understand the appropriate precautions and contraindications. Febrile illness is generally a contraindication since the immunization may result in an increased fever. In situations where the child always appears with a cold, however, the academy suggests that the immunizations be given anyway. Certain chronic diseases may also be contraindications or at least precautions to immunizations of specific types. The package insert should be studied carefully in this regard.

In general, any child with a chronic illness should have a physician's order for immunization. This is particularly important in any central nervous system disorders in a child who needs a DPT immunization. Although uncommon, pertussis vaccine has caused permanent and severe brain damage in such individuals, and the nurse must take an extremely detailed neurological history before giving a pertussis vaccine. This should include questions concerning past convulsions (including febrile convulsions), fainting spells, tremors, and twitching, as well as a discussion of any reaction to a previous DPT. Open skin lesions of any kind, but particularly eczema in the child or any one else in the house, are contraindications to the use of smallpox vaccine. In general, any kind of immunologic deficiency state including cancer of the lymphatic system is a contraindication, particularly to the live-virus vaccines, as is immunosuppressive therapy such as with corticosteroids, at least without a physician's explicit order.

Specific allergies to the substance the vaccine was grown on, such as dog embryo or chick embryo (which are listed on the packet insert), are contraindications to its use. In some vaccines an antibiotic may have been used in preparation, such as the neomycin in polio and rubella vaccines; in this case, the nurse must question the patient carefully concerning allergic reactions to this substance. Much more unusual is an allergy to the preservative used in the vaccine, such as mercury.

Another question which arises when considering contraindications is the question of simultaneous administration of live vaccines. There is some controversy concerning this. There is a theoretical argument against this practice, since it would be possible for the antibody responses of the two organisms to interfere with each other. For this reason many advise leaving an interval of 6 to 8 weeks between live-vaccine injections. Krugman (1973) states that, theoretically at least, the worst interval would be between 2 days and 2 weeks; so if it were impossible to wait for 6 weeks, it would be better to give them either together or one 2 weeks after the other. More and more clinical evidence seems to be accumulating, however, to indicate that this argument may be only theoretical, and several studies show that individuals immunized with two live vaccines on the same day do become immune to both diseases (Weibel et al., 1972; Korchner et al., 1971). There are some combination vaccines on the market now, such as mumps-rubella and mumps-measles-rubella, which are given as one injection in one syringe. These vaccines have been thoroughly researched and are in fact effective in this form. This does not necessarily mean, however, that separate injections of mumps, measles, and rubella vaccines which are not marketed as one injection would be effective if given together. The American Academy of Pediatrics at this time still recommends an interval of at least 1 month between injections of live vaccines; it is possible that this recommendation will change in the near future.

Basic Immunizations

Although it must be changed to meet various special circumstances, the general schedule for basic immunizations recommended by the American Academy of Pediatrics is shown in Table 3-1.

Table 3-1 Recommended Schedule for Active Immunization and Tuberculin Testing of Normal Infants and Children

Age	Immunization or test
2 months	DTP—trivalent OPV
3 months	DTP
4 months	DTP—trivalent OPV
6 months	Trivalent OPV
12 months	Tuberculin test—live measles vaccine
15-18 months	DTP—trivalent OPV—smallpox vaccine
4-6 years	DTP—trivalent OPV—smallpox vaccine
12-14 years	Td—smallpox vaccine—mumps vaccine
Thereafter	Td every 10 years—smallpox vaccine every 3-10 years—rubella vaccine

Source: The Report of the Committee on Infectious Diseases, Evanston, Ill.: American Academy of Pediatrics, 1970, p. 5.

DPT Probably the most commonly known of the "baby shots" is the DPT (sometimes called DTP) or combination of diphtheria, pertussis, and tetanus vaccines. Although this immunization has been used for many years and the diseases are not as prevalent as they were earlier in the history of this country, a need for this immunization continues today. Although diphtheria, for instance, is uncommon in the United States today, local outbreaks in various parts of the country do continue to appear, and when they do, they carry a 10 percent fatality, primarily in children. The immunization will not prevent the carrier state, but completely immunized children will be adequately protected against the disease itself. The need for protection against tetanus also continues. In 1970, 148 cases of tetanus were reported in the United States, and over 60 percent of these were fatal. The tetanus organism is ubiquitous, and there is no natural immunity against it; therefore artificial immunization is imperative for protection. Most of the reported cases occurred in the Southern states, with a rate for minorities four times higher than that for other groups, and a 3:2 ratio of males to females.

Pertussis, too, remains an important disease. Because there is little or no maternal transfer of antibodies to the young infant, it is possible to give this vaccine rather early. In fact, some researchers have attempted to give it at birth although the American Academy of Pediatrics continues to recommend its administration at 2 months. Pertussis is an extremely serious disease in young infants and children, with a high rate of morbidity and mortality. In older children the disease is not so devastating, and the vaccine is not recommended after age 6, since at this point the dangers of the vaccine outweigh those of the disease.

Various preparations of the vaccines both separate and combined are available. The combined form (Wyeth's triple antigen or Lederle's Triimmunol) is most commonly used. This is a depot type of preparation and should be given intramuscularly, preferably in the lateral thigh. It should not be given with a current febrile illness, since a fever may result from the injection and be superimposed on the preexisting one. In the case of a mild upper respiratory infection in children who may not return to the clinic when it is over or who are always seen at their well-baby check-ups with a cold, it is advisable to give the DPT anyway. In any case, the mother should be warned that a fever may follow in 24 to 48 hours, and the nurse should be sure that the mother has some type of acetaminophen preparation (e.g., Tempra, Tylenol, or Liquiprin) at home and knows how to give it properly. It may be given prophylactically immediately after the shot; this is particularly wise if the child has had fevers with previous DPTs. The mother should also be warned that a lump may continue to persist for several months but that it will eventually disappear without problems. The most dangerous ingredient of the DPT is the pertussis vaccine; cases have been recorded in which pertussis encephalopathy has resulted from the shot and the child has been permanently brain-damaged or has died. For this reason, a thorough history of any central nervous system illness (convulsions, epilepsy, etc.) must be obtained, and the decision for immunization should be left to a physician if any of these problems exist. A careful history of the child's reaction to the last DPT should also be evaluated. If a reaction was particularly severe, it may be wise to reduce the dose from 0.5 to 0.25 and double the number of injections. The three vaccines can also be given separately although there are few indications for this. Pertussis vaccine is available as a fluid vaccine without any adjuvant for use in epidemics when very rapid absorption is necessary; it is also available as a depot vaccine with alum, aluminum phosphate, or aluminum hydroxide added. Diphtheria vaccine is similarly available either as a fluid toxoid or as a depot injection but is seldom needed unless a specific contraindication to diphtheria and pertussis exists. Tetanus vaccine is also available in fluid form for more rapid absorption, but again is seldom needed. It is available in adjuvant form as well, and in this form is commonly used for prophylaxis in wound management when more than 5 years has elapsed since the last booster or DPT or DT. A booster is all that is needed as long as the patient has received at least two injections from the primary series. If the child has received less than two of these or if the wound has been untended for more than 24 hours, it is necessary to provide passive protection in the form of tetanus antitoxin (a horse serum product) or tetanus immune globulin (a human product). As stated previously, horse serum injections are highly undesirable and should never be preferred to human products; nor should they ever be the responsibility of the nurse. Tetanus immune globulin, therefore, should be used in case of an injury which has been neglected for more than 24 hours if the previous tetanus booster was more than 10 years before or in a child with less than two of the primary injections. Tetanus toxoid can and should be given simultaneously to induce active protection; the immune globulin will not interfere with the child's antibody production; the two immunizations should be given at different sites. Table 3-2 is a schedule for wound prophylaxis with tetanus immunization recommended by Krugman.

Table 3-2 Schedule for Tetanus Immunizations

History of tetanus immunization (doses)	Clean, minor wounds		All other wounds	
	Td	TIG	Td	TIG
Uncertain	Yes	No	Yes	Yes
0–1	Yes	No	Yes	Yes
2	Yes	No	Yes	No*
3 or more	No†	No	No‡	No

* Unless wound more than 24 hours old.

† Unless more than 10 years since last dose.

‡ Unless more than 5 years since last dose.

Source: Saul Krugman and Robert Ward, *Infectious Diseases of Children and Adults,* St. Louis: Mosby, 1973, p. 436.

DT can be of either the adult or the pediatric type. The adult type has less diphtheria toxoid in it and should be used for children over 6 years. The pediatric type has the same amount of tetanus and diphtheria toxoids in it as the DPT, but has no pertussis protection. It is used in situations in which there is a question of sensitivity to the pertussis component in children under 6. In no case should DPT be given to children over the age of 6 since the complications from the pertussis component are more serious by this age than the actual disease.

Polio The next most commonly known childhood immunization procedure in this country is against polio. Immunization has been tremendously effective in eliminating polio epidemics here. A few cases do continue to appear each year in the United States, however, and it is much more common in certain other countries. There are two types of polio vaccines, the killed or Salk vaccine, which is given in injection form, and the live or Sabin, which is given in oral preparations. The Salk was the first preparation available, but it is no longer available. Although it had an advantage over the oral type in that it eliminated the carrier state as well as susceptibility to the disease and never itself caused a case of polio, it also had several disadvantages in that it had to be given by injection and required a booster every 2 years. The Sabin vaccine is an oral attenuated preparation available in either the trivalent or monovalent forms. The trivalent contains organisms of all three types of polio in one solution and is generally preferred. The monovalent has only one type in each solution, and it is recommended that it be given in the sequence of type I, type III, and the type II, with a booster of trivalent. In practice, this would probably be useful only in cases of epidemics in which the type of polio prevalent was known. Sabin vaccine is reported to have an effectiveness of over 90 percent and does protect against the carrier state as well as the actual disease. There have been rare cases of vaccine-caused polio in the vaccinee or close contacts within the first 2 months after vaccination. Chances of this occurrence are 1 in 1 million with type III, 1 in 5 million with type I, and almost no chance at all with type II. For this reason, vaccination of individuals over 18 years of age (i.e., those in whom the disease would be less devastating) is no longer routinely advised. Pregnancy is not a contraindication, although it is no longer considered to be a specific indication either. The vaccine should not be given in cases of lowered resistance such as lymphoma, leukemia, or other malignancy or when the patient is receiving drugs such as antimetabolites or steroids or radiation. There is some research indicating that in many women who breast feed, polio antibodies will be transmitted to their child through their milk and thus invalidate the immunization procedure; there is a somewhat lesser possibility that this is also true for cow's milk derived from polio-immune cows. However, the schedule recommended for infants by the American Academy of Pediatrics takes this fact into consideration, and immunity should be completely achieved by breastfed infants on this schedule. The academy recommends that infants receive polio drops at 2, 4, and 6 months, 1 year following the third dose, and immediately before entrance into school. It is recommended that older children and adolescents receive the first two immunizations 6 to 8 weeks apart and the final one 3 to 12 months later. Care must be taken with the storage of the presently available vaccines; they should be maintained at freezing temperature in a freezer cold enough to freeze ice. Once in the refrigerator, the solution must be used within 30 days and within 7 days if the container has been opened.

Measles Measles (rubeola) vaccine is a less well-known but extremely important immunization available today. Although many parents have considered measles an innocuous childhood disease, this is not true. The rate of measles encephalitis is 1 in 1,000 and often results in permanent mental retardation, brain damage, or death. Bronchopneumonia and middle-ear infections are other complications of the disease. The original measles vaccine was an inactivated type which is no longer available. It conferred short-term immunity only, and when children who had received this vaccine later contracted the disease, it was often manifested in a very serious atypical form. Children who have received such a vaccination previously need to receive the new live type now available. Actually two live measles vaccines are now on the market, the Edmonston or attenuated type and the further attenuated strain (Schwartz or Attenuvax). The Edmonston is grown on either chick embryo or dog embryo and should usually be given simultaneously with measles immune globulin in separate sites; with this regime, 15 percent will experience side effects; if the measles immune globulin is not used, the percentage of side effects will increase to about 30 percent (*Report of the Committee on Infectious Diseases,* 1970). If side effects do occur, they will generally be noticed about 7 to 10 days after the injection and usually consist of a fever and in some cases a rash. Anticipatory guidance concerning handling of fever should be given. In normal situations, the measles vaccine should not be given until 12 months of age since earlier administration may encounter interference from maternal antibodies. Several studies have shown that many children who were originally immunized before 1 year of age were not adequately protected later in life (Lerman and Gold, 1971). In cases of epidemics it may be wise to immunize sooner, but in this case another injection should then be given after 1 year of age. Vaccines are 95 percent effective if given after the first year. Vaccines are effective if given within 2 days after exposure to measles; they can be given later without harmful effect but will not protect the child from the previous exposure. Measles immune globulin can also be given after exposure in the dosage of 0.1 mg/lb as soon as possible to mitigate the severity of the disease. The Schwartz vaccine is essentially the same as the Edmonston except that it has been further attenuated and for that reason should not have the measle immune globulin administered with it. This, of course, has the advantage of eliminating one shot. The inactivated or killed vaccine is no longer available.

It had several disadvantages. One of these was that it conferred short-term immunity only; more important, however, was the fact that when children who had been vaccinated with the killed vaccine later contracted the disease, they manifested an atypical form of measles which was much more dangerous than the usual type. For this reason, any child who has previously been given the killed vaccine should now receive either the attenuated or further attenuated types. In this situation, an edematous local reaction may result in the area of the injection site, and the parents should be warned of this possibility.

Precautions and contraindications to receiving the measles vaccine are similar to those pertaining to most live vaccines: it should not be given in the presence of febrile illness, immunologic deficiencies, sensitivity to the specific vaccine ingredients listed on the package insert (usually either dog or egg products or neomycin), or pregnancy since it is unknown what effect the vaccine might have on the fetus. Because it is known that the actual measles wild virus can exacerbate tuberculosis, it is theoretically possible that the vaccine might do the same thing. For this reason, in routine care, a tine test to eliminate the possibility of measles should be administered prior to the measles vaccine. It is also known that the measles vaccine can give false negative results in tuberculosis testing. In situations of epidemics or emergencies, however, the American Academy of Pediatrics advises to give the measles vaccine even without prior tuberculosis screening.

Rubella Rubella vaccine is a fairly recently available immunization of great importance. Although rubella is generally a benign disease in children and even in adults, its results are devastating to the fetus of a pregnant woman who contracts the disease. In the 1964 rubella epidemic, 20,000 infants were born permanently handicapped because their mothers had contracted the disease during pregnancy. The cost of rehabilitative care to these children has been over 2 billion dollars (Krugman, 1971). The major reservoir of rubella is the group of children in their early school years (about 5 to 9 years old), and generally these children should have first priority if a shortage of the vaccine exists. Ideally, however, every child from 1 year to puberty should receive this protection. Earlier than 1 year, it is possible that maternal antibodies will interfere with immunity. Past puberty, each situation should be evaluated individually. It is important not to immunize women during or immediately before pregnancy, since it is known that the vaccine does produce a viremia and is transmitted to the fetus and there is a very real possibility that the fetus may be damaged in the same way by the vaccine as by the disease. For this reason, a hemaglutin antibody screening test (an HAI titer) should be drawn before administering the vaccine to this age group. Approximately 80 percent of these women will be found to be already immune, and it should be explained to them that there is then no need for the vaccine. In the remaining 20 percent, the vaccine should be given only after making sure that the woman is not at the time pregnant and that she understands the importance of not becoming pregnant for the next 2 to 3 months and is willing to take some precautionary measures in this regard. These same guidelines apply to postpartum women who have been tested during their pregnancy and found to be unprotected. Although the long-term immunity from this vaccine is not yet established, the immediate effectiveness is 96 to 100 percent and has lasted since the vaccine has been released. Although reinfection can occur both in previous vaccinees and in previous disease victims, the reinfection is not accompanied by viremia and thus presents no danger to a fetus. Side effects of rash, fever, lymphadenopathy, and occasionally arthritis, arthralgia, and even paresthesia occurs in approximately 5 to 15 percent of recipients of the vaccine. Side effects are much more common with the vaccine grown on dog kidney, and for this reason, that preparation is less desirable than the others. Symptoms, when occuring, may occur anywhere from 2 to 10 weeks after vaccination, and the recipient should be warned of this possibility. Although one case has been recorded in which the symptoms actually lasted for 103 days, the majority of them are quite mild and short-lived and none have been permanent (Lerman, 1971). Virus shedding from the nasopharynx has been noted in about half of the vaccinees for periods ranging from 1 to 4 weeks, but there has been no documentation that any vaccinee has infected another person with this shed, apparently because it is quantitatively much less than that which occurs in the actual disease (Krugman, 1971). Precautions and contraindications are basically the same as those of other live vaccines.

Mumps Another recently available vaccine is that for mumps. Although mumps is generally a mild disease in childhood, complications can arise from spread to the testicles, epididymis, ovaries, prostate, labyrinthes, brain, vulvovaginal glands, spleen, thymus, heart, liver, pancreas, thyroid, cranial nerves, spinal cord, and mammary glands. About 20 percent of adult men who contract mumps suffer the complication of orchitis 3 to 7 days after the parotid swelling subsides. Only 35 percent of these suffer any testicular atrophy, and only 10 percent of these are bilateral; sterility is actually quite rare. However, 85 percent of these men suffer epididymitis, and although it seldom has permanent effects, it is extremely painful. Less often complications of arthritis (occuring in about 0.4 percent of individuals and lasting from a few days to 3 months), thyroiditis (usually subacute and usually in women), myocarditis (extremely rare), and certain central nervous system problems such as meningitis or meningoencephalitis (which although rarely fatal, does have frequent residual effects and occurs both in children and adults) do occur. For these reasons, the mumps vaccine is a welcome addition to the armamentarium of preventive vaccines.

The mumps vaccine now available is grown on chick embryo and contains neomycin so that sensitivity to these two ingredients may be a contraindication to its use. In addition the usual precautions and contraindications to live viruses, hold, i.e., immunosuppressant therapy, decreased antibody response, pregnancy (on theoretical grounds), febrile illnesses, and children under 1 year of age, since maternal antibodies appear to interfere with the action of this vaccine. Since the presently used mumps vaccine induces immunity rather slowly, it is not effective after exposure to the disease. Although a mumps immune globulin is available, it does not appear to be very effective either.

Less Common Immunizations

Rabies The rest of this chapter will discuss vaccines which are less commonly used than those previously discussed but are important in certain specific situations. Many of these will not usually be the responsibility of the nurse, but she should keep informed concerning them. Rabies is the first to be considered here. The incidence of rabies has greatly decreased in the last several decades. In 1940, there were 22 reported cases; this has dropped to 1 or 2 a year in the 1970s. Rabies in domestic animals appears to have decreased, but that found in wild animals has increased; this is especially true of skunks, foxes, raccoons, and bats; in 1971, 70 percent of the rabies cases were from wild animals. In spite of the drop in incidence of this disease, 50,000 individuals continue to receive the vaccine each year in this country since most clinicians prefer to be safe and give the vaccine (Krugman, 1973). There are two types of active immunization available at this time: the Semple (NTV) type and the duck embryo vaccine (DEV) type. The Semple form is grown on rabbit brain and reaches higher levels of antigenicity although these levels begin later than with the DEV. The DEV grown on duck embryo has lower but adequate antigenicity. It is highly preferable since its rate of neurological complications is much lower than that seen with the NTV type. Local reactions of pain erythema and pruritis are common with both types of vaccine, although they do not usually occur until after the 5th day. They are not sufficient reason to discontinue the vaccine. The more serious complications are those of the central nervous system, much more commonly seen with the NTV vaccine. Encephalitic reactions can occur between 6 and 54 days after the first dose. Paralytic reactions, usually in the form of a flaccid paralysis of the lower extremities may occur gradually, seldom beginning before the 5th day. These are seldom fatal, but about 35 percent result in permanent residual damage (Krugman, 1973). Prophylactic schedules of antirabies vaccine can be given to those in high-risk categories, such as veterinarians, spelunkers (cave explorers who may come into frequent contact with bats), and laboratory workers involved in work concerning rabies organisms. To maintain immunity, boosters are necessary every 1 to 3 years. This schedule is not 100 percent effective and so titers must be drawn to make sure the individual is protected. If such an immunized person is bitten, five doses of vaccine with a booster 20 days later is recommended, but no antiserum is necessary. If the individual is exposed without being bitten (for instance in a laboratory situation), only one dose is required. If a nonimmunized person is exposed through either a bite or other type of exposure, the regime in Table 3-3 is recommended. It can be seen that the exact amount needed depends on what type of exposure exists. Passive vaccination with horse serum will usually be required as well as active immunization. Because this is horse serum, all the precautions discussed concerning horse serum apply here. Wound care is also important, and the wound should be flushed with quarternary ammonium (zephiran) after a soap-and-water washing. Care must be taken to thoroughly rinse the soap first since soap can inactivate zephiran. Up to half of the antiserum is then used to infiltrate the wound area. In most situations the decision for rabies prevention will not be the responsibility of the nurse although she will often be assisting in this care.

Influenza Influenza vaccines are not recommended for routine use but may be important in certain parts of the population which are at risk; these include young infants; patients with chronic pulmonary, metabolic, neurologic, cardiac, and renal problems; institutionalized children; and the elderly. This is especially true in epidemic years. The main difficulty with this vaccine is that epidemics of influenza are characteristically caused by different strains of the virus. By the time an adequate vaccine is developed to one strain, the next epidemic appears, caused by a different strain. There are basically two types of vaccine available: the polyvalent with many different strains in it, and the bivalent with only two strains in it. Generally the bivalent is preferred since it allows heavier concentration of the currently

Table 3-3 Postexposure Antirabies Guide*

Animal and its condition		Treatment	
		Kind of exposure	
Species	**Condition at time of attack**	**Bite†**	**Nonbite†**
Wild Skunk Fox Raccoon Bat	Regard as rabid	S + V[1]	S + V[1]
Domestic	Healthy	None[2]	None[2]
Dog	Escaped (unknown)	S + V	V[3]
Cat	Rabid	S + V[1]	S + V[1]
Other	Consider individually		

* These recommendations are only a guide. They should be used in conjunction with knowledge of the animal species involved, circumstances of the bite or other exposure, vaccination status of the animal, and presence of rabies in the region.

† See text definitions.

V = Rabies vaccine; S = Antirabies serum; 1 = discontinue vaccine if fluorescent antibody (FA) tests of animal killed at time of attack are negative; 2 = begin S + V at first sign of rabies in biting dog or cat during holding period (10 days); 3 = 14 doses of DEV.

Source: Saul Krugman and Robert Ward, *Infectious Diseases of Children and Adults,* St. Louis: Mosby, 1973, p. 447.

infective strain. Frequent systemic reactions (as many as 50 percent) of malaise and fever are encountered. The primary series consists of two subcutaneous doses 6 to 8 weeks apart with a booster every year after. For those who have previously had an influenza immunization which contained the Hong Kong variety (any vaccine received since 1968), only a booster is needed. Central nervous system complications have been reported but are rare.

Smallpox Smallpox immunization, although formerly common, is now recommended only for foreign travel to certain countries in which smallpox is endemic. At present smallpox is endemic in only eight countries, and in the near future, it will probably not be endemic anywhere. However, the vaccine probably should continue to be given to hospital personnel. The last confirmed case in the United States was in 1949. Since that time there have been no cases of the disease, but the vaccine itself has caused many problems each year. In 1968, there were reported 16 cases of vaccine-induced encephalitis, 11 cases of vaccinia necrosum, 126 cases of eczema vaccinatum, and 9 fatalities (Krugman, 1973). In other words, at this time in this country, the risk from the vaccine is greater than the risk from the disease. Presently there are two types available: one grown on calf lymphatic tissue, which is the more stable, and the avianized form, which gives milder reactions but confers as potent protection as does that grown on calf lymph. The precautions discussed for all live vaccines apply to smallpox vaccine. It is particularly important not to give the vaccine during pregnancy since there have been cases in which the fetus has suffered from vaccinia when the mother was immunized during pregnancy. Egg-sensitive individuals should not receive the avianized type, and any person with a skin rash, particularly eczema, or who comes in contact with such a person should not receive the vaccine.

There are three basic methods of injection: puncture, pressure, and jet injection. In the multiple-puncture method, the skin is cleansed with water only and dried; a sterilized bifurcated needle with a droplet of vaccine is held perpendicular to the skin, and punctures are made deep enough for a drop of blood to appear. Only 5 punctures are needed for primary immunization; 15 are recommended for revaccination. The multiple-pressure technique begins with the same cleansing of the skin; a drop of vaccine is then placed on the skin, and the needle is held tangentially toward the skin and used to make pressure marks 1/8 in. deep into the skin covered by the droplet. For the primary vaccination, 10 pressure marks are needed, for revaccination, 30 are needed. When many individuals are to be given the vaccine at one time, a jet injection gun may be used with intradermal injection. The vaccination should be read 6 to 8 days after it is given. A vesicle is expected with a primary series, and either a vesicle or pustule or at least an area of palpable induration is expected with a secondary immunization.

Anything less than this is considered equivocal and the vaccination should be redone.

Rocky Mountain Spotted Fever Rocky Mountain spotted fever vaccination is needed prophylactically only by laboratory personnel working with this organism and by certain individuals who are expected to have occupational exposure; it is not recommended for recreational exposure. The vaccine available does not prevent the disease, but does limit its severity. Side effects are generally local in the form of slight pain, tenderness, erythema, and induration; less often systemic fever and malaise occur. The vaccine is grown on chick eggs, and egg-sensitive individuals should not receive it. For children under 12, the primary series consists of three subcutaneous injections of 0.5 ml at 7- to 10-day intervals followed by a booster of 1 ml a year later. For children 12 years or older and adults the original series consists of three 1.0-ml subcutaneous doses at 7- to 10-day intervals.

Cholera Cholera vaccination is needed only by travelers to certain parts of the world. Cholera is endemic in South and Southeast Asia, the Middle East, Africa, and part of Europe, but even in these regions it is unlikely to be contracted in the tourist areas where food and water are carefully monitored since this is the route of transmission. Some countries require evidence of a complete primary series or a booster within the preceding 6 months, although infants under 5 years of age are not usually required to have it. Reactions consist of local tenderness for 1 or 2 days and, at times, fever, malaise, and headache; more serious reactions are extremely rare.

Plague A vaccine against the plague is also available although its effectiveness has never been accurately measured. The plague is endemic in some parts of South America, Africa, and Asia; vaccination is recommended for all travelers going to Vietnam, Cambodia, and Laos since the plague is most severe there. A few cases are reported each year in the Western United States, where wild rodents have it, but vaccination is recommended only if an individual's occupation brings him or her into frequent contact with these rodents. As with cholera, mild local reactions of pain, swelling, and erythema may be encountered, as may systemic reactions of malaise, headache, and fever, particularly with repeated doses.

Yellow Fever Yellow fever vaccination is recommended only for travelers to sub-Sahara Africa and South America and for laboratory personnel working with this organism. This vaccine requires special handling and can be given only at yellow fever vaccination centers listed with the World Health Organization. After reconstitution with normal saline, the vaccine is good for only 1 hour. There are two types available. The Dakar or French neurotropic type is associated with a high incidence of meningoencephalitic reactions and is not recommended. The 17D type is better and has not been associated with significant complications. Although 5 to 10 percent of vaccinees suffer from mild headache, aching muscles, and a slight fever, less than 0.2 percent have to curtail their typical activities. In the United States, of the 34 million vaccinations given, only 2 cases of encephalitis have been reported. All the usual precautions to live vaccines apply. Since it is grown on chick embryo, egg-sensitive individuals should not receive it.

Typhus Although a vaccine is available for typhus, it is seldom necessary. The United States has not had a case of typhus since 1922 although it is possible that typhus might become a problem in time of war or disaster if louse infestation became prevalent. Vaccination is not recommended for travel to any of the usual areas although it may be desirable for travel to certain mountainous highland areas where louses are prevalent; this might be true, for instance, in remote mountains of Asia, Peru, Bolivia, Mexico, Ecuador, Burundi, Ethiopia, and Ruanda. It is suggested for scientific investigators in these areas, for medical personnel caring for patients in these areas, and for laboratory personnel working with this organism. Effectiveness of this vaccine has not been adequately tested although clinical impressions seem to indicate that it does help. It protects only against louse-borne typhus, not against the scrub or murine types. Local tenderness may occur and rarely is a systemic reaction encountered. The vaccine is grown on embryonated eggs, and egg-sensitive individuals should not receive it.

Typhoid Typhoid is another vaccine available although not recommended for routine use. It is, however, recommended if a known exposure to a carrier exists, if there is a community or group outbreak, and for foreign travel. Effectiveness ranges from 50 to 90 percent. Because of possible febrile reaction, this vaccine should not be given in the presence of febrile illness.

Other Certain other vaccines which are generally considered dangerous and of questionable effectiveness are available and should be used only at the physician's discretion. Examples are the vaccines for gas gangrene, botulism, and parathyphoid A and B.

Certain other vaccines are currently under study and may bc released in the future. Examples of these are vaccines to protect against gonorrhea, syphilis, and meningococcal disease.

In summary, immunizations are one of the most important advances in preventive health we have today, but they cannot be considered without danger; the nurse working in ambulatory pediatrics should be familiar with the nature of the commonly used vaccines and know where to get information when presented with an unfamiliar one. Appropriate precautions must be taken when making decisions concerning vaccine administration.

CHILDHOOD SAFETY

Anyone involved in health care of children is painfully aware of the tremendous problem posed by accidents of all kinds in this age group. From 1 month to 24 years, accidents are the leading cause of death and are second only to acute infections in accounting for morbidity and visits to the doctor's office. Every year about 15,000 fatal accidents occur to children and about 17 million which are nonfatal (Green and Haggerty, 1968). Three out of every ten children under the age of 1 experience accidents serious enough to visit the physician or to restrict activity (Green and Haggerty, 1968). Although some of these accidents are minor, many result in lifelong disabilities of a very serious nature. In New York, children under the age of 5 experience a death rate from accidents six times higher than that from meningitis, tuberculosis, encephalitis, measles, rheumatic fever, poliomyelitis, whooping cough, chicken pox, scarlet fever, and diphtheria all combined (Einhorn and Jobziner, as quoted in Barnett, p. 302). Generally, accidents are more common in boys than girls, and the incidence is higher in summer than winter. Specific types of accidents also vary with particular age groups. Mechanical suffocation is the most frequent type of accident encountered in children under 1 year of age, while burns are the most common accidental problem of children from 1 to 4 years. From 5 to 14 years, drowning is the most common accident for boys, while it ranks fourth for girls; automobile accidents rank first for girls and second for boys. See Table 3-4.

Poisonings

Poisonings are an extremely important type of accident with which the nurse working in ambulatory pediatrics will be intimately involved. Every year in this country it is estimated that between 500,000 and 2,000,000 poisonings

Table 3-4 Accident Frequencies at Various Ages

	Death rate per 100,000					
	Males			Females		
Type of accident*	Ages 5–14	Ages 5–9	Ages 10–14	Ages 5–14	Ages 5–9	Ages 10–14
All types	25.1	22.9	27.5	10.9	13.1	8.5
Motor vehicle	10.4	10.5	10.3	5.2	6.1	4.3
Drowning†	5.5	4.8	6.3	1.2	1.1	1.3
Firearm	1.8	0.9	2.7	0.3	0.3	0.3
Fire and explosion	1.7	2.2	1.1	2.3	3.5	1.0
Falls	0.8	0.8	0.9	0.3	0.3	0.2

* According to rank among males.

† Exclusive of deaths in water transportation.

Source: "Reports of the Division of Vital Statistics, National Center for Health Statistics," *The Statistical Bulletin,* Metropolitan Life Insurance Company, September 1964.

occur; of these about 500 are fatal. According to the National Clearinghouse for Poison Control, 90 percent of the victims are children under 5 years of age, and 75 percent of them are between 1 and 3 years; the highest 6 month incidence is from 18 to 24 months. It is interesting to note that 95 percent of these poisonings occurred while the child was under the supervision of the parents or other adults. In general, the younger children tend to be poisoned by household products while older children more frequently ingest medicines—perhaps an indication of their growing awareness that medicines are for swallowing. The 1972 bulletin of the National Clearinghouse for Poison Control lists the following as the most commonly ingested substances:

1. Aspirin
2. Soaps, detergents, cleaners
3. Plants (not including mushrooms and toadstools)
4. Vitamins
5. Antihistamines and cold medicines
6. Disinfectants and deodorizers
7. Miscellaneous internal medicines
8. Perfume and toilet water
9. Bleach

Many investigators have attempted to study children who ingest nonfood substances, and a controversy exists over the characteristics of these children. Margolis (1971) finds that childhood poisoning victims tend to have more behavior problems than children who have not ingested poisons; specific examples of the types of behavior problems which he found to be more common in these children are hyperactivity, destructiveness, stubbornness, fighting and temper tantrums, and more aggressive, demanding, and generally negative behavior. Homes in which these children live are more likely to harbor marital conflict, recent loss of family members, and mental and physical illness. Not all agree with Margolis's analysis of the situation, but these findings certainly do indicate clues for the nurse to use in assessing the social situation of poisoning incidents. Jones has also shown (1969) that a child who has had one poisoning is nine times as likely to become a victim of a second poisoning. Again the implications for counseling are clear.

Probably the three biggest sources of poisons in the home are medicines, household products, and plants. A survey by Roney in 1966 showed that the number of different medicines in the home varied from 3 to 88, with an average of 30. These present a particular danger to the child under 5 years (the one who is commonly told that medicines are candy). Saving of old medicines must be discouraged, and safe storage of those medicines in the house should be discussed. A survey in 1961 showed that 22 percent of the homes in this country had no medicine chest; and where medicine chests did exist, they very seldom had adequate locks and could be reached by children of climbing age. Jones had investigated the problem of locks for medicine chests and has found that the two types shown in Fig. 3-1 are the most child-proof. Although medicine cabinets of this type are made by all the major manufacturers and have been available since 1964, they are seldom used. Jones suggests that it might be helpful to make such chests mandatory in federal housing and homes bought with FHA and GI financing. In the absence of such chests, however, a fishing tackle box with a lock or a small suitcase with adequate lock is probably the best storage place for medicine in a home where small children live. It must be emphasized, however, that no matter how adequate the storage place, it does not help if the medicines are not replaced there after use. The large majority of poisonings take place when the medicine is not in its usual storage place. Purses are a particular hazard and frequently contain many types of medication. Previously the largest number of childhood poisonings were caused by aspirins.

Certainly the best approach to the problem of poisonings is prevention. Some measures of prevention must be taken by society and some by the individual. It is important that the nurse be involved in both approaches. On a national level, the most effective approach in this area has been the legislation for safety packaging. According to the Poison Prevention Child-Resistant-Packaging Act of December 1970, all oral prescription drugs are required by law to be packaged in child-resistant packages unless a specific prescription is written by the physician (for instance, in the case of the elderly or crippled who may not be able to open such packages easily). By 1972 this included all products containing aspirin; all narcotics, barbiturates, and amphetaminelike drugs; all preparations containing more than 5 percent oil of wintergreen; and all liquid furniture polish containing more than 10 percent petroleum distillates such as mineral oil. In 1972 the American Academy of Pediatrics further recommended that all prescription drugs, proprietary drugs, drain cleaners, kerosine, turpentine, paint thinners, charcoal lighter fluids, household pesticides, bleach products, and high-pH deter-

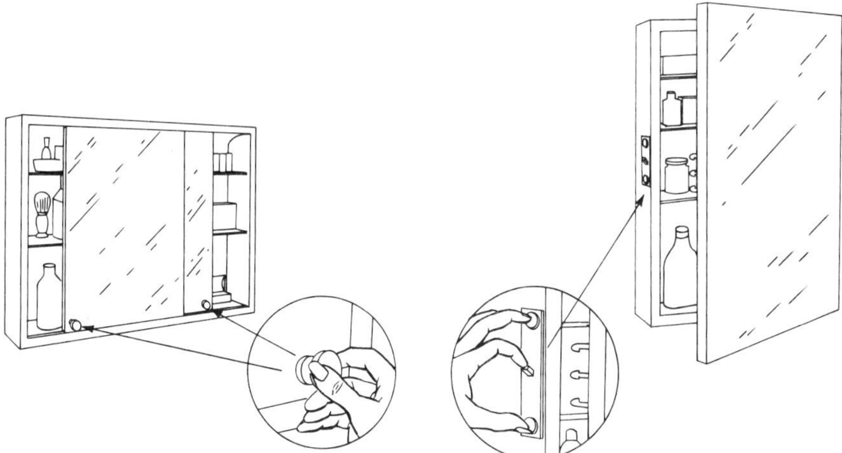

Figure 3-1 Safe medicine chests. *(Source: Jerry Jones, "Preventing Poisoning Accidents in Children," Clinical Pediatrics, vol. 8, no. 8, p. 484.)*

gents be included in this law. It is interesting to note, however, that a great many such drugs are still in the traditional screw-top containers. This is probably partially due to lack of enforcement of the law and to the lack of specification in the law since it does not specify types of containers which are "child-proof." Some interesting research has been done on the effectiveness of various types of safety containers (Done et al., 1971), and the three types of containers found to be the most child-proof were the Screw-Loc, Palm 'N Turn, and unit packaging with pressure-release bubbles (Fig. 3-2). It has been suggested that unit packaging might be even more effective if a bad-tasting substance were incorporated into the packaging since the only way young children seem able to open these packages is by chewing them open. In counseling, the nurse must remember to explain the importance for insisting on such packaging when buying medicines and also for reclosing the containers correctly.

A national approach to the treatment of poisoning is the establishment of regional poison control centers, first begun in 1953. These are generally housed in public hospitals and consist of a central collection of information on all types of products and their ingredients, antidotes, and treatments. The center is usually staffed by physicians familiar with these resources who will look up any question asked by consumers or physicians who call. This service is gradually being computerized, and it is now possible for a private physician to purchase a periodically updated computerized program covering about 40,000 commercial products. Cities will soon be able to purchase such programs with information on over 100,000 products, and the clinics and offices in that city will be able to hook up to the central system.

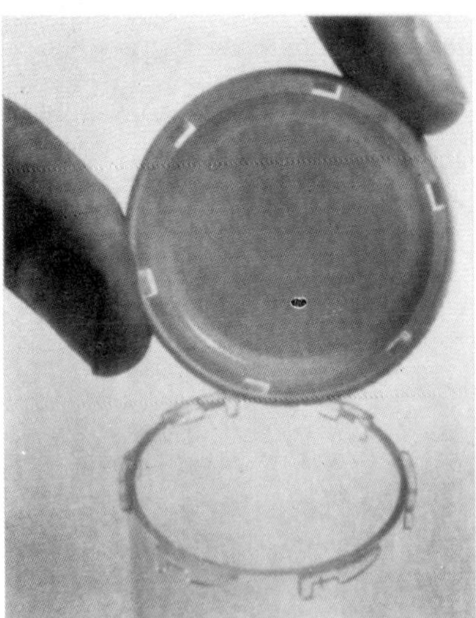

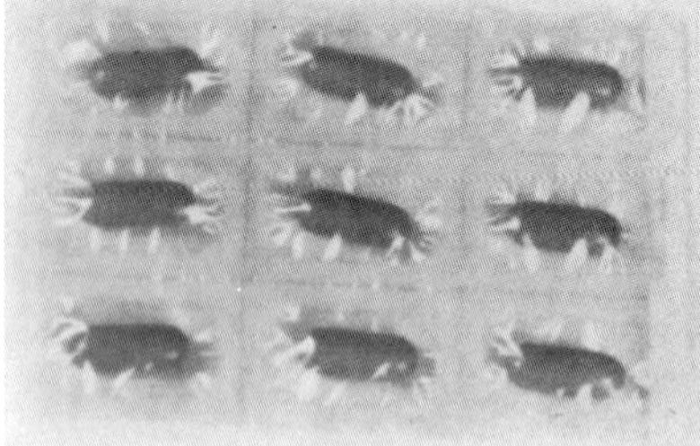

Figure 3-2 Safe medicine containers. *(Source: Jerry Jones, "Preventing Poisoning Accidents in Children," Clinical Pediatrics, vol. 8, no. 8, p. 487.)*

The nurse working in ambulatory settings will also have many occasions to contribute to poison prevention on an individual basis. Developmental counseling with parents is essential here. It is important that parents be taught to anticipate the child's next developmental step *before* it arrives and prepare the environment to be safe for a child at that developmental level. Medicines should be removed from low cabinets *before* the child learns to manipulate the cabinet handle. A lock must be put on the medicine cabinet *before* the child learns to climb.

Specifics for poison-proofing a house should be discussed with all parents of young children. Most children suffering from poisoning obtain the poisons in their own homes, and parents must be helped to see which parts of their homes are dangers to their children. Fourteen percent of the items ingested by children under 5 years of age are polishing agents. Turpentines, paints, petroleum products, cosmetics, and pesticides each constitute 5 percent of the total ingested substances in this age group (Jones, 1969). In the average American household, 41 percent of the cleaners in kitchens are in the open while in bathrooms 52 percent of the cleaning agents are in the open (Jones, 1969). Table 3-5 lists household substances that are nontoxic, and Table 3-6 lists household poisons and their effects and treatments. Certain kinds of household and garden plants are also toxic and evaluation of these is part of poison-proofing a home. Table 3-7 lists some of these poison sources and discusses their effects.

Table 3-5 Frequently Ingested Nontoxic Household Products

Adhesives (most)	Mucilage and paste
Ballpoint pen inks	Paint, indoor (less than 1 percent lead)
Bathtub floating toys	Pencil, (lead-graphite and coloring)
Battery (dry cell) (1/5 MLD of mercury chloride)	Play-Doh and modeling clays
Bubble bath soaps (detergents)	Polaroid picture coating fluid
Candles (beeswax or paraffin)	Porous-tip ink-marking devices (felt tip markers)
Caps (toy pistol) (potassium chlorate)	Putty (less than 2 or 3 oz.)
Chalk (calcium carbonate)	Sachets (essential oils and powder)
Cigarettes or cigars (nicotine)	Shampoos (liquid)
Cosmetics (most)	Shaving creams (soap, perfume, and menthol)
Contraceptive pills	Silly putty (silicones and 1 percent boric acid)
Crayons (marked A.P., C.P.)	Soaps (may cause vomiting)
Dehumidifying packets (silica or charcoal)	Sweetening agents (Saccharin)'
Detergents (most—not electric dishwasher)	Teething rings (water—?sterility)
Deodorants	Thermometer (mercury)
Fish bowl additives	Toothpaste
Golf ball (fluid core can cause mechanical injury)	Vitamins with or without fluoride
Ipecac syrup	Writing ink (blue, black) (ferrous sulfate, tannic acid, gallic acid)
Matches (potassium chlorate)	

Source: Alan Done, "Poisonings from Common Household Products," *The Pediatric Clinics of North America*, vol. 17, no. 3, Aug. 30, 1970, p. 572.

Table 3-6 Household Poisons

Toxicity	Product	Toxic ingredient or effect	Treatment*
		Deodorizers and disinfectants	
High	Naphthalene deodorizer (bathroom, toilet, garbage can)	Irritation, coma, convulsions, hemolysis, kidney damage	Supportive; alkalinize urine; transfuse as needed
	Acid disinfectant (boric, chloroacetic, formic, salicylic, etc.)	Corrosive, plus systemic effects of anion	Supportive and as caustic burn
	Phenolic disinfectant	Phenols; hexachlorophene (gastrointestinal irritation, shock, coma; corrosion or kidney damage possible)	Treat as caustic burn or anticipate renal failure
Medium to high†	Alkali disinfectant (sodium or ammonium hydroxides)	Potentially caustic	Demulcents; treat as caustic burn
	Benzalkonium and other QAC‡ disinfectants	Gastrointestinal irritation, convulsions, coma, respiratory distress, collapse	Supportive; demulcents; mild soap solution or milk
	Pine oil disinfectant	Gastrointestinal and genitourinary irritation; depression and weakness	Supportive; demulcents
	Halogen disinfectants	Hypochlorites or chlorinated hydrocarbons (irritation; excitation)	Demulcents; treat as caustic burn: sedation as needed
Medium	Wick deodorizers	Formaldehyde and hydrocarbons (gastrointestinal irritation, abdominal pain, shock, hematuria, coma, convulsions)	Supportive; demulcents
	Deodorizing cleansers	Pine oil or QAC‡	(See above)
	p-Dichlorobenzene or sodium bisulfate deodorizer (bathroom, toilet, garbage can)	Irritation, abdominal pain, narcosis; liver, kidney damage possible	Supportive; demulcents; sodium bicarbonate
Low	Iodophor disinfectant	Detergent-iodine complex (gastrointestinal irritation)	Demulcents
Nil	Spray deodorizers	(Variable)	Symptomatic
	Refrigerator deodorizer	Charcoal (inert)	None

* In addition to evacuation of stomach (except with caustic burn) or removal from skin, when indicated.
† Depending upon constitution and concentration.
‡ Quaternary ammonium compounds.

Table 3-6 Household Poisons *(Cont'd)*

Toxicity	Product	Toxic ingredient or effect	Treatment*
	Soaps, detergents, cleaners, and bleaches		
High	Electric dishwasher granules§	Caustic (may be severe)	Treat as caustic burn§
	Ammonia§	Caustic; coma and convulsions	As caustic;§ supportive
	Bleach, commercial	Boric acid or oxalate poisoning	Milk; calcium; supportive
	Bleach, oxygen	Boric acid poisoning	Supportive
Medium	Bleach, chlorine	Gastrointestinal irritation, some causticity	Demulcents; treat as caustic burn
	Borax	Boric acid poisoning	Supportive
	Water softeners§ (soluble)	Some caustic; hypocalcemia and acidosis possible	Milk; as for caustic;§ supportive
	Liquid general cleaners:		
	Kerosine	Pneumonia, systemic toxicity	As for petroleum distillates†
	Pine oil	Gastrointestinal and genitourinary irritation; depression and weakness	Supportive; demulcents
	Detergent granules§ for laundry, dishes and general use	Gastrointestinal irritation to causticity (some frankly caustic and have higher toxicity)	Demulcents; treat as caustic burn†
Low	Detergent powders§	Gastrointestinal irritation (causticity possible, but unlikely)	Demulcents, soap; treat as caustic burn§
	Liquid detergents	Gastrointestinal irritation	Demulcents, soap
	Toilet soap	Gastrointestinal irritation	Demulcents
	Fabric softeners	None	None
	Window cleaners (liquid)	Alcohol	
Inhalation hazard	*Chlorine bleach mixed with:*		
	Strong acid (bowl cleaner)	Chlorine gas (intense respiratory irritation)	Bicarbonate aerosol; oxygen
	Ammonia	Chloramine fumes (respiratory irritation, nausea)	Terminate exposure; supportive

§ Products threatening caustic effects will be identified with a *caution* label.

Table 3-6 Household Poisons *(Cont'd)*

Toxicity	Product	Toxic ingredient or effect	Treatment*
		Cosmetics	
High	Permanent wave neutralizer	May contain either: Perborate (boric acid poisoning) Bromate (irritation, collapse, hemolysis, kidney damage)	Supportive For boric acid poisoning Sodium thiosulfate by mouth; demulcent; consider dialysis early
	Fingernail polish remover	Toluene; aliphatic acetates (irritation; central nervous system depression)	Supportive
Medium	Fingernail polish	Same as fingernail polish remover	Supportive
	Hair dye, metallic	Metal salts, pyrogallol (metal poisoning; corrosive)	For metal (if severe); demulcents
	Permanent wave lotion	Thioglycolate (irritation; possible hypoglycemia)	Supportive; demulcent
	Bath oil	Perfume; sulfated castor oil	Demulcent (milk)
	Shaving lotion	Alcohol	Supportive
	Hair tonic	Alcohol, others (variable)	Supportive;¶ demulcents
	Cologne; toilet water	Alcohol, essential oils	Supportive;¶ demulcents
Low	Perfume	Alcohol, essential oils (irritation; possible hypoglycemia)	Supportive;† demulcents
	Shampoo	Anionic detergent (irritation)	Demulcent (milk)
	Bubble bath	Sodium lauryl sulfate (gastrointestinal irritation)	Demulcent (milk)
	Depilatories	Thioglycolate (see above)	Supportive; demulcent
	Hair straightener	Glycols and alcohols; may be caustic	Supportive; as for caustic
	Hair dye, oxidation	Various amines, etc. (gastrointestinal irritation; ?methemoglobinemia)	Demulcent; methylene blue for severe methemoglobinemia.
	Deodorants	Alcohol; aluminum or zinc salts (gastrointestinal irritation; hypoglycemia possible)	Supportive;¶ demulcents
	Shaving cream	Soaps	Milk
	Bath salts	Polymeric phosphate; borax	For causticity or boric acid poisoning

¶ Ethyl alcohol, in addition to being a depressant, may produce hypoglycemia in young children. Related alcohols, with the exception of methanol, have qualitatively similar effects; none of the above contains methanol.

Table 3-6 Household Poisons *(Cont'd)*

Toxicity	Product	Toxic ingredient or effect	Treatment*
		Cosmetics	
Nil	Make-up, liquid Eye make-up Hair dye, vegetable (henna, indigo) Cleansing or conditioning cream Hair dressing (nonalcoholic) Hand lotion or cream Lipstick, tube rouge	None	None

Source: Alan Done, "Poisonings from Common Household Products," *Pediatric Clinics of North America*, vol. 17, no. 3, Aug. 30, 1970, p. 572.

Table 3-7 Toxicity of Common Plants

	Symptoms and signs	Treatment
Autumn crocus (colchicum)	Abdominal cramps, severe diarrhea, CNS depression, and circulatory collapse. Occasionally, oliguria and renal shutdown. Delirium or convulsions occur terminally.	Fluid and electrolyte monitoring. Abdominal cramps may be relieved with meperidine or atropine.
Caladium (arum family) Dieffenbachia, calla lily, dumbcane	Burning of mucous membranes and airway obstruction secondary to edema caused by calcium oxalate crystals.	Accessible areas should be thoroughly washed. Corticosteroids relieve airway obstruction. Apply cold packs to affected mucous membranes.
Castor bean plant	Mucous membrane irritation, nausea, vomiting, bloody diarrhea, blurred vision, circulatory collapse, acute hemolytic anemia, convulsions, uremia.	Fluid and electrolyte monitoring. Saline cathartic. Forced alkaline diuresis will prevent complications due to hemagglutination and hemolysis.
Foxglove and cardiac glycosides	Nausea, diarrhea, visual disturbances, and cardiac irregularities (e.g., heart block).	If ECG is normal, treat symptomatically. If abnormal, give potassium chloride to protect against irritability of cardiac muscle. (Do not use potassium if renal function is impaired.) Quinidine, procainamide, or calcium disodium edathamil may be useful in treating marked arrhythmias. Epinephrine may precipitate ventricular tachycardia.

Table 3-7 Toxicity of Common Plants *(Cont'd)*

	Symptoms and signs	Treatment
Larkspur (Delphinium)	Nausea and vomiting, irritability, muscular paralysis, and CNS depression.	Symptomatic. Atropine may be helpful.
Monkshood (Aconitum)	Numbness of mucous membranes, visual disturbances, tingling, dizziness, tinnitus, hypotension, bradycardia, and convulsions.	Activated charcoal, oxygen. Atropine is probably helpful.
Oleander (dogbane family)	Nausea, bloody diarrhea, respiratory depression, tachycardia, and muscle paralysis.	Symptomatic. Atropine may be helpful. Dipotassium edathamil chelates calcium, decreasing cardiac toxicity of oleandrin.
Poison hemlock	Mydriasis, trembling, dizziness, bradycardia, CNS depression, muscular paralysis, and convulsions. Death is due to respiratory paralysis.	Symptomatic. Oxygen and cardiac monitoring equipment are desirable. Assisted respiration is often necessary. Give anticonvulsants if needed.
Rhododendron	Abdominal cramps, vomiting, severe diarrhea, muscular paralysis, CNS and circulatory depression. Hypertension with very large doses.	Atropine can prevent bradycardia. Epinephrine is contraindicated. Antihypertensives may be needed.
Rosary pea (jequirity bean)	Nausea, vomiting, abdominal and muscle cramps, hemolysis and hemagglutination, circulatory failure, respiratory failure, and renal and liver failure.	Symptomatic. Renal failure can be prevented by alkalinizing the urine. Gastric lavage or emetics are contraindicated because the toxin is necrotizing. Saline cathartics are indicated.
Yellow jessamine (active ingredient related to strychnine)	Restlessness, convulsions, muscular paralysis, and respiratory depression.	Symptomatic. Because of the relation to strychnine, forced acid diuresis and diazepam (Valium) for seizures would be worth trying.

Source: Jack Ott, "Poisoning," in C. Henry Kempe et al., *Current Pediatric Diagnosis and Treatment,* Los Altos, Calif.: Lange, 1972, p. 817 (Table 30-5).

Certainly the best individual approach to the prevention of poisonings in children consists of a good rapport between nurses and parents and sound counseling based on adequate knowledge. A pediatric nurse practitioner has prepared teaching aids which she finds useful in counseling parents about poison prevention (Fig. 3-3). One of these consists of a list of questions with space for answering which can be given to the patient before the interview and then used to highlight the areas of counseling most appropriate to a specific patient. The second teaching aid presents specific information about children at various developmental levels. These information sheets can be given out to parents or used by the nurse as a guide in counseling. (Permission is not needed to reproduce or modify these forms for clinical use.)

---

1. Do you have any syrup of ipecac at home?

2. Do you ever refer to medicine as candy?

3. Where do you store aspirin, laxatives, vitamins, sleeping pills, and other medicines?

4. Do you keep old drugs prescribed for previous illnesses?

5. Where do you store paints, paint thinners, cleaning fluid, kerosine, gasoline, garden sprays, and insecticides?

6. Do you keep harmful substances in their original containers?

7. What do you store under the sink in the kitchen and bathroom?

8. Do you have a closet or cabinet with a lock that could be used for the storage of medicines and other harmful household products?

9. Do you carry any medicines (aspirin, birth control pills, laxatives, tranquilizers) in your purse?

10. Has anyone in your home ever accidentally taken any medicine or poison?

Figure 3-3 (*a*) Questionnaire for poison prevention—A teaching device. *(Developed by Ms. Glennis Pagano, Pediatric Nurse Practioner.)*

The First 6 Months

This is a time when the infant is under a great deal of supervision and the need and opportunity for safety education is great. This is also the time when the infant is more likely to be seen more frequently in the office and intensive prevention efforts can be made. The average infant by 6 months can roll over, sit with or without support, reach for objects, and put things in the mouth. General rules to give parents:

1. In the first months your baby will be sucking on everything within reach—make sure furniture and toys are finished with lead-free paint.
2. Give infants and young children drugs only as directed by your physician.
3. Never leave the baby alone in the house.
4. Always read the labels on all products and keep all pesticides, household bleaches, detergents, cleansers, furniture polish, and *all medicine* under lock.
5. Keep all aerosol containers away from children.
6. Cosmetics can be potential poisons—keep nail polish, perfumes, and facial creams out of the reach of children.
7. Keep all products in original containers—*never* place kerosine, antifreeze, paints, or solvents in cups, glasses, milk bottles, or pop bottles.
8. Have ipecac at home.

7 to 12 Months

This is the age of the crawler. At this creeper stage the baby's curiosity is developing. Crawlers go after objects not in their reach. They learn to crawl, pull to a stand, and walk holding on. They put everything in the mouth, and while they have learned to pull themselves up, they pull everything else down. General suggestions for parents:

1. All household cleaning agents, polishes, and poisons (bug killers, weed sprays and powders, etc.) as well as medicines should be *locked up* and put back immediately after use.
2. Store medicines separately from cleaning agents; store both away from edible products.
3. Bureau drawers with anything potentially dangerous should be locked.
4. Remember that the crawler's world is the low places—the floor and low storage areas. Crawlers relate containers with food and too often find poisons in bottles, jars and other containers.
5. Never allow your child to play with "empty" containers for pesticides, detergents, furniture polish, and similar products. Never reuse the empty container yourself.
6. Have ipecac at home.

1 to 3 Years

The toddlers have the highest accident rate of any group. Their world now includes the tops of tables, desks, kitchen counters—wherever they can reach above eye level. At 15 months they are walking and by 18 months can maneuver stairs. By 19 months to 3 years they begin to run better, imitate, and are in the dependency-versus-independency stage. Their curiosity is full-blown and again everything goes into the mouth. General suggestions for parents:

1. Children often explore with taste and they should be allowed to taste something unpleasant, such as vinegar, with the warning that they will not like it. They may learn that not everything is pleasant to eat.
2. Reminder: All medicines, even aspirin can cause poisoning. *Keep them locked up.*
3. When possible buy bottles with safety closures.
4. Some medicines taste good—be careful when administering these. *Never* describe medicine as candy. Refer to medicines by their proper names. Safeguard those medicines which are candied; children will eat them like candy.
5. Never leave your purse around where a child can reach it. A purse may contain medicine, and is a ready source of poison for the curious child who seeks gum, candy, and other treasures.
6. Follow all suggestions given previously.

3 to 5 Years

This is the age of the climber. Even the 2-year-old can reach the high, "safe" places—cabinets, shelves, and medicine chests. Motor development increases greatly to riding tricycles, jumping, and throwing balls. The desire to please and conform is great, and preschool begins. As children venture out into the neighborhood, their world expands rapidly and the danger of accidents in general increases. They ask "why" to everything, and instructions in safety should begin. They begin to understand what is dangerous. General suggestions for parents:

1. Remember again: Take another look at where you store poisons—drugs, harmful household substances, garden insecticides, and fertilizer. *Lock Up!* Even if you must leave the room for only an instant, remove the container to a safe spot.
2. Dispose of poisons (rat poison, roach paste or powders) as much as possible.
3. Warn small children not to eat or drink drugs, chemicals, plants, or berries they find without your permission, and insist on it.
4. Have ipecac at home.
5. Follow all previous suggestions.

The above material can be adapted and added to, to assist in counseling and provide handout material for parents. The addition of the following general rules should be made:

1. Discard old unused medicine and hazardous substances by flushing down the drain; then rinse and throw away the container out of reach of children and pets.
2. Do not take medicine from an unlabeled bottle; transparent tape can be applied over the label to protect it. Replace all torn labels.

3. Read all labels—directions and caution statements—before giving medicine.
4. Never give medicine in a darkened room, and when measuring drugs, pay close attention to what you are doing.
5. Always shake the bottle thoroughly before measuring liquid medicine.
6. Give medicine only to the person it was prescribed for and only in the amount directed.
7. Mark each drug carefully with the name of the person it was prescribed for, and date all drug supplies when you buy them.
8. Clean out the medicine cabinet periodically and weed out leftovers, especially any prescription drug that your doctor ordered for a particular illness.
9. When purchasing drugs, ask your pharmacist for child-resistant safety closures. Do the same with your grocer when buying household cleaning and polishing supplies; ask which ones have safety packaging.
10. Learn to use the special child-resistant packaging and be certain to resecure the safety feature after use.
11. Do not take medicines in front of children.
12. Remove cleaning aids, polishes, kerosine, lye, etc., from under the sink and *lock up*.
13. Read all labels on such supplies and carefully follow "caution" statements. Even if a chemical is not labeled "poison", incorrect use may render it dangerous.
14. Be sure all poisons are clearly marked by sealing with adhesive tape or using a special marker.
15. Household chemicals in aerosol spray cans or bottles with very small openings are safer because less of the harmful substance can get out at one time.
16. Do not allow food or food utensils to become contaminated when using insect sprays, aerosol mists, rat poisons, weed killers, or cleaning agents.
17. Follow the directions for protecting eyes and skin when using insect poisons, weed killers, solvents, and cleaning agents. Be sure to wash thoroughly after using these things and remove contaminated clothing.
18. Use cleaning fluids in adequate ventilation only—never in baby's room—and avoid breathing vapors.
19. Never eat or serve foods that smell or look abnormal, and remember that they may also poison animals.
20. Remove all poisonous plants from your home.
21. Check your yard to see if there are any plants with poisonous leaves or berries and remove them.
22. Have ipecac at home and remember to call your doctor, hospital, or poison control center immediately *before using* in the case of an accidental poisoning.

Figure 3-3 (*b*) Developmental counseling form for poison control. *(Developed by Ms. Glennis Pagano, Pediatric Nurse Practitioner.)*

Burns

Burns are another very common and very serious hazard to young children. Burns and scalds are the third most frequent cause of accidental deaths (falls have the highest rate, primarily because of the elderly, and poisonings have the second highest rate). One-half of the burn incidents in this country affect children under 4 years of age (Wilkinson, 1970), and burns constitute 10 percent of the total accidental mortality rate. They are more common in the lower socioeconomic classes and are usually associated with a lack of supervision. There are two distinguishable types of accidental burns: scalds and flame burns. Scalds resulting from burning liquid are most common between the ages of 13 and 24 months, happen most frequently in the kitchen, and usually occur in the morning. Steam vaporizers and electric cords attached to electric appliances which hang over a counter edge are hazards, as are pots whose handles extend over the stove edge in such a way that a toddler can reach them and tip over the contents. Flame burns tend to be more serious and occur most often in the 3- to 5-year-old groups, with a female/male death ratio of 31:1 (Smith, 1968). This ratio is due primarily to the difference in clothing, with little girls more commonly attired in loose-fitting flammable clothes. More than half of these deaths involve clothing which catches fire. In over 50 percent of the cases the source of the flame is a furnace, fireplace, heater, or stove. Playing with matches and cigarette lighters and trial smoking are the second most frequent cause (White, 1971).

The death rate from burns is so high and the morbidity so serious that it is obvious that prevention is the only acceptable approach to this problem. Again there are two important approaches: individual counseling and federal legislation. Individual counseling is important in helping parents realize the magnitude of the problem and understand which aspects of their own homes may present hazards. Careful monitoring of all open-flame sources, covering of electric outlets with safety plugs, protection from hot radiators in older homes, purchase of kitchen appliances with buttons out of reach of children, and care in using matches, cigarette lighters, and burning liquids are all important aspects of discussion in accident prevention counseling.

Federal legislation is important in this area, particularly in the area of fabric flammability. As mentioned previously, a large cause of the seriousness of burns is the flammability of children's clothing. The nurse should be aware of some important aspects of fabric and clothing construction which affect their flammability and of legislation current in this area. This is important both for her own input to legislation and for counseling of parents. In general, contrary to popular opinion, fabrics of vegetable fibers such as cotton and rayon are more flammable than most synthetics. Silk, wool, and animal hair fabrics are the least flammable. Although some synthetics such as modacrylic are inherently flame-retardant and some can be chemically treated to be flame-retardant, others, although they burst into flame less readily, are of serious concern because as they melt from the intense heat of the flame, they turn into a burning hot syrup, scalding the skin. The most dangerous fabric, however, is a combination of synthetic and natural fibers since the natural fibers will flame and cause the synthetic fibers to melt and scald. Other qualities of clothing construction also affect flammability. Naps and piles greatly increase flammability, as do loose weaves and loose design (the classic firetrap is the billowy cotton nightgown worn so often by little girls). Public concern about these hazards has prompted legislation concerning fabric flammability. This began in 1945, triggered by an epidemic of burns caused by certain highly piled so-called torch sweaters and highly flammable cowboy chaps. By 1953 legislation prohibited extraordinary flammability in fabrics sold across state lines; it did not, however, affect the flammability of more common types of clothing. In 1967 the Flammable Fabrics Act was amended to include household fabrics and items such as hats and shoes, but still included only extraordinarily flammable items. In 1973, a further step was taken, and children's sleepwear up to size 6X was required to be flameproof. Flameproofing cuts down even the more common degree of flammability which is responsible for most burns; it requires that when the cloth is exposed to a flame for 3 seconds, the fire must self-extinguish with an area no larger than 7 inches becoming charred. Flameproofing does increase the cost of the product about 30 percent and makes the texture less attractive and the wearing qualities of the cloth poorer. However, these disadvantages seem well worth the increase in safety for the child. It is expected that by the time this book is published, legislation will cover clothing through size 12X as well.

Falls

Falls are also an important cause of home injuries although they are probably more significant in the elderly population. About 4 percent of childhood accidents consist of falls, particularly from the age of 6 months, when the baby first learns to roll over, until about 5 years. The ratio of male to female victims is about 2:1 in the older children; this sex differential is less marked in the younger children. Ninety percent of the most serious falls, i.e., those which resulted in death or hospitalization, were falls from windows or fire escapes, usually in the lower socioeconomic areas of cities and usually from May to September (Bergner, 1971). Gregg (1971) reports that fully 50 percent of children fall from relatively high surfaces (i.e., dressing tables and other furniture) at least once before 1 year of age.

The nurse working in ambulatory pediatrics must be alert to all opportunities to counsel and help prevent accidental falls. Developmental guidance may help parents know that although their 5½-month-old child may not roll off a couch today, he or she may very well be able to by tomorrow. Gates across stairways and open doors are important for crawling children who cannot yet safely navigate stairways. Windows should open from the top. Window guards are available at about $200 per window as are window bars at about $20 per window.

Drownings

Drowning presents another threat to the safety of children. It is the fourth leading cause of accidental death in the United States and is predominant in preschoolers, especially toddlers. Each year 7,000 drownings occur in the United States (American Academy of Pediatrics statement, 1968). Preventive efforts can be directed toward making the environment safer by eliminating or supervising such hazards as unattended back yard swimming pools, birdbaths, and decorative garden pools, by encouraging supervision near all sources of water including the bathtub, and by beginning swimming lessons early.

Traffic Accidents

Traffic hazards are certainly one of the most common safety concerns in large metropolitan areas of industrial countries such as the United States. Accidents occur to pedestrians, to children on bicycles, and to those riding in automobiles. The nurse working in this area must be knowledgeable about all these hazards. In 1967, 9,400 pedestrians died in traffic accidents; of these, 2,740 were children (Burg, 1970). Most of these accidents occurred at night and most in the dark winter months. Certainly children must be supervised and taught to cross streets at the corner, look both ways before crossing, and not play in the street. It has also been found (Campbell, 1968; Hazlett and Allen, 1967) that reflectorized materials are seen more quickly by drivers than nonreflectorized materials, and Campbell (1968) found a decrease in accidents when reflectorized license plates were used. Reflectorized patches for children's clothing and bicycles are available and it might be well to provide parents with this information.

Bicycles Bicycles also present a traffic hazard to children of all ages. There are two common types of bicycle injuries: spoke injuries and handlebar injuries. Spoke injuries occur mostly to toddlers riding in toddler seats behind the adult driver. Eighty percent of these injuries were in children under 6 years of age, and most of them were in the summer months. It is extremely important to encourage parents to purchase adequate toddler seats if they intend to have their small children ride with them. Such a toddler seat must have foot braces and straps to restrain the feet in these braces (actually as of this writing, few models are available with these straps and generally the parents will have to buy them separately). In Britain bicycles are manufactured with a guard covering the top half of the front wheel; guards on both wheels would be ideal, but as of now they are not available in this country. Certainly guards would prevent children slipping their feet out of the foot braces and through the spokes of the moving cycle.

With older children who are riding their own bicycles, it is important to impress on them the seriousness of the "rules of the road." Smaller wheels are safer since the center of gravity is better for purposes of control. It is important also that the front wheel be equipped with a lock (few models at this time are so equipped). The most common injury is a genital injury caused by loss of control in which the front wheel continues to spin around resulting in injury from the handlebars. A lock would stop such spinning before the handlebars could injure the genital area.

Automobiles The most devastating of accidents in this country are surely automobile accidents. In general, children are much more vulnerable when involved in an automobile accident and in addition, they are usually provided with less extrinsic protection that adults. Because small children do not have pelvic girdles which have developed to the point where they can safely use adult safety belts, they must be provided with adequate substitutes. The most dangerous position a child can be in when an accident occurs is in an adult's lap. It is important to help parents realize how to adequately protect their children while they are automobile passengers. In a recent telephone survey (Pless, 1972) it was discovered that less than one-fifth of those interviewed had used any type of safety device at all, and in an observational study by the same author it was found that in only 11 percent of 200 situations with children as passengers in automobiles were all the rules of safety obeyed. Furthermore, only 3 percent of the pediatricians polled stated that they always discussed seat belts with parents, and only 55 percent said they ever discussed it. Yet in most years, automobile deaths are far more numerous in the pediatric age group than deaths from all types of cancer. It is important that the nurse working in ambulatory pediatrics be aware of which types of safety devices are adequate for which age children and where they can be purchased. There are many flimsy useless seats currently on the market, and it is important to help parents avoid these. Table 3-8 summarizes the specific devices recommended by the American Academy of Pediatrics for children of various ages. For infants up to 12 lbs

Table 3-8 A Summary of Safe Automobile Devices

Size of child	Device
Up to 12 lbs	Car bed or infant carrier
12 to 24 lbs	Infant harness or toddler seat
24 to 50 lbs	Child seat (shield type)
More than 50 lbs, less than 55 in.	Adult belt—no shoulder harness
More than 55 in.	Adult belt with shoulder harness

Source: Frederic Burg, John Douglass, Eugene Diamond, and Arnold Siegel, "Automotive Restraint Devices for the Pedicatric Patient," *Pediatrics*, vol. 45, no. 1, part I, January 1970, p. 49.

(about 9 months), an infant carrier is the most protective device available. There are many types on the market, and at the publication date of this book, there is as yet no federal safety code covering minimum requirements for such a carrier. It should have heavy padding on both sides and back, restraint belts at least 1½ in. wide, and holes through which the car safety belt can be threaded to hold the carrier securely in the seat. It must provide adequate protection to head and shoulders, and should be placed in a semi-upright position facing the rear of the car, preferably in the middle of the back seat. See Fig. 3-4(*a*).

An alternative for the infant is an infant bed covered with heavy padding and deep enough so the child cannot roll out. It should be placed crosswise in the rear seat and fastened with the middle front and rear seat belts and covered with a strong net over the top. The child's feet should be toward the front. See Fig. 3-4(*b*).

When a child reaches 12 to 24 lbs the American Academy of Pediatrics recommends either a toddler seat or a harness. The toddler seat allows less freedom but many children are happy with it [Fig. 3-4(*c*)]. The law now requires that any seat made after April 1, 1971, must meet federal regula-

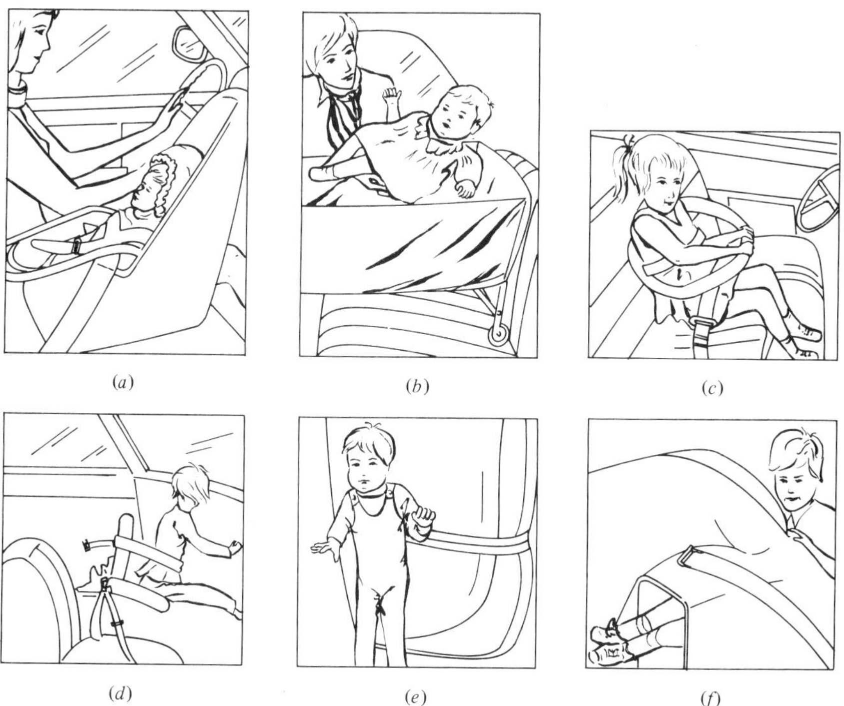

Figure 3-4 Automobile restraining devices: safe and unsafe. *(Source: American Academy of Pediatrics, Committee on Accident Prevention Statement, Feb. 1, 1972.)*

tions and should be stamped with the date of the manufacture, the recommendation for height and weight, which makes of cars and which seats in the car will adequately accommodate it, and the fact that it conforms to the Federal Motor Vehicle Standard 213. Seats should have adequate head support and thick, protective padding. Flimsy seats which hook over the top of the seat or which have bendable metal parts, toys or steering wheels attached, buckles which the child can undo, and restraining belts less than 1½ in. wide should be avoided [Fig. 3-4(*d*)].

Some parents and children prefer harnesses which allow the child more freedom. Again, those made since 1969 must conform to Federal Motor Vehicle Standard 209. They should have both pelvic and chest straps, sometimes with netting in between; these straps must be checked to see that they cover only the pelvic and chest areas; they must not ride up or down across the abdomen. It is best to anchor these harnesses directly to the floor; this is particularly important if the car has a hinged seat without a lock. It is acceptable but less adequate to have a strap which loops around to the back of the seat and attaches to the floor [Fig. 3-4(*e*)]. For the child who weighs between 25 and 50 lbs the best seat now available is the shield type, although it has a major disadvantage in that it limits the child's view [Fig. 3-4(*f*)].

When a child reaches 50 lbs, an adult lap belt should be used; it is important not to use the shoulder strap until the child is at least 55 in. high, however, since there is a chance of strangulation. As is true with adults, a child should never wear only a shoulder belt.

NUTRITION

Certainly one of the most important parts of well-child management with which the nurse in ambulatory pediatrics will be concerned is infant and childhood nutrition. This section will discuss some basic information about which nutrients are important to consider in dietary counseling and also what common foods and commercial products are available to supply these nutrients.

In general, proteins, fats, carbohydrates, vitamins, and minerals are the essential ingredients of any diet. The nurse working in this area should be aware of what is known about these nutrients in regard to the pediatric age group and the meaning of the recommendations that are usually made concerning them. It is useful to be familiar with certain terms used in this regard. A nutrient's *requirement* is defined as the least amount of that nutrient which will promote optimal health. This is really never known exactly since it varies with the racial group, age, and other individual characteristics. It can only be estimated. The *recommended daily allowance* (RDA) is a recommendation made by the Food and Nutrition Board of the National Academy of Science of the National Research Council. It is intended as a recommendation for broad groups consisting of various age levels and individual characteristics. It is purposely set high enough that it will cover all individuals in that group, and consequently allows a rather large margin of safety. The term *advisable intake,* on the other hand, indicates the recommendation for an individual rather than a group. In order to allow for error, it is approximately two times the requirement except where the range of safety is small (for instance, in the case of calories, fluoride, vitamin A, and vitamin D, an excess would be reached if this much margin were left, and the excess itself could do damage).

Proteins

Proteins are an important part of the diet. They are of two types: essential (such as arginine, isoleucine, leucine, lysine, methionine, phenylalanine, threonine, tryptophan, valine, and histidine), which cannot be synthesized in the body, and nonessential amino acids, which can be synthesized in the body (i.e., tyrosine, which can be made from phenylalanine, and cystine, which can be made from methionine). There are two primary types of milk proteins: casein, which is found predominantly in the curd of cow's milk, and whey, which is the main protein in human milk. Lactalbumin is the major constituent of whey, and commercial formulas attempt to duplicate the higher percentage of lactalbumin in breast milk. There is no evidence, however, that duplicating the exact ratio of whey or casein ensures that the infant absorbs a similar ratio. In general, it is recommended that 9 percent of the infant's calories be received as protein.

Fats

Fats are another important part of the child's diet. There is currently a great deal of discussion concerning the fat content of diets, particularly in reference to later atherosclerosis. To date, there is no definite proof that early feeding of certain types of fat leads to atherosclerosis in later life although the issue is certainly not settled yet. In 1961 Pikering et al. did some experimental work with monkeys in which early introduction of fats was not associated with later atherosclerosis. Fat content is just as high in breast milk as in cow's milk. There are only two essential fatty acids, linoleic and arachidonic. These are necessary in very small amounts for growth and for skin maintenance. Otherwise, the primary use of fat is for energy and for absorption of the fat-soluble vitamins. There are two basic types of fats: the saturated type, which has no double bonds and consequently solidifies at room temperature, and the polyunsaturated type, which is characterized by double bonds and remains liquid at room temperature. The fats in all types of milks and commercial formulas are polyunsaturated. Generally, a child's diet should contain between 20 and 50 percent fats. If the fat content is less than 20 percent, either the protein intake is too high, resulting in an increased solute load, or the disaccharide intake is too high, resulting in diarrhea. The most easily absorbed fat is human fat; the next best are corn and soy oil;

coconut oil is also fairly easily absorbed but it lacks linoleic acid. Animal fat is less well absorbed. This is why commercial formulas generally replace the animal fat in cow's milk with a vegetable oil. The fat intake of low-birth-weight infants must be watched particularly, since these babies often tend to have an increased amount of fecal fat loss, sometimes carrying with it important fat-soluble vitamins such as A, D, E, and K, as well as certain minerals such as calcium.

Carbohydrates

Carbohydrates are another essential component of any diet. In infants, the carbohydrate intake is mostly in the form of mono- and disaccharides, while in adults, polysaccharides such as the starches predominate. This is due primarily to the maturation of the sugar-splitting enzyme systems of the body. Human milk derives 37 percent of its calories from carbohydrate; cow's milk derives 29 percent of its calories from this source; and commercial formulas vary between 32 and 51 percent. A commonly encountered problem in pediatric nutrition is the situation in which disaccharides are not absorbed, either because there is too much of them in the diet or because of some enzyme deficiency. If disaccharides are not absorbed from the gastrointestinal tract, they become osmostic and draw water out from the body, causing diarrhea and potential dehydration.

Vitamins

Vitamins are an essential nutrient which were discovered more recently than fats, carbohydrates, and proteins, and less is known about them. This chapter will discuss some specific vitamins which are likely to be important in pediatric diets. Vitamin A, or retinol, is a well-known fat-soluble vitamin found only in animal sources such as liver, eggs, and milk fats. Its precursor, carotene, however, is found in yellow and orange plant sources such as carrots and squash. The human body can utilize this precursor to supply enough vitamin A for its needs. The exact requirement is unknown. Vitamin A is stored well, and therefore daily intake is not as important as an average intake. Suggested daily averages are:

Birth to 6 years: 1,000 IU
7 to 9 years: 1,500 IU
10 to 12 years: 2,000 IU
13 to 15 years: 2,700 IU
16 to 19 years: 3,200 IU
Adults: 3,700 IU
Pregnant women: 4,200 IU
Lactating women: 5,200 IU

Vitamin A Deficiencies of vitamin A are most common in underdeveloped countries. Because of the high levels of this vitamin contained in meat and milk and because of the frequently used supplements, deficiency of this vitamin is rare in developed countries. However, deficiency is possible, particularly in the underprivileged groups in this country or among those on special diets, such as the fad diets of adolescence or any diet in which the fat content is severely restricted. This may be the case also in the generally unwise decision to put 6- to 12-month-old babies on skim milk for purposes of weight reduction. Babies of this age are often taking unreliable amounts of fats from other sources, and it is possible to cause a fat-deficient diet in which the intake of the fat-soluble vitamins may be inadequate. Symptoms of such deficiency may be seen as failure to thrive; dry, scaly skin; corneal changes; poor dark adaptation of vision; and even mental retardation. Much more likely in this country, however, is the danger of overdose. Until fairly recently, it was thought that it took doses of 75,000 to 500,000 IU per day for 3 to 12 weeks to result in an overdose (Foman, 1974). With the new aqueous solutions, however, Persson (1965) reported that 18,500 IU for 3 months in one child and 22,500 IU for 1 to 1½ months in three children under 6 months of age resulted in symptoms of overdose. This is one reason it is so important that mothers who are feeding commercial formulas (all of which are adequately fortified with vitamins) must be told *not* to give other vitamin supplements. Even in hospitals, women on the postpartum ward are frequently sent home with samples of vitamin drops and feel that this implies that such supplementation is necessary even though the baby is receiving supplemented formula. This is even more likely to be a problem when the baby begins baby foods which are also heavily supplemented with vitamins. Symptoms of vitamin A overdose include rash, fissured lips, painful swollen long bones, alopecia, irritability, pruritis, constipation, failure to gain weight, and increased intercranial pressure (with such the accompanying signs and symptoms of bulging fontanelle, nausea, vomitting, and headache). Another situation leading to possible overdose is the treatment of acne in adolescence with extremely large doses of vitamin A (a practice which has never been proven to do any good, and which has proven to be a significant risk for vitamin A overdose). Popular writer Adelle Davis has suggested large doses of this vitamin for general health, creating a rather large popular demand for high-dosage capsules. Realizing the danger, Congress has recently introduced a bill to require a prescription for the larger doses of vitamin A. It is hoped that this will limit the potential danger of overdose. It is important to keep in mind the distinction between preformed vitamin A and its precursor carotene, however. It is impossible to cause a vitamin A overdosage by excessive intake of carotene. Such intake may result in carotenemia, presenting as yellow to orange coloration of the skin (but not of the sclera as would occur in jaundice), but this is a relatively innocuous and reversible situation.

Vitamin D Vitamin D is another fat-soluble vitamin which is necessary to absorb calcium and phosphorus. In the United States it is now added to almost all milks, many breakfast drinks, cereals, milk flavorings, margarines, and certain breads. Certain infants' foods are extremely high in it, particularly egg yolk and tuna fish, which contain 200 IU/100 gm. It is also available from sunlight through the skin. People with dark pigmentation have more difficulty making use of this source, and rickets is much more likely to be found in Black individuals than in those of fair skin. The requirement is 100 to 200 IU for all ages and the advisable daily intake is 400 IU, largely because storage of this vitamin is very poor. Deficiency of vitamin D is still reasonably common in the United States (Foman, 1974) although it is more common in Canada where the milk is not always fortified. It has become much less common in this country since the law now requires that almost all types of milk be fortified with 400 IU per quart.

As with vitamin A, overdoses of this vitamin are possible, and the law now requires a prescription for large doses of this vitamin also. There is much controversy concerning what constitutes overdosage of vitamin D. Selig feels that even the 400 IU required by law is too much. One study did show that when a group received 200 IU per day, another group 135 IU per day, and a third group 400 IU per day, the poorest growth was in the group receiving 200 IU per day and the best was in the group receiving 400 IU per day. It is further possible that overdose may cause permanent kidney damage. The evidence regarding the role of vitamin D in idiopathic hypercalcemia is confusing. The symptoms of this disease are failure to thrive, vomiting, mental retardation, hypertension, aortic stenosis, renal failure, and elfin facies; it is possible, but has not been proven, that this disease begins in utero. The vast majority of information which we have concerning this syndrome comes from the British experience in the 1950s. During 1953 and 1954, many of the commonly used foods in Britain were highly fortified with vitamin D, and it was estimated that children could easily be ingesting as much as 3,000 to 4,000 IU per day from ordinary diets. An extraordinary number of cases of idiopathic hypercalcemia were reported during these years—about 100 new cases per year. On the premise that the large amount of vitamin D supplementation of common foods might be responsible for the number of idiopathic hypercalcemic children being seen, the government changed its legislation relating to this fortification, and supplementation was severely reduced. In 1956 and 1957 another survey of idiopathic hypercalcemia was taken and it was discovered that, just as hoped, the number had dropped dramatically since the supplementation of foods had been lessened. No increase in the incidence of rickets was found when the amount of supplementation was decreased. At first this was taken as support for the idea that the heavy supplementation had caused the cases of idiopathic hypercalcemia. Unfortunately, however, the evidence became less clear when several years later it was discovered that the incidence of hypercalcemia was again increasing even though the fortification had remained the same. So it is difficult to know exactly what the risks of overdose with this vitamin are, but it is clear that doses in excess of 400 IU per day are not necessary and show some signs of being harmful.

Vitamin E Vitamin E, another fat-soluble vitamin, is important in parts of the reproductive process and in certain blood functions. It is found in almost all foods and practically never requires supplementation except in situations where there is a problem with inadequate fat intake or absorption, such as occurs in children with cystic fibrosis or in certain premature infants who have not received much fat store from their mothers and may have a diet low in fat and an increased fecal fat loss. It is becoming more clear that vitamin E deficiency is in some way associated with certain types of anemia. This occurs most frequently in the premature infant. No specific danger of overdose is known at this time, but it is certain that the advertisers' claims that large doses of vitamin E will increase the sexual drive are without foundation.

Vitamin K Vitamin K, another fat-soluble vitamin, plays a very crucial role in pediatrics, particularly in the case of the newborn. Most infants normally become deficient in vitamin K 2 to 3 days after birth. About 1 in 400 will manifest clinical symptoms of such deficiency in the form of bleeding, i.e., "hemorrhagic disease of the newborn." Breastfed children are more susceptible to this than artificially fed infants, as are children whose mothers have been on coumadin during their pregnancy. For this reason, every newborn should receive 0.5 to 1.0 mg of vitamin K parentally after birth and perhaps more if the mother has been receiving coumadin. For a while, many physicians attempted to give the required amount to the mother prenatally, but the exact absorption was too unpredictable, and it is now considered better to give it directly to the infant. After the newborn period, there is generally little problem with vitamin K deficiency since it is available in most foods. One situation did occur several years ago when certain soy, meat base, and casein hydrolysate formulas contained inadequate amounts of vitamin K. This is not true today, however, and in general the only time one must be particularly careful is in the case of very-low-fat diets.

Vitamin C The first of the water-soluble vitamins, vitamin C, is well known to every one. It is needed for maintenance of mucous membranes and for certain other organic functions. Because it is water-soluble, an adequate supply must be taken in daily since the body is unable to store it from day to day. Most formulas contain it, and it will come through in breast milk if mother receives an adequate daily supply herself. Fruit juices and many of the baby foods, particularly baby bananas are highly fortified with it. Even the fruit drinks are usually quite highly fortified today, and deficiency in this country is not common although it still occurs. It is ironic that its concentration in this country is confined primarily to the South and Southeast, areas with the greatest crop of citrus fruit (Foman, 1974). Beginning symptoms consist of apathy, irritability, and anorexia. Later the irritability increases and tenderness of the legs, even extending to pseudoparalysis, may occur. Finally, costochondrial beading and hemorrhages of the skin and mucous membranes, particularly around erupting teeth, occur. Caffey (1961) and Greward (1965) conclude that symptoms of such a deficiency first become evident at about 3 months of age and are seldom apparent after 12 months of age. Because vitamin C is water-soluble and the body can rid itself of excess, there is no danger of overdosage in the sense that large quantities are stored in the body. Some people, however, feel that excess amounts may cause irritation to the bladder mucosa since such strong concentrations are excreted in the urine.

Vitamin B Complex Another group of water-soluble vitamins is the B complex. Again, because the B vitamins are water-soluble, daily intake is important, and the danger of overdose is minimal. Vitamin B_1, or thiamine, is important in the metabolism of carbohydrate, and its requirement is proportional to the carbohydrate intake of the diet. Only two cases of infant deficiency have been reported in the United States, and both of these children were on soy formula which had apparently lost its thiamine content in the production process, which involved exposure to high temperatures. This problem has now been corrected, however. There is a current controversy concerning whether thiamine stimulates appetite; the available information does not seem to indicate that it does.

Cobalamin, or vitamin B_{12}, is needed to utilize folic acid, and deficiency of this vitamin may result in megaloblastic anemia. It is plentiful in animal foods such as kidney, liver, milk, eggs, and cheese, and most normal diets in the United States will not be deficient in this vitamin.

Pyridoxine, or vitamin B_6, is another of the B complex which is important in metabolism, this time in protein metabolism. Its requirement varies with the amount of protein in the diet. Its importance became well known in 1954 when the heat process used in the manufacture of certain infant formulas destroyed it and many infants developed the symptoms of weakness, ataxia, abdominal pain, irritability, and finally convulsions. This problem has been corrected today, and all presently available formulas contain vitamin B_6 in sufficient quantities. Normal requirements vary with the amount of the protein in the diet and are raised by some medications such as isoniazid as well as by certain disease entities. A specific hereditary defect is seen in some infants who are vitamin B_6-dependent at birth and will die without administration of vitamin B_6. Symptoms of this problem usually begin 3 to 7 hours after a birth marked by meconium staining. Apnea and hyperirritability are the primary symptoms. A positive family history for this disease usually exists.

Folic acid is the final vitamin of the B complex to be discussed. It is found widely in such foods as liver, kidney, and meats in general as well as in yeast and deep-green leafy vegetables. Vitamin C is necessary for its utilization, and deficiency of either may cause megaloblastic anemia while excess may mask a pernicious anemia (because of this the FDA requires that large doses be available only by prescription). The most common situation presenting this difficulty includes a child who is on goat's milk which has a type of folic acid that is not fully utilized by human beings. Other B vitamins exist, such as B_2 (riboflavin), biotin, PABA, niacin, and lipoic acid, but difficulties in childhood which are known to derive from a deficiency or excess of these vitamins are not known.

Minerals

Minerals are another category of nutrients which have been discovered more recently. Less is known about them than about proteins, fats, and carbohydrates. The most abundant in the body are sodium, chloride, potassium, calcium, phosphorus, magnesium, and sulfur. The requirements for each mineral are influenced by the presence of other minerals (for instance, an individual needs more magnesium when more calcium and phosphorus are in the diet), by the presence of certain nonminerals (for instance, if there is too much fat present in the diet, the increased fecal fat loss may carry with it some of the calcium, and the required intake of calcium may be increased), and by the chemical form of the mineral (certain forms are better absorbed than others). The renal solute load is an important consideration when evaluating mineral content of the diet. From 75 to 89 percent of the renal solute load is composed of sodium, potassium, and chloride, and these are the major mineral intakes that must be looked at when there is a question of overload. Although there is quite a bit of phosphorus in milk (which can also cause an overload), there is practically none in other food; therefore the amount of phosphorus is generally ignored. The renal solute load of breast milk is approximately half that of cow's milk, and most commercial formula companies attempt to manipulate the solute load in their product to resemble that in human milk. Danger from renal overload is most likely in the first 2 weeks of life when children are unable to concentrate their urine adequately to meet their bodies' needs. After this, unless they suffer from renal disease or diabetes insipidus, they will generally be able to adjust their own solute load as long as they are getting enough water. Problems may arise later if renal disease exists, if there is very scant fluid intake (i.e., under 100 ml/kg/day), or if there are increased extrarenal losses such as those which may occur in fever or diarrhea. Weaning is a particularly vulnerable time as far as decreased fluid intake is concerned; it may be wise during this time to stress low-solute solids like fruits. When a child has diarrhea, a particular danger in terms of renal solute load exists. Some people prescribe fluids such as Lytren or salt solutions, but mistakes in mixing the salt solution can be so catastrophic that it is probably best to avoid homemade mixtures. Dilution of the formula (or whole or skim milk, if that is what the child is on) is probably best. It is most important to avoid the practice of boiling the skim milk, which just increases the renal solute load. Another instance in which renal solute load demands careful attention is when a high-calorie diet is desired, such as in certain cardiovascular, central nervous system, or gastrointestinal problems. In such cases, it is important to ensure that the high concentration of calories is not associated with a higher concentration of the renal solute load.

Seven minerals will be considered as major dietary minerals in this chapter: sodium, calcium, phosphorus, magnesium, chlorine, potassium, and sulfur.

Sodium Sodium is a well-known mineral, and most people are aware of the argument which states that the large amounts of sodium which exist in baby foods, may eventually result in an increased incidence of hypertension in adulthood. To date this has been supported only in rat studies, but it does seem a reasonable hypothesis. Almost all baby foods except fruits and juices contain sodium; sodium chloride content is also extremely high in adult soup concentrates, particularly Campbells', and the common practice of substituting these for junior foods should be discouraged.

Calcium, Phosphorus, and Magnesium The need for calcium, phosphorus, and magnesium is closely interrelated. The best ratio of calcium to phosphorus is not exactly known although many try to duplicate the ratio in breast milk. Some researchers feel that if the amounts of calcium and phosphorus are not equal, whichever is in excess will draw the other out of its deposition in bone or teeth. Again, there is no definitive proof concerning this. Although the exact relationship is unknown, it is known that the need for magnesium increases as the amount of calcium and phosphorus increases. All three are needed for building bone and teeth and for effective functioning of muscle contraction. Neonatal tetany is a particular concern in this regard. It is more common in premature infants, in infants born after dystocia, and in infants born of diabetic mothers. It is never seen in breastfed babies, and the incidence is higher in those infants on unaltered cow's milk, probably because the increased phosphorus levels may interfere with the calcium absorption and because the higher fat level may result in some amount of staetorrhea, which removes the calcium with it.

Chlorine Chlorine is another major dietary mineral important in fluid-electrolyte balance, in acid-base balance, and for maintaining gastric acidity. Its primary source is table salt, and few individuals suffer from a deficiency in this regard.

Potassium Potassium is also an important mineral, particularly in regard to muscle activity, protein systhesis, fluid-electrolyte balance, and again the acid-base balance. It is found in such sources as meats, poultry, and fish, as well as fruits, vegetables, and whole grain cereals.

Sulphur Sulphur is also considered a major dietary mineral and is important as an ingredient of protein and for its function in activating enzymes. It is found in most protein foods.

Other Essential Minerals Other minerals are necessary in much lesser quantities than the major dietary minerals, but are still essential in the diet. Most well known of these is iron. Iron deficiency is the most common mineral deficiency of childhood. Particularly at risk for this deficiency are low-birthweight infants, premature infants, infants who have lost excessive blood either during the birth process or during a circumcision or other early surgical situation, those born of iron-deficient mothers, and those in whom a twin-to-twin or fetomaternal tranfusion took place prenatally. [These latter two are controversial and the American Academy of Pediatrics (1969) has stated that these conditions do not predispose to anemia.] It is generally considered that between 5 and 20 percent (on the average 10 percent) of the iron taken into the body is absorbed, although premature infants have been shown to absorb as much as 32 percent (a similar percent has been shown to be absorbed from medicinal iron when a child is suffering from iron deficiency). Deficiency is associated with frequent upper respiratory infections although the exact nature of this association is uncertain; it may also be associated with milk allergies which are manifested by blood loss through the gastrointestinal tract (this is assumed to be a causal association); worm infestations, particularly of hookworm, are also known to contribute to iron deficiency. Certain situations, on the other hand, are known to contribute to increased absorption of iron. Presence of vitamin C is one of these, as is the local condition in which the soil is high in iron and the plant products grown in that soil are also high in iron. Cooking acid food in iron pots may increase the amount of iron content: from 30 to 100 times what was originally present in the food. In 1971 the American Academy of Pediatrics officially recommended the fortification of baby formulas with iron, a stance which is still controversial. The reason for the recommendation was the large number of infants in this country who developed iron-deficiency anemia from birth through their second year. The academy recommended that 1.0 mg/kg up to a maximum of 15 mg/day be given to normal full-term infants and that 2.0 mg/kg be given to low-birthweight infants (1969). It felt that although the amount of iron taken in the first 4 to 5 months had little effect immediately (except in premature infants), it was possible that this iron was being stored for future use and might prevent later anemia. The academy felt that this form of medicinal iron should not increase feeding problems and that there was no risk of overload unless there existed a chronic anemia like thalassemia major, where there was an increased iron absorption. In general, supplements are better absorbed in ferrous form than in ferric form (examples are ferrous sulfate, ferrous gluconate, ferrous fumarate, ferrous succinate, and ferrous lactate) since these forms appear to dissociate better, leaving the iron available for use by the body. Baby cereals have long been fortified, and if infants absorb the average 10 percent of the iron available in these products, they should be taking in a sufficient amount if they eat 3 tablespoons dry or 30 to 45 ml reconstituted for the first 6 months and 5 to 6 tablespoons dry or 60 to 90 ml reconstituted after that time. There has recently arisen some controversy, however, as to whether the iron present in these baby cereals is actually available to the infants. This issue has yet to be firmly decided by well-controlled research. Although it is impossible to receive an overdose of iron from dietary sources, it is quite possible to reach toxic levels medicinally. This most commonly occurs when a child gets into a bottle of medicinal iron. As few as five 10-gr tablets can cause death, and any time a child (or more commonly, a pregnant mother) is on medicinal iron, this danger should be explained to the mother.

Although little is known about zinc, another of the essential trace minerals, it is felt that zinc functions in some way in skin keratinization and muscle growth. Iodine is essential for thyroid functioning. Although symptoms of iodine deficiency do occur in older children, they are uncommon in infants. A diet high in organic sulfurs, which may be found in foods like cabbages and beans, may predispose to iodine deficiency. Molybdenum, manganese, cobalt, and copper are all known to be essential, but very little else is known about them. They are not generally a matter of concern in pediatric diets.

Nonessential Minerals Another group of trace minerals is generally considered nonessential; this group includes chromium, selenium, aluminum, boron, cadmium, and fluoride. Of these the most likely to be a matter of concern in children's diets is fluoride. Although technically considered to be nonessential since the body can function without it, it must certainly be considered extremely important for optimal dental health. Studies of fluoridation of the local water supply have shown a 50 to 60 percent decrease in the caries of a community (Dunning, 1965). Medicinal supplements are also effective in this regard (Hennon et al., 1966), although it is not known if they work as well as fluoridation of the water. Certainly it is most important that the child receive adequate fluoride while the enamel is being formed (from the 3d to 4th prenatal month to at least 7 or 8 years). It is recommended that 1 ppm be added to the community water supply, and nurses involved in ambulatory pediatrics in communities without such fluoridation should certainly exert pressure to correct this situation. Fluoride does cross the placental wall, and if a woman drinks an adequate amount of fluoridated water, the infant should be well supplied while beginning to form enamel. If this is not possible, supplements of fluoride are usually suggested during the last two trimesters of pregnancy. In fluoridated areas, infants fed on concentrated liquid formulas which are diluted with half water or on homemade formulas of evaporated milk and water will receive an adequate amount of fluoride. This may not be true, however, of an infant who is being breastfed or fed ready-to-serve formula to which no water is added. Since not much fluoride gets through in the breast milk (Foman, 1974), it is sometimes wise to consider supplementation in this situation. Approximately 1.0 to 2.5 ppm in the water supply is considered beneficial to teeth. The level of 3 ppm may result in a mottling of the teeth, which is cosmetically unappealing although not structurally damaging to the teeth. Tea, fish, bone meal, and certain baby foods are also high in fluoride. It is recommended that a child in an area without fluoridated water or who is not drinking sufficient quantities of this water, as in the case of the infant receiving breast milk or ready-to-serve formula, be supplemented with 0.5 mg from 6 months to 3 years and 1.0 mg thereafter. For exact supplementation, see Table 3-9.

Breast Feeding versus Bottle Feeding

The question of how to supply the essential nutrients to an infant or young child can be answered by various alternatives. The primary choice is between breast feeding and bottle feeding. Advantages and disadvantages of both should be discussed with the mother prenatally so that she has sufficient accurate information upon which to base her decision. There are many differences between human and cow's milk. Cow's milk, for instance, has more protein and electrolytes than does human milk, resulting in a higher solute load than is the case with human milk. This can be a problem, but as explained previously, generally it is a problem only during the first 2 weeks when the kidneys are immature. Breast milk is more acidic than cow's milk because of its higher lactose content. Since breast milk has a higher carbohydrate content (primarily due to the larger amount of lactose), the basic bowel process consists of fermentation of carbohydrate rather than a putrefaction of protein as is the case with cow's milk, which contains a higher percent of protein. This gives stools of breastfed infants their particular odor and characteristics and also accounts for the fact that it is virtually impossi-

Table 3-9 Fluoride Supplements

	Fluoride concentration of water supply, ppm			
Milk or formula	**<0.3**	**0.3–0.7**	**0.8–1.1**	**>1.1**
Breast milk	0.5	0.5	0.5	0
Cow's milk	0.5	0.25	0.25	0
Commercially prepared liquid	0.5	0.25	0	0
Evaporated milk formula	0.5	0.25	0	0
Commercially prepared powder	0.25	0	0	0

Source: Samuel Foman, *Infant Nutrition,* Philadelphia: Saunders, 1967, p. 184.

ble for a breastfed infant to become constipated (due to the high carbohydrate content) even though going for as long as 7 days without a bowel movement. In general, the frequency of bowel movements of breastfed infants is much more unpredictable than that of bottle-fed infants, sometimes being much more frequent, sometimes much less frequent. Breast milk has certain other chemical differences from cow's milk: it has a higher percentage of whey protein, while cow's milk has more casein proteins; breast milk has more unsaturated fatty acids and a higher percentage of the essential fatty acids (i.e., linoleic and arachnidonic) and is generally higher in fat and lower in protein than cow's milk. Furthermore breast milk contains fat that is better absorbed than that in cow's milk, which is more likely to leave the body through the bowel, taking with it a certain amount of calcium. Infant formula companies have attempted to modify cow's milk to make it correspond more closely with human milk. It is difficult to evaluate these results. In certain situations, the companies have attempted to replicate the specific chemical constituents of human milk only to find that the infant absorbed less of the various artificially mixed nutrients; thus even though the formula contained amounts of nutrients that were similar to those found in human milk, what was actually absorbed into the child's body was, in fact, quite different. Breast feeding has certain definite advantages over bottle feeding. It does seem to be true that breastfed infants suffer fewer infections, are less likely to die of sudden infant death syndrome, and are less likely to gain excessive weight. It is also true that breast feeding confers a certain limited type of birth control by suppression of ovulation, but it is important that the mother not consider this a 100 percent reliable means of birth control. Many feel that breast feeding is also cheaper, more convenient (no bottles to warm), and more conducive to a close mother-infant relationship. When considering the extra nutrients that mother must consume, however, and the necessary supplemental vitamins (breast milk does not transmit sufficient vitamin D, and the vitamin C content will depend on the mother's diet), it may not be very much cheaper. The question of convenience is also a matter of opinion since although no bottles need to be warmed, there is certainly a time, at least during the first few weeks, when the baby will need to be fed much more often if the mother's milk is to be stimulated properly. The idea that breast feeding is more conducive to a close mother-child relationship is also not well proven, since a bottle-fed infant can be held and played with in much the same way, not only by mother but by others in the family as well. There are some advantages to bottle feeding also. Breast milk jaundice cannot occur in these babies, many women find it more convenient, and other members in the family can also enjoy feeding the baby. The important point is that there are both advantages and disadvantages to each type of feeding, and basically the decision should be the parents'; the nurse's job is only to make available the information with which they can make that decision. Both breast- and bottle-fed babies can grow up to happy, healthy children.

Forms of Milk

Because milk is such a large part of the child's diet, the nurse working in ambulatory pediatrics must also be familiar with the various forms of milk now on the market. There are two basic processes to which milk is subjected: pasteurization (sterilization) and homogenization (the process of breaking up the curds into finer pieces). Pasteurization is now required by law for most milks sold commercially, and homogenization, although not required by law, is usually performed for consumer appeal.

Fluid whole milk is by far the most familiar type of milk and is usually both pasteurized and homogenized although a raw form that has had no heat treatment and must be boiled at home is available in certain locales. Other types of fluid milk are skim fluid milk and 2 percent fluid milk. These are familiar products in almost all parts of the country. They are exactly the same as whole fluid milk except for their fat content. Skim milk has only about 1 percent fat content, while 2 percent milk has 2 percent fat content; whole milk has about 3 percent fat content. All three types are usually fortified with vitamin D. Cultured milks are also available in fluid form. Buttermilk is usually made from fresh skim milk with added lactic acid. This is particularly useful when a child is receiving an antibiotic such as ampicillin which denudes the bowel of lactobacillus since it can replace much of the normal flora and pH. Yogurt is a similar form of milk but of solid consistency. Acidophilus milk is a similar type of cultured milk but is available in very few places in the United States. Certified milk may be either raw or pasteurized and is certified as to its cleanliness. It is sometimes fortified with vitamin D, but not universally; it is presently sold in only a very few places in the United States. Evaporated milk is canned milk from which half the normal amount of water has been evaporated. Both whole and skim evaporated milk is available, and both are fortified with vitamin D. One advantage is that no refrigeration is required until the can is open. This is the type of milk usually used when parents decide to make their own baby formula. Condensed milk is also sold in cans, and it is important to warn mothers not to mistake it for evaporated milk and make formula with it. It has far more sugar and far less protein than evaporated milk. Concentrated milk is seen in some parts of the United States although it is not common. It is made by removing two-thirds of the water from whole milk; it must be kept near freezing and should not be kept longer than 6 weeks. Dry milk comes in powder form with all the water removed from either the whole or skim milk. Most dry milk is made from skim milk since the fat particles present a problem in storage. Dry whole milk is also available, however. Vitamin D supplementation is present in almost all dry milks.

Milk Substitutes

Milk substitutes are now appearing in certain parts of the United States. They fall into two main categories: filled milks and imitation milks. Filled milks are a combination of true milk solids with a nonmilk fat; usually these have all the nutrients of regular milk, but may have a higher carbohydrate content. When coconut oil is used as the nonmilk fat, the nutrient linoleic acid may be missing. Filled milk may or may not be fortified with all the vitamins of regular milk. It is not recommended for infants, but is probably acceptable for older children who are receiving adequate linoleic acid from other dietary sources. Imitation milk is quite different. At the present time it is available in very few states (at the time of this writing, Arizona, New York, and California). It is usually much cheaper than regular milk but is also nutritionally inferior to milk, generally being lower in calcium and phosphorus and often lacking the vitamin supplementation. It should not be used as a replacement for milk for infants or children, although it is acceptable for use as an additional fluid and probably better than soda pop.

Infant Formulas

The nurse working in ambulatory pediatrics area must be familiar with the various types of milk that are available to be used by young infants. Human and cow milk have already been discussed. As mentioned previously, cow's milk has many disadvantages for young infants; consequently, when it is used as the primary food for infants, certain modifications aimed at making it more like human milk are advised. These can either be made by the mother herself or be purchased ready-made by various commercial formula companies. The formula made by mother at home (Table 3-10) consists basically of cow's milk modified by adding water and sugar. Most often this is made by mixing evaporated milk with water and corn syrup in the proportions of 13:19:3, that is, 13 oz. (one can) of evaporated milk, 19 oz. of water, and 3 tablespoons of corn syrup. A similar product can be based on whole milk instead of evaporated milk, although this is slightly more allergenic. In this situation less water is needed and the formula is 28:4:3, that is, 28 oz. of milk, 4 oz. water, and 3 tablespoons of corn syrup. The water and corn syrup are gradually decreased until the infant is about 6 months old, at which time the corn syrup is eliminated entirely and equal amounts of evaporated milk and water are used. This is the same as whole milk, and many mothers prefer to switch to whole milk. Either light or dark corn syrup may be used, and table sugar is sometimes substituted. Vitamins A, C, and D and iron are usually inadequate with this mixture and should be supplemented. The amount of calories, nutrients, and fluid needed for the infant and a sample of the calculation used to arrive at the 13:19:3 formula are shown in Table 3-11. The butterfat in this homemade formula may increase the fat excretion, but this is rarely of importance except in an occasional baby in the first 2 weeks or in the low-birthweight baby.

Most commercial formulas are based on skimmed cow's milk with added vegetable oil and carbohydrate. Examples of this type are Similac, Enfamil, and Modilac.

Another group of formulas also based on nonfat cow milk attempt to duplicate the whey/casein ratio (60:40) of human milk. Two examples are SMA S-26 and Similac PM 60/40. These products have a lower solute load which, although not necessary in the usual situation, may be important for children who need a very concentrated formula, for instance, those with congestive heart problems.

There are other milk-based formulas made for very specialized situations. Probana is low in fat and lactose content and is used in cases of significant diarrhea, coeliac disease, and cystic fibrosis. Supplements of vitamins C, E, and K are usually used if steatorrhea is present. Lonalac is another specialty product useful with children with cardiac conditions because of its low sodium content. It should not be concentrated any further than it is in its prepared form, however, since this will increase the renal solute load above an acceptable limit. Portagen is a medium-chain triglyceride product manufactured for use in cases of chyluria, steatorrhea, or intestinal lymphagiecturia.

Allergies Surprisingly frequently, allergies arise in children and force a modification of the milk in the diet. Allergies can be specific to the beta-lactoglobulin, alpha-lactoglobulin, bovine serum albumin, or bovine gamma globulin of the milk. Since both the bovine serum albumin and the bovine gamma globulin are quite heat-sensitive, children who are allergic to these elements may be able to tolerate evaporated milk but not whole milk since the evaporation process entails exposure to high heat. Neither beta-lactoglobulin nor alpha-lactoglobulin are affected by heat, and a child who is allergic to these will have trouble with either evaporated or whole milk. Furthermore, children who are allergic to these elements in cow's milk are most often allergic to them in goat's milk as well. This means that generally a child who can tolerate neither whole nor evaporated cow's milk will not tolerate goat's milk either. All proteins have the potentiality of antigenicity, but this is not true of amino acids. Probably the reason many infants have allergies which they later outgrow is that their digestive system is somewhat immature and not all proteins are adequately broken down into amino acids. As the child matures, this situation corrects itself.

To avoid allergies, five possible courses of action can be taken. One can substitute protein in cow's milk with protein of another mammal like the goat; one can substitute the protein of a vegetable like soybean or almond; one can substitute a meat protein like lamb or beef; one can treat the cow protein by heat as is done in the evaporation process; or one can hydrolyze the casein. All these processes have been used in various allergic formulas. Soy bean protein formulas are the most common type of allergic formula. Examples are Neo-Mull-soy and Soyalac, Nursoy, Prosobee, and Isomil. Soy formulas must be checked carefully for vitamin content since some of them have lacked various vitamins: deficiencies of thiamine and vitamin A as well

Table 3-10 Calculations for Homemade Formulas

Weight, lbs	Total formula for the day, oz.	Evaporated milk formula		Formula using homogenized or pasteurized whole milk		How to divide the formula
Birth to 6 weeks						
6	16–18	Evaporated milk	6 oz.	Whole milk	12 oz.	2¼–2½ oz. in 7 bottles, or
		Water	10–12 oz.	Water	4–6 oz.	2½–3 oz. in 6 bottles
		Sugar or syrup	2 tablespoons	Sugar or syrup	2 tablespoons	
7	19–21	Evaporated milk	7 oz.	Whole milk	14 oz.	2¾–3 oz. in 7 bottles, or
		Water	12–14 oz.	Water	5–7 oz.	3–3½ oz. in 6 bottles
		Sugar or syrup	2 tablespoons	Sugar or syrup	2 tablespoons	
8	22–24	Evaporated milk	8 oz.	Whole milk	16 oz.	3–3½ oz. in 7 bottles, or
		Water	14–16 oz.	Water	6–8 oz.	3½–4 oz. in 6 bottles or
		Sugar or syrup	2 tablespoons	Sugar or syrup	2 tablespoons	4½–5 oz. in 5 bottles
9	24–27	Evaporated milk	9 oz.	Whole milk	18 oz.	3½–4 oz. in 7 bottles, or
		Water	15–18 oz.	Water	6–9 oz.	4–4½ oz. in 6 bottles, or
		Sugar or syrup	2 tablespoons	Sugar or syrup	2 tablespoons	5–5½ oz. in 5 bottles
10	25–30	Evaporated milk	10 oz.	Whole milk	20 oz.	3½–4½ oz. in 7 bottles, or
		Water	15–20 oz.	Water	5–10 oz.	4–5 oz. in 6 bottles, or
		Sugar or syrup	2 tablespoons	Sugar or syrup	2 tablespoons	5–6 oz. in 5 bottles
11	28–32	Evaporated milk	11 oz.	Whole milk	22 oz.	4–4½ oz. in 7 bottles, or
		Water	17–21 oz.	Water	6–10 oz.	4½–5¼ oz. in 6 bottles, or
		Sugar or syrup	2 tablespoons	Sugar or syrup	2 tablespoons	5½–6½ oz. in 5 bottles
12	30–36	Evaporated milk	12 oz.	Whole milk	24 oz.	5–6 oz. in 6 bottles, or
		Water	18–24 oz.	Water	6–12 oz.	6–7 oz. in 5 bottles
		Sugar or syrup	2 tablespoons	Sugar or syrup	2 tablespoons	

13	32–36	Evaporated milk Water Sugar or syrup	13 oz. 19–23 oz. 2 tablespoons	Whole milk Water Sugar or syrup	26 oz. 6–10 oz. 2 tablespoons	$5\frac{1}{4}$–6 oz. in 6 bottles, or $6\frac{1}{2}$–7 oz. in 5 bottles
			6 weeks to 4 months			
8	20–24	Evaporated milk Water Sugar or syrup	8 oz. 12–16 oz. 3 tablespoons	Whole milk Water Sugar or syrup	16 oz. 4–8 oz. 3 tablespoons	$3\frac{1}{2}$–4 oz. in 6 bottles, or 4–5 oz. in 5 bottles
9	23–27	Evaporated milk Water Sugar or syrup	9 oz. 14–18 oz. 3 tablespoons	Whole milk Water Sugar or syrup	18 oz. 5–9 oz. 3 tablespoons	4–$4\frac{1}{2}$ oz. in 6 bottles, or $4\frac{1}{2}$–$5\frac{1}{2}$ oz. in 5 bottles
10	25–30	Evaporated milk Water Sugar or syrup	10 oz. 15–20 oz. 3 tablespoons	Whole milk Water Sugar or syrup	20 oz. 5–10 oz. 3 tablespoons	4–5 oz. in 6 bottles, or 5–6 oz. in 5 bottles, or 6–$7\frac{1}{2}$ oz. in 4 bottles
11	25–33	Evaporated milk Water Sugar or syrup	11 oz. 14–22 oz. 3 tablespoons	Whole milk Water Sugar or syrup	22 oz. 3–11 oz. 3 tablespoons	4–$5\frac{1}{2}$ oz. in 6 bottles, or 5–$6\frac{1}{2}$ oz. in 5 bottles, or 6–8 oz. in 4 bottles
12	27–36	Evaporated milk Water Sugar or syrup	12 oz. 15–24 oz. 3 tablespoons	Whole milk Water Sugar or syrup	24 oz. 3–12 oz. 3 tablespoons	$4\frac{1}{2}$–6 oz. in 6 bottles, or $5\frac{1}{2}$–7 oz. in 5 bottles, or 7–9 oz. in 4 bottles

Table 3-10 Calculations for Homemade Formulas *(Cont'd)*

Weight, lbs	Total formula for the day, oz.	Evaporated milk formula		Formula using homogenized or pasteurized whole milk		How to divide the formula
			6 weeks to 4 months			
13	30–36	Evaporated milk Water Sugar or syrup	13 oz. 17–23 oz. 3 tablespoons	Whole milk Water Sugar or syrup	26 oz. 4–10 oz. 3 tablespoons	6–7 oz. in 5 bottles, or 7½–9 oz. in 4 bottles
14	31–36	Evaporated milk Water Sugar or syrup	13 oz. 18–23 oz. 3 tablespoons	Whole milk Water Sugar or syrup	28 oz. 3–8 oz. 3 tablespoons	6–7 oz. in 5 bottles, or 7½–9 oz. in 4 bottles
Over 14	30–36	Evaporated milk Water Sugar or syrup	13 oz. 17–23 oz. 3 tablespoons	Whole milk Water Sugar or syrup	30 to 36 oz. None 3 tablespoons	6–7 oz. in 5 bottles, or 7½–9 oz. in 4 bottles
			5 months			
12	24–30	Evaporated milk Water Sugar or syrup	12 oz. 12–18 oz. 1–2 tablespoons	Whole milk Water Sugar or syrup	24 oz. 0–6 oz. 1–2 tablespoons	5–6 oz. in 5 bottles, or 6–7½ oz. in 4 bottles, or 8–9 oz. in 3 bottles

13	26–32	Evaporated milk Water Sugar or syrup	13 oz. 13–19 oz. 1–2 tablespoons	Whole milk Water Sugar or syrup	26 oz. 0–6 oz. 1–2 tablespoons	5–6¼ oz. in 5 bottles, or 6¼–8 oz. in 4 bottles, or 8–9 oz. in 3 bottles
14	26–32	Evaporated milk Water Sugar or syrup	13 oz. 13–19 oz. 1–2 tablespoons	Whole milk Water Sugar or syrup	28 oz. 0–4 oz. 1–2 tablespoons	5–6¼ oz. in 5 bottles, or 6¼–8 oz. in 4 bottles, or 8–9 oz. in 3 bottles
Over 14	26–32	Evaporated milk Water Sugar or syrup	13 oz. 13–19 oz. 1–2 tablespoons	Whole milk Water Sugar or syrup	26–32 oz. None 1–2 tablespoons	6¼–8 oz. in 4 bottles, or 8–9 oz. in 3 bottles
6 months and over						
Over 13	26–32	Evaporated milk Water Sugar or syrup	13 oz. 13–19 oz. None	Whole milk Water Sugar or syrup	26–32 oz. None None	6¼–8 oz. in 4 bottles, or 8–9 oz. in 3 bottles

Source: Henry K. Silver, C. Henry Kempe, Ruth Kempe, and Grover Powers, *Healthier Babies, Happier Parents,* Sausalito, Calif.: Purposeful Publications, 1957, pp. 32–33.

Table 3-11 Calories and Fluid in Formulas for Various Ages

Age, months	0	1	2	3	4	5	6	7	8	9	10	11	12
Calories per day*	130–100/kg (60–45/lb)					110–100/kg (50–45/lb)				100–90/kg (45–40/lb)			
Fluid per day, ml	130–200/kg (2–3 oz./lb)				130–165/kg (2–2½ oz./lb)						130/kg (2 oz./lb)		
No. of feedings per day†	6 or 7		4 or 5				3 or 4					3	
Ounces per feeding	2.5–4	3.5–5	4–6	5–7	6–8	7–9							
Milk: Evaporated / Whole	65 ml/kg (1 oz./lb) up to a total of 13 oz. (1 can) daily / 130 ml/kg (2 oz./lb) up to a total of 28–32 oz. daily												
Sugar per day	1–1.5 oz. (30–45 gm)						‡	None					

* The larger amount should be used for the younger infant.

† Will vary somewhat with individual babies.

‡ Decrease sugar by ½ oz. (15 gm) every 2 weeks.

Source: Henry K. Silver, C. Henry Kempe, and Henry B. Bruyn, *Handbook of Pediatrics*, Los Altos, Calif.: Lange, 1965, p. 65.

as iodine have been reported in infants receiving soy formulas in the past. All soy products marketed at the time of this writing are adequately fortified with vitamins and minerals. Although extensive studies are not available, those growth studies which have been done (Kane, 1957; Kay et al., 1960; Omans et al., 1963) seem to indicate that the growth curve of children receiving soy formulas is similar to that of children receiving cow's fomula. These formulas are usually used in situations where the child is allergic and sometimes will be used prophylactically when there is a great deal of allergy in the family. They may also be useful in lactase deficiency, and some people feel they are helpful for 2 to 3 weeks after severe diarrhea, since a lactase deficiency frequently persists in such situations.

Certain nonsoy allergic formulas are also marketed. One of these is made from beef heart with added carbohydrate. Although there is some galactose present, the amount seems to be clinically insignificant. The second product now available is Nutramigen, which is prepared from a digest of casein and is used for galactosemia as well as for allergic children. It has an unpleasant taste, at least to adults, and very thin stools should be expected when using this formula. There have been two studies of Nutramigen (Hill, 1953; Hartmann, 1942), both utilizing very small samples, but they seem to indicate that both growth patterns and nitrogen retention remain adequate in children receiving this formula. Another formula made from a digest of casein is Lofenalac, but this formula is generally considered to be for children with PKU rather than allergy problems. Goat's milk is also available, but as mentioned before, there is a high cross-allergenicity between cow's milk and goat's milk. It must be remembered that goat's milk does not supply sufficient amounts of vitamin B_{12}, and a folic acid supplement should be given with it.

Intolerance to Milk Allergies are one problem that the nurse may encounter in regard to milk-based formulas. Another is the child with an intolerance. Sometimes this is due to a deficiency of amylases, which is commonly present the first 3 months of life. In this situation, the child may not digest the starches, simply excreting them in an undigested form, causing diarrhea. In other situations there is a deficiency of the enzyme needed for digestion of disaccharides (this may occur rarely with the enzyme for digestion of monosaccharides). Most often the enzyme involved is for the digestion of lactose or sucrose. This may occur as a congenital deficiency or as an acquired problem after difficulty with diarrhea. The most common example of this is lactase deficiency, which seems to be a racially determined trait in most nonwhite groups (American Indians, Blacks, Asiatics) and in some percentage of the white population. It is generally not present in infants, but becomes apparent as children mature. These children have great intolerance to milk and some milk products. This problem should certainly be considered in situations such as school lunch programs in which children of all races are required to finish their pint of milk or in prenatal clinics in which mothers of all races are strongly urged to drink a quart of milk daily. Symptoms associated with such lactose deficiency are flatus, a bloating sensation, diarrhea, and other gastrointestinal disturbances. Such deficiencies can also be secondary to injury to the gastrointestinal tract as occurs in coeliac disease, severe diarrhea, and kwashiorkor. One practice is to test the stool for acidity after a bout with diarrhea; if it remains acid in reaction, disaccharides should be eliminated from the diet.

Malabsorption Another similar situation is malabsorption, a condition in which the child passes frequent, pale, bulky, foul-smelling, semisolid, greasy stools. This may be the result of a low level of pancreatic lipase and trypsin as occurs in cystic fibrosis or from lack of bile salts as occurs in hepatitis or from infection, starvation, or coeliac disease. These children also need specially formulated diets.

Solid Baby Foods

Baby food solids are another important aspect of infant and child nutrition. The trend in this country in recent years has been to begin the introduction of solids earlier and earlier. Today, Beal (1970) has shown that 6-month-olds are getting about one-third of their calories from solids. Some practitioners start solids as early as the 2d or 3d day of life; others not until the 6th month. Nutritionally, infants do not actually need anything except milk for the first 6 months or until the supply of iron they were born with runs out.

Conceivably an iron-fortified formula would be sufficient for even longer. Most infants want solid food by this time, however, and enjoy the chewing motion. There is no good scientific evidence on the best time to start solid foods although most people in this country now begin around 2 to 3 months. Neither is there any good scientific evidence concerning which food should be started first, although most practitioners tend to be quite dogmatic in their beliefs. It probably makes little difference, and certainly the desires of the mother should be respected in this regard. At the present time, there are three manufacturers of baby foods: Heinz, Gerbers, and Beechnut. Both Heinz and Gerbers make available a listing of all their foods with the exact ingredients and nutritional contents, and any nurse involved in ambulatory pediatrics should have these lists. New ones should be obtained periodically since the recipes change often. Gerbers also puts out lists of which foods can be safely used in situations of the more common allergies (i.e., foods that are wheat-free, gluten-free, citrus-free, or egg-free). It is interesting to note that about 200 of the 362 varieties of baby food are free of the common alergens.

In general, solid foods have about 1½ to 3 times as many calories as milk; however, plain vegetables, some strained dinners, and some strained breakfasts have fewer calories. Baby foods are lower in calories than comparable products prepared at home simply because of their higher water content. These are important things to be aware of when weight control is being considered.

Strained and junior foods of the same name are nutritionally similar and differ only in their particle size. It is useful to know the sizes of serving: all juices are presently sold in 4½-oz. jars; all other infant foods are sold in either 4½- or 3¾-oz. jars except meat and egg yolks, which are sold in 3½-oz. jars. Junior foods are all 7½ to 7¾ oz. except meats, which are 3½ oz. and high meat dinners, which are 4½ to 4¾ oz.

It is helpful to be aware of some additional specific facts about the different types of foods. Surprisingly, for instance, baby fruits and desserts of comparable names are made from almost exactly the same recipe. Sugar is added to both, usually in the form of tapioca. All fruit juices except apple and orange are mixtures, and they are all higher in calories than the adult counterparts because of the added dextrose and sucrose.

Vegetables are available in two varieties: creamed and plain. Sucrose is added to the Heinz and Beechnut plain varieties but not to those made by Gerbers. The creamed vegetables have additional milk solids and corn starch and are consequently higher in calories. Many soups and dinners are available, and the variety can be confusing to the consumer. When the meat name precedes the vegetable name, the meat is the principle ingredient, although there is still only one-sixth the protein found in the pure meat products. When the vegetable name precedes the meat name, negligible meat nutrients are available. The so-called high meat dinners have about three times the amount of protein as the other dinners but still only half the protein found in the pure meats.

The meat products are relatively more expensive if measured per unit of volume, but not necessarily more expensive per gram of protein. They contain both less fat and less protein than a similar product made at home, again because of the higher water content. Meat sticks have a lower water content and are higher in calories, protein, carbohydrate and fat than meat sold in jar. Canadian baby foods contain a much higher fat content than those made in the United States.

The protein content of baby foods is highest in the plain meats and egg yolks and slightly less high in the high meat dinners; it is medium in soups and dinners and low in fruits and desserts. Fat content is again highest in meats, egg yolks, and high meat dinners (again slightly less in these), is medium in the various soups and dinners, and is lowest in fruits, vegetables, and desserts. Carbohydrate content is high in all baby foods except egg yolks, meats, and high meat dinners. Iron is found in smaller amounts than would be true of comparable products prepared at home except in the case of the dry baby cereal to which it is added (it is *not* added to the moist baby cereal packaged in jars). As mentioned before, however, controversy now exists over whether this iron is in a form unavailable to the human body. A large amount of sodium is present in almost all baby foods, and the question has arisen about whether this may predispose to future hypertension. No definitive research exists on this subject. The renal solute load is relatively high in meats, egg yolks, and high meat dinners, but fairly low in juices, fruits, desserts, and puddings.

Nutrition of the Older Child

As children grow older, their diet becomes more and more similar to that of those around them. Most babies begin to try some table foods by 6 months and by 1 year eat primarily the same foods as adults. Probably one caution that should be mentioned to parents is to try to avoid difficult-to-chew foods such as peanuts and popcorn since the aspiration rate for these foods is high. Otherwise the same basic principles of adult nutrition apply to children, except they are probably more important here since lifelong patterns are being formed. Early counseling on snacking and "empty calories" as well as caries-forming foods is appropriate at this time. A 1-year-old may worry parents because of a suddenly decreased appetite. This is an expected part of growth and development since the tremendous physical growth of the previous year is also slowing. Besides this, the child's interest in walking is increasing, and frequently, the addition of many "finger-foods" which children can eat while walking and on which they can practice their eye-hand coordination may help to keep the diet balanced. By 2 years, if not earlier, children usually have very special preferences, and most often these can be respected without undue harm to a well-balanced eating pattern (with the exception, of course, of those children who have been exposed to too many high-carbohydrate foods like candy). Common at about 2½ and again at 4 years old are "food jags" in which the child will insist on repetitious servings of a limited number of foods day after day. These are ritualistic ages, and usually the situation is best handled by paying as little attention to it as possible. Again, children seldom carry these jags to the point where they develop nutritional problems. By the time children are 5 years old, their eating habits will be those of their family; later their habits will be influenced by their school friends. These food patterns usually remain fairly stable until adolescence, when food habits like everything else are likely to be rebelled against. Particularly for girls, this period presents a potential nutritional hazard. The tremendous power of peer influence and the frequent parties and gatherings with the many "empty calorie" high-carbohydrate snacks of candy and potato chips present a real problem. Besides this, there is a natural increase in appetite during the adolescent growth spurt, but often the habits are formed and cannot be broken at the end of this growth spurt (usually about 4 years after menses). Increased concern with appearance and body image can lead to many unbalanced crash diets. Studies of the actual diets of teenagers have shown that they are likely to be low in vitamins A and C, iron, and calcium (Clark, 1969; Hampton et al., 1967; Wharton, 1963). In polls asking what foods were most liked and least liked by this age group, adolescents said they preferred milk, ice cream, steak, roast beef, hamburger, pork chops, ham, chicken, turkey, orange juice, oranges, apples, fries, corn, peas, bread, cake, and pie in that order. These foods would supply all the necessary nutrients with the exception of vitamin A. Least liked foods were liver, spinach, and squash (Schorr, 1972; Einstein, 1970; Kennedy, 1952; Schuck, 1961). Girls are at a nutritional disadvantage when their menses begins since the need for iron increases and this is one of the nutrients found to be frequently deficient in adolescent diets. Another risk in adolescent girls is that of pregnancy. A girl who becomes pregnant before the end of her growth spurt (which averages around 17 in the United States) has an increased risk for a variety of pregnancy complications, including toxemia, iron deficiency anemia, fetopelvic disproportion, a long labor, and an infant who is either premature or of low birthweight or both. Also, a girl with nutritional difficulties resulting in a low level of folic acid is probably at risk for third trimester bleeding and premature rupture of the membranes (Van de Mark and Wright, 1972). It can easily be seen, then, that the nurse in ambulatory pediatrics must pay particular attention to the adolescent diet.

Other Issues

There are a number of miscellaneous questions that occur sporadically in the literature concerning pediatric nutrition, and some of these will be briefly discussed at this point. One of these is the question of radioactivity, particularly how much radioactivity is present in both cow and human milk.

This subject has really not been fully researched, but the American Academy of Pediatrics (1963) has reviewed what is known about this situation and has stated that at this point the amount of radioactivity is probably not sufficient to present a problem. Atherosclerosis is another topic sometimes alluded to in the literature. The question here is whether infant and child diets high in cholesterol will predispose to atherosclerosis in later life. There is as yet no proof that this is the case, but many authorities suggest that restriction of cholesterol might be worthwhile in children who have Type II hyperlipoproteinemia in their blood (a hereditary condition) (American Academy of Pediatrics, 1972). A similar question is also mentioned: Will an increased amount of sodium in the diet of infants and children predispose to later hypertension? Again, there have been no long-term studies, and the answer to this question is simply not known. At one time the question arose as to whether any harm was done to a child by the androgens and estrogens injected into certain animals which were later killed for foods. Again, reviewing the information at that time, the American Academy of Pediatrics in 1960 said it felt this presented no problem. One final nutritional question which will be encountered on some occasions concerns the presence of nitrates in foods. It is known that nitrates can change to nitrites and cause methahemaglobinemia since the nitrate oxidizes the ferrous ion into a ferric ion, thus rendering the hemoglobin incapable of combining with oxygen. Probably fetal hemoglobin is more susceptible to this problem; it is also known that a gastric pH of over 4 is needed, and this exists primarily in the infant under 10 days old. The cases that have been recorded have been in young infants drinking contaminated water either from a well or from the run-off of farms which were using nitrogen fertilizer. Although there are large amounts of nitrites present in spinach and beets, commercial baby foods are processed in such a way that these amounts present no problem; it is possible, however, that if there were a mistake in home processing of these foods, difficulty might be encountered (American Academy of Pediatrics, 1970). It is felt by some that sufficient quantities of vitamins C and K may be protective against methahemaglobinemia.

It is certainly clear that nutrition is a very important subject for nurses working in ambulatory pediatrics, and it is necessary for them to keep up with all the current research done in this field.

BIBLIOGRAPHY

Childhood Immunizations

Ashcroft, M. T., B. Singh, C. C. Nicholson, et al.: "A Seven-Year Field Trial of Two Typhoid Vaccines in Guyana," *Lancet,* vol. 2, 1967, pp. 1056-1059.

Baratta, R. O., M. C. Ginter, M. A. Price, et al.: "Measles (Rubeola) in Previously Immunized Children," *Pediatrics* vol. 46, 1970, pp. 397-402.

Bauer, D. J., L. St. Vincent, C. H. Kempe, et al.: "Prophylaxis of Smallpox with Methiazone," *American Journal of Epidemiology,* vol. 90, 1969, pp. 13-145.

Berg, J. M.: "Neurologic Complications of Pertussis Immunization," *British Medical Journal,* vol. 2, 1958, pp. 24-27.

Bradford, W. L.: "The Bordetella Group," in Dubos and Hirsch, *Bacterial and Mycotic Infections of Man,* 4th ed., Philadelphia: Lippincott, 1965, pp. 742-751.

Brody, J. A., J. L. Sever, R. McAlister, et al.: "Rubella Epidemic on St. Paul Island in the Pribilofs, 1963, I. Epidemiologic, Clinical, and Serologic Findings," *Journal of the American Medical Association,* vol. 191, 1965, pp. 83-87.

Burmeister, R. W., W. D. Tigertt, and E. L. Overhold: "Laboratory Acquired Pneumonic Plague," *Annals of Internal Medicine,* vol. 56, 1962, pp. 789-800.

Burruss, H. W., and M. C. Hargett: "Yellow Fever Vaccine Inactivation Studies," *Public Health Reports,* vol. 62, 1947, pp. 940-956.

Buynak, E. B., R. E. Weibel, and J. E. Whitman, Jr.: "Combined Live Measles, Mumps, and Rubella Virus Vaccines," *Journal of the American Medical Association,* vol. 207, 1969, pp. 2259-2262.

Carpenter, C. C. J.: "Cholera Enterotoxin—Recent Investigations Yield Insights into Transport Processes," *American Journal of Medicine,* vol. 50, 1971, pp. 1-7.

Caten, J. L., and L. Kartman: "Human Plague in the United States," *Journal of the American Medical Association,* vol. 205, 1968, pp. 333-336.

Cavanaugh, D. C., H. G. Dangerfield, D. H. Hunter, et al.: "Some Observations on the Current Plague Outbreak in the Republic of Vietnam," *American Journal of Public Health,* vol. 58, 1968, pp. 742-752.

Center for Disease Control: *Influenza-Respiratory Disease of Surveillance Report,* no. 87, December 1971.

———: *Annual Poliomyelitis Summary—1969,* June 15, 1970; *Annual Poliomyelitis Summary—1970,* Sept., 30, 1971.

———: *Morbidity and Mortality Weekly Report,* vol. no. 38, Sept. 25, 1971, pp. 339-345.

Cohen, R. J., and J. I. Stockard: "Pneumonic Plague in an Untreated Plague-vaccinated Individual," *Journal of the American Medical Association,* vol. 22, 1967, pp. 365-366.

Cooper, L. Z., and S. Krugman: "The Rubella Problem," *DM* 1969, pp. 31-38.

Cvjetanovic, B. and K. Uemura: "The Present Status of Field and Laboratory Studies of Typhoid and Paratyphoid Vaccine," *Bulletin of the World Health Organization,* vol. 32, 1965, pp. 29-36.

Davis, W. J., H. E. Larson, J. P. Simsarian, et al.: "A Study of Rubella Immunity and Resistance to Infection," *Journal of the American Medical Association,* vol. 215, 1971, pp. 600-608.

Donovick, R., and R. W. G. Wyckoff: "The Comparative Potencies of Several Typhus Vaccines," *Public Health Report,* vol. 60, 1945, pp. 605-612.

Ecke, R. S., A. G. Gilliam, J. C. Snyder, et al.: "The Effect of Cox-type Vaccine on Louse-borne Typhus Fever. An Account of 61 Cases of Naturally Occurring Typhus Fever in Patients Who Had Previously Received One or More Injections of Cox-type Vaccine," *American Journal of Tropical Medicine,* vol. 25, 1945, pp. 447-462.

Eckmann, L. (ed.): "Principles on Tetanus," *Proceedings of the International Conference on Tetanus, Bern, July 15-19, 1966,* Bern: Huber, 1967.

Eickhoff, T. C.: "Immunization against Influenza: Rationale and Recommendations," *Journal of Infectious Diseases,* vol. 123, 1971, pp. 446-454.

———, I. L. Sherman, and R. E. Serfling: "Observations on Excess Mortality Associated with Epidemic Influenza," *Journal of the American Medical Association,* vol. 176, 1961, pp. 776-782.

Eldering, G: "Some Laboratory Aspects of a Pertussis Surveillance Program," *Proceedings of the Fifth Annual Immunization Conference, San Diego, California,* U.S. Department of Health, Education, and Welfare, PHS, HSMHA, National Communicable Disease Center, 1968, pp. 91-95.

"Evidence on the Safety and Efficacy of Live Poliomyelitis Vaccines Currently in Use, with Special References to Type 3 Poliovirus," *Bulletin of the World Health Organization,* vol. 42, 1970, pp. 925-945.

Farrar, W. E., Jr., A. R. Warner, Jr., and S. Vivona: "Pre-exposure Immunization against Rabies Using Duck Embryo Vaccine," *Military Medicine,* vol. 129, 1964, pp. 960-965.

Foege, W. H., S. O. Foster, and J. A. Goldstein: "Current Status of Global Smallpox Eradication," *American Journal of Epidemiology,* vol. 93, 1971, pp. 223-233.

Francis, T., Jr.: "Epidemic Influenza: Immunization and Control," *Medical Clinics of North America,* vol. 51, 1967, pp. 781-790.

Fulginiti, V. A., L. A. Winograd, M. Jackson, et al.: "Therapy of Experimental Vaccinial Keratitis," *Archives Opthalmology,* vol. 74, 1965, pp. 539-544.

Gangarosa, E. J., and G. A. Faich: "Cholera; The Risk to American Travelers," *Annals of Internal Medicine,* vol. 74, 1971, pp. 412-415.

———, and W. H. Mosley: "Asiatic Cholera," in W. H. Tice, *Practice of Medicine,* 1970, vol. III, chap. 28.

Gilliam, A. G.: "Efficacy of Cox-type Vaccine in the Prevention of Naturally Acquired Louse-borne Typhus Fever," *American Journal of Hygiene,* vol. 44, 1946, pp. 401-410.

Gordon, J., and R. L. Hood: "Whooping Cough and Its Epidemiological Anomalies," *American Journal of the Medical Sciences,* vol. 222, 1951, pp. 333-361.

Gordon, J. E.: Ten years in the Epidemiology of Mumps," *American Journal of the Medical Sciences,* 1949, pp. 338-359.

Gottlieb, S., M. Martin, F. X. McLaughlin, et al.: "Long-Term Immunity to Diphtheria and Tetanus: A Mathematical Model," *American Journal of Epidemiology,* vol. 85, 1967, pp. 207-219.

Greenberg, M., and J. Childress: "Vaccination against Rabies with Duck-Embryo and Semple Vaccines," *Journal of the American Medical Association,* vol. 173, 1960, pp. 333-337.

Groot, H., and R. B. Riberio: "Neutralizing and Hemagglutination-Inhibition Antibodies to Yellow Fever 17 Years after Vaccination with 17D Vaccine," *Bulletin of the World Health Organization,* vol. 27, 1962, pp. 608-707.

Habel, K: "Rabies Antiserum Interference with Antigenicity of Vaccine in Mice, *Bulletin of the World Health Organization,* vol. 17, 1957, pp. 933-936.

Hardy, G. E., C. C. Hopkins, C. C. Linnemann, Jr., et al.: "Trivalent Oral Poliovirus Vaccine: A Comparison of Two Infant Immunization Schedules," *Pediatrics,* vol. 45, no. 3, part I, 1970.

Hargett, M. V., H. W. Burruss, and A. Donovan: "Aqueous-Base Yellow Fever Vaccine," *Public Health Report,* vol. 58, 1943, pp. 505-512.

Harris, R. W., C. D. Turnbull, P. Isacson, et al.: "Mumps in a Northeast Metropolitan Community," *American Journal of Epidemiology,* vol. 88, 1968, pp. 224-233.

Heiner, G. G., N. Fatima, P. K. Russell, et al.: "Field Trials of Methisazone as a Prophylactic Agent against Smallpox," *American Journal of Epidemiology,* vol. 94, 1971, pp. 435-449.

Hejfec, L. B., L. A. Levina, M. L. Kuz'minova, et al.: "Controlled Field Trials of Paratyphoid B Vaccine and Evaluation of the Effectiveness of a Single Administration of Typhoid Vaccine," *Bulletin of the World Health Organization,* vol. 38, 1968, pp. 907-915.

Henderson, D. A., J. J. Witte, L. Morris, et al.: "Paralytic Disease Associated with Oral Polio Vaccines," *Journal of the American Medical Association,* vol. 190, 1964, pp. 41-48.

Hopkins, C. C., W. E. Dismukes, T. H. Glick, et al.: "Surveilance of Paralytic Poliomyelitis in the United States," *Journal of the American Medical Association,* vol. 21, 1969, pp. 694-700.

Hilleman, M. R., E. B. Buynak, R. E. Weibel, et al.: "Live, Attenuated Mumps-Virus Vaccine," *New England Journal of Medicine,* vol. 278, 1968, pp. 227-232.

Horstmann, D. M.: "Enterovirus Infections of the Central Nervous System. The Present and Future of Poliomyelitis," *Medical Clinics of North America,* vol. 51, 1967, pp. 681-692.

———, H. Liebhaber, G. L. LeBouvier, et al.: "Rubella: Reinfection of Vaccinated and Naturally Immune Persons Exposed in an Epidemic," *New England Journal of Medicine,* vol. 283, 1970, pp. 771-778.

Ispen, J.: "Circulating Antitoxin at the Onset of Diphtheria in 425 Patients," *Journal of Immunology,* vol. 54, 1946, pp. 325-347.

"International Conference on Hong Kong Influenza," *Bulletin of the World Health Organization,* vol. 41, 1970, pp. 335-748.

Johnson, H. N.: "Rabies Virus," in Horsfall and Tamm, *Viral and Rickettsial Infections of Man,* 4th ed., Philadelphia, Lippincott, 1965, pp. 814-840.

Kilbourne, E. D.: "Influenza 1970: Unquestioned Answers and Unanswered Questions," *Archives of Environmental Health,* vol. 21, 1970, pp. 286-292.

———: "Influenza: The Vaccines," *Hospital Practice,* vol. 10, 1971, pp. 103-114.

Krugman, S.: "Present Status of Measles and Rubella Immunization in the United States: A Medical Progress Report," *Journal of Pediatrics,* vol. 78, 1971, pp. 1-16.

———, and R. Ward: *Infectious Diseases of Children and Adults,* 5th ed., St. Louis: C. V. Mosby, 1973.

———, G. Muriel, and J. U. Fontana: "Combined Live Measles, Mumps, Rubella Vaccine," *American Journal of Diseases of Children,* vol. 121, 1971, pp. 380-381.

LaForce, F. M., L. S. Young, and J. V. Bennett: "Tetanus in the United States (1965-1966): Epidemiologic and Clinical Features," *New England Journal of Medicine,* vol. 280, 1969, pp. 569-574.

Lambert, H. J.: "Epidemiology of a Small Pertussis Outbreak in Kent County Michigan," *Public Health Report,* vol. 80, 1965, pp. 365-369.

Landrigan, P. J., and J. I. Conrad: "Current Status of Measles in the United States," *Journal of Infectious Diseases,* vol. 124, 1971, pp. 620-622.

Lane, J. M., F. L. Ruben, E. Abrutyn, et al.: "Deaths Attributable to Smallpox Vaccination 1959 to 1966, 1968," *Journal of the American Medical Association,* vol. 212, 1970, pp. 441-444.

———, ———, J. M. Neff, et al.: "Complications of Smallpox Vaccination, 1968. National Surveillance in the United States," *New England Journal of Medicine,* vol. 281, 1969, pp. 1201-1208.

———, ———, ———, et al.: "Complications of Smallpox Vaccination, 1968. II. Results of Ten Statewide Surveys." *Journal of Infectious Diseases,* vol. 122, 1970, pp. 303-304.

Langmuir, A. D., D. A. Henderson, and R. E. Serfling: "The Epidemiological Basis for the Control of Influenza," *American Journal of Public Health,* vol. 54, 1964, pp. 563-571.

LeHane, D. E., N. R. Newberg, and W. E. Beam: "Evaluation of Rubella Herd Immunity during an Epidemic," *Journal of the American Medical Association,* vol. 213, 1970, pp. 2236-2239.

Lerman, S. J., and E. Gold: "Measles in Children Previously Vaccinated Against Measles," *Journal of the American Medical Association,* vol. 216, May, 1971, pp. 1311-1314.

Mallory, A., E. Belden, and P. Brachman: "The Current Status of Typhoid Fever in the United States and a Description of an Outbreak," *Journal of Infectious Diseases,* vol. 119, 1969, pp. 673-676.

McCormack, W. M., A. M. Chodwhury, N. Jahangir, et al.: "Tetracycline Prophylaxis in Families of Cholera Patients," *Bulletin of the World Health Organization,* vol. 38, 1968, pp. 787-792.

Meyer, H. M., and P. D. Parkman: "Rubella Vaccination: A Review of Practical Experience," *Journal of the American Medical Association,* vol. 215, 1971, pp. 613-619.

Meyer, K. E.: "Pasteurella and Francisella," in Dubos and Hirsch, *Bacterial and Mycotic Infections of Man,* 4th ed., Philadelphia: Lippincott, 1965, pp. 659-697.

Naiditch, M. J., and A. G. Bower: "Diphtheria: A Study of 1,433 Cases Observed during a Ten-Year Period at the Los Angeles County Hospital," *American Journal of Medicine,* vol. 17, 1954, pp. 229-245.

National Communicable Disease Center: *Diphtheria Surveillance Report,* no. 9, Mar. 24, 1969.

———: *NCDC Zoonoses Surveillance,* Annual Rabies Report, 1970.

Neff, J. M., J. M. Lane, J. H. Pert, et al.: "Complications of Smallpox Vaccination. I. National Survey in the United States, 1963," *New England Journal of Medicine,* vol. 276, 1967, pp. 125-132.

———, R. H. Levine, J. M. Lane, et al.: "Complications of Smallpox Vaccination, United States, 1963, II. Results Obtained by Four Statewide Surveys," *Pediatrics,* vol. 39, 1967, pp. 916-923.

Peck, F. B., Jr, H. M. Powell, and C. G. Culbertson: "A New Antirabies Vaccine for Human Use," *Journal of Laboratory and Clinical Medicine,* vol. 45, 1955, pp. 679-683.

Peebles, T. C., L. Levine, M. C. Eldred, et al.: "Tetanus-Toxoid Emergency Boosters: A Reappraisal," *New England Journal of Medicine,* vol. 280, 1969, pp. 575-581.

Phillipines Cholera Committee: "A Controlled Field Trial of the Effectiveness of

Cholera and Cholera El Tor Vaccines in the Philippines," *Bulletin of the World Health Organization,* vol. 32, 1965, pp. 603-625.

"Plague in the Americas," Pan American Health Organization, Scientific Publication, no. 115, 1965, pp. 114-117.

Polish Typhoid Committee: "Controlled Field Trials and Laboratory Studies on the Effectiveness of Typhoid Vaccines in Poland, 1961-64: Final Report," *Bulletin of the World Health Organization,* vol. 34, 1966, pp. 24-222.

Pollitzer, R.: *Plague,* World Health Organization Monograph Series, no. 22, Geneva, 1954, pp. 1-698.

———: "A Review of Recent Literature on Plague," *Bulletin of the World Health Organization,* vol. 23, 1960, pp. 313-400.

"Report of Special Advisory Committee on Oral Poliomyelitis Vaccines to the Surgeon General of the Public Health Service: Oral Poliomyelitis Vaccines," *Journal of the American Medical Association,* vol. 190, 1964, pp. 49-51.

Rosenzweig, E. G., R. W. Babione, and C. L. Wisseman, Jr.: "Immunological Studies with Group B Arthropod-borne Viruses. IV. Persistence of Yellow Fever Antibodies Following Vaccination with 17D Strain Yellow Fever Vaccine," *American Journal of Tropical Medicine,* vol. 12, 1963, pp. 230-235.

Rubbo, S. D.: "New Approaches to Tetanus Prophylaxis," *Lancet,* vol. 2, 1966, pp. 449-435.

Ruben, F. L., and J. M. Lane: Ocular Vaccinia, an Epidemiologic Analysis of 348 Cases," *Archives of Ophthalmology,* vol. 84, 1970, pp. 45-48.

Sabin, A. B.: "Commentary on Report on Oral Poliomyelitis Vaccines," *Journal of the American Medical Association,* vol. 190, 1964, pp. 52-55.

Sadusk, J. F.: "Typhus Fever in the United States Army Following Immunization. Incidence, Severity of Disease, Modification of the Clinical Course and Serologic Diagnosis," *Journal of the American Medical Association,* vol. 133, 1947, pp. 1192-1199.

Scheibel, I., M. W. Bentzon, P. E. Christensen, et al.: "Duration of Immunity to Diphtheria and Tetanus after Active Immunization," *Acta Pathologica et Microbiologica Scandinavica,* vol. 67, 1966, pp. 380-392.

Schroeder, S.: "The Interpretation of Serologic Tests for Typhoid Fever," *Journal of the American Medical Association,* vol. 205, 1968, pp. 839-840.

Sever, J. L., J. A. Brody, G. M. Schiff, et al.: "Rubella Epidemic on St. Paul Island in the Pribilofs, 1963. II. Clinical and Laboratory Findings for the Intensive Study Population," *Journal of the American Medical Association,* vol. 191, 1965, pp. 88-90.

Sikes, R. K.: "Guidelines for the Control of Rabies," *American Journal of Public Health,* vol. 60, no. 6, June 1970.

Smadel, J. E., E. B. Jackson, and J. M. Campbell: "Studies on Epidemic Typhus Vaccine," *Arch. Inst. Past Tunis,* vol. 36, 1959, pp. 481-499.

Smith, H. H., H. Calderon-Cuervo, and J. P. Leyva: "A Comparison of High and Low Subcultures of Yellow Fever Vaccine (17D) in Human Groups," *American Journal of Tropical Medicine,* vol. 21, 1941, pp. 579-587.

Smithburn, K. C., C. Durieux, R. Koerber, et al.: "Yellow Fever Vaccination," WHO Monograph Series, no. 30, Geneva, 1956.

Strode, G. K. (ed.): *Yellow Fever,* 1st ed., New York: McGraw-Hill, 1951.

Stuart-Harris, C. H.: *Influenza and Other Virus Infections of the Respiratory Tract,* 2d ed., Baltimore: Williams and Wilkins, 1965.

Tasman, A., H. P. Lansberg: "Problems Concerning the Prophylaxis, Pathogenesis, and Therapy of Diphtheria," *Bulletin of the World Health Organization,* vol. 16, 1957, pp. 939-973.

Tierkel, E. S., and R. K. Sikes: "Preexposure Prophylaxis against Rabies," *Journal of the American Medical Association,* vol. 201, 1967, pp. 911-914.

Topping, N.H.: "Typhus Fever. A Note on the Severity of the Disease among Unvaccinated and Vaccinated Laboratory Personnel at the National Institutes of Health," *American Journal of Tropical Medicine,* vol. 24, 1944, pp. 57-62.

"Typhoid Vaccines,"*Lancet,* vol. 2, 1967, pp. 1075-1076.

U.S. Public Health Service Advisory Committee on Immunization Practices: "Recommendation of the Public Health Service Advisory Committee on Immunization Practices: Diphtheria, Tetanus, and Pertussis Vaccine—Tetanus Prophylaxis in Wound Management," *Morbidity and Mortality Weekly Report,* vol. 15, no. 48, Dec. 3, 1966, pp. 416-418.

Volk, V. K., R. Y. Gottshall, H. D. Anderson, et al.: "Antigenic Response to Booster Dose of Diphtheria and Tetanus Toxoids: Seven to Thirteen Years after Primary Inoculation of Noninstitutionalized Children," *Public Health Report,* vol. 77, 1962, pp. 185-194.

Wehrle, P. F.: "Immunization against Poliomyelitis," *Archives of Environmental Health,* vol. 15, 1967, pp. 485-490.

———, J. Posch, K. H. Richter, et al.: "An Airborne Outbreak of Smallpox in a German Hospital and Its Significance with Respect to Other Recent Outbreaks in Europe," *Bulletin of the World Health Organization,* vol. 43, 1970, pp. 669-679.

———, E. B. Buynak, J. Stokes, Jr., et al.: "Measurement of Immunity following Live Mumps (5 Years), Measles (3 Years), and Rubella ($2\frac{1}{2}$ Years) Virus Vaccines," *Pediatrics,* vol. 49, 1972, pp. 334-341.

White, W. G., G. M. Barnes, A. H. Friffith, et al.: "Duration of Immunity after Active Immunization against Tetanus," *Lancet,* vol. 2, July 12, 1969, pp. 95-96.

Wissman, C. L., Jr.: "The Present and Future of Immunization against the Typhus Fevers," in *First International Conference on Vaccines against Viral and Rickettsial Diseases of Man,* Pan American Health Organization, Scientific Publication, no. 147, 1967, pp. 523-527.

———, and B. H. Sweet: "Immunological Studies with Group B Arthropodborne Viruses. III. Response of Human Subjects to Revaccination with 17D Strain Yellow Fever Vaccine," *American Journal of Tropical Medicine,* vol. 11, 1962, pp. 570-575.

Witte, J. J., and A. W. Karchmer: "Surveillance of Mumps in the United States as Background for Use of Vaccine," *Public Health Report,* vol. 83, 1968, pp. 95-100.

———, G. Case, et al.: "Epidemiology of Rubella," *American Journal of Diseases of Children,* vol. 118, 1969, pp. 107-111.

World Health Organization: "Diphtheria and Pertussis Vaccination, Report of Conference of Heads of Laboratories Producing Diphtheria and Pertussis Vaccines, Part I—Diphtheria," WHO Technical Report Series, no. 61, 1953.

———: "A Revised System of Nomenclature for Influenza Viruses," *Bulletin of the World Health Organization,* vol. 45, 1971, pp. 119-124.

———: "Expert Committee on Plague, 3rd Report," WHO Technical Report Series, no. 165, 1959.

———: "Fifth Report of the Expert Committee on Rabies," WHO Technical Report Series, no. 321, 1966.

———: *Weekly Epidemiological Record,* vol. 45, 1970, pp. 453-458.

———: *Weekly Epidemiological Record,* vol. 47, 1972, pp. 17-25.

Yugoslav Typhoid Commission: "A Controlled Field Trial of the Effectiveness of Acetone-dried and Inactivated and Heat-phenol-inactivated Typhoid Vaccines in Yugoslavia," *Bulletin of the World Health Organization,* vol. 30, 1964, pp. 623-630.

Childhood Safety

Armstrong, George D.: "Vitamin Ingestions," *Bulletin of the National Clearinghouse for Poison Control Centers,* April-June 1972, pp. 1-6.

Barich, Donald P.: "Steam Vaporizers—Therapy or Tragedy?" *Pediatrics,* vol. 49, January 1972, pp. 131-132.

Barnako, Donna: "Flammable Fabrics," *Journal of the American Medical Association,* vol. 221, no. 2, July 10, 1972, p. 189.

Bergner, Lawrence, Shirley Mayer, and David Harris: "Falls from Heights: A Childhood Epidemic in an Urban Area," *American Journal of Public Health,* vol. 61, no. 1, 1971, pp. 90-95.

Berry, Teresa, Fredric D. Burg, and Harvey Kravitz: "The Toddler as a Bicycle Passenger," *Pediatrics,* vol. 49, no. 3, March 1972, pp. 443-446.

Birch, John R.: "Flammable Fabrics and Human Burns," *The Canadian Journal of Surgery,* vol. 14, May 1971, pp. 177-178.

Burg, Frederic D., "Reflectorization: A New Defense Mechanism against Automobile Injury to Pedestrians," *Pediatrics,* 1970, p.775.

———, John M. Douglass, Eugene Diamond, and Arnold W. Siegel, "Automotive Restraint Devices for the Pediatric Patient," *Pediatrics,* vol. 45, no. 1, part I, January 1970, pp. 49-53.

Campbell, B. J., and W. S. Rouse: "Reflectorized License Plates and Rear-End Collisions at Night," *Research Review,* June 1968, p.72.

Cashman, Thomas M., and Harvey C. Shirley: "Emergency Management of Poisoning," *Pediatric Clinics of North America,* vol. 17, August 1970, pp. 525-534.

Committee on Accident Prevention: "Perils of the Water: The Problem of Drowning and the Child," *AAP Newsletter Supplement,* Mar. 15, 1968, pp. 886-887.

———: "Investigation of Fabrics Involved in Wearing Apparel Fires," *Pediatrics,* November 1964, pp. 728-733.

Crikelair, George F.: "Burn Prevention," *The Journal of Trauma,* April 1972, pp. 363-364.

Cullinan, T. R.: "Children at Risk of Accident," *Community Health,* vol. 2, no. 4, January/February 1971, pp.175-178.

Done, Alan K., "Poisoning from Common Household Products," *Pediatric Clinics of North America,* vol. 17, August 1970, pp. 569-581.

———, August L. Jung, et al.: "Evaluations of Safety Packaging for the Protection of Children," *Pediatrics,* vol. 48, no. 4, October 1971, pp. 613-628.

Green, M., and R. Haggerty: *Ambulatory Pediatrics,* Philadelphia: W. B. Saunders Company, 1968.

Haggerty, Robert J.: "Childhood Poisoning: An Overview," *Pediatric Clinics of North America,* vol. 17, August 1970, pp. 473-475.

Hanes, Lee N.: "Safeguarding Children in Automobiles," *American Journal of Diseases of Children,* vol. 125, February 1973, p. 163.

Hazlett, R. D., and J. A. Merrill: "The Ability to See a Pedestrian at Night, the Effects of Clothing Reflectorized, and Driver Intoxication," *American Journal of Optometry,* vol. 44, 1967, p. 246.

Jones, Jerry G.: "Preventing Poisoning Accidents in Children," *Clinical Pediatrics,* vol. 8, no. 8, August 1969, p. 484-491.

Julyan, M., and Jan A. Kuzemka: "Parents and Their Children in Accidental Poisoning," *The Practitioner,* vol. 208, February 1972, pp. 252-253.

Kravitz, Harvey: "The Roll-up Garage Door," *Clinical Pediatrics,* November 1970, p. 641.

Lawrence, Ruth A., and Robert J. Haggerty: "Household Agents and Their Potential Toxicity," *Modern Treatment,* vol. 8, August 1971, pp. 511-527.

Maragos, George D., et al.: "Household Plant Emergencies," *Nebraska State Medical Journal,* vol. 55, November 1970, pp. 653-654.

Margolis, J. A.: "Psychosocial Study of Childhood Poisonings," *Pediatric Annals,* vol. 2, January 1973, pp. 54-59.

Martin, Helen L.: "Antecedents of Burns and Scalds in Children," *British Journal of Medical Psychology,* 1970, pp. 39-47.

McCaughey, Helen: "The Ability of Children to Obtain Tablets from Different Containers," *The Medical Journal of Australia,* Nov. 22, 1969, pp. 1076-1077.

Michelinakis, E.: "Safety-Belt Syndrome," *The Practitioner,* vol. 207, July 1971, pp. 77-80.

Mofenson, Howard C., and Joseph Greensher: "Acute Childhood Poisoning," *Pediatric Annals,* vol. 2, January 1973, pp. 54-59.

Oglesbay, Floyd B.: "The Flammable Fabrics Problem," *Childhood Injuries,* 1970, pp. 827-832.

Pless, Ivan B., Klaus Roghmann, and Paula Algranati: "The Prevention of Injuries to Children in Automobiles," *Pediatrics,* vol. 49, no. 3, March 1972, p. 420.

Polk, Lewis D.: "Best Age for Smallpox Vaccination,"*Clinical Pediatrics,* vol. 9, no. 3, March 1970, pp. 126-127.

Quentzel, David: "Choosing the Safest Car Seat (or Carrier or Harness) for Your Child," *Institute/Engineering.*

Repath, Elizabeth: "Home Accidents: A Socio-medical Problem," *Community Health,* vol. 2, no. 1, July/August 1970, pp. 12-17.

Report of the Committee on Accident Prevention: "Seat Belts in the Prevention of Automobile Injuries," *Pediatrics,* vol. 30, no. 5, November 1962, pp. 841-843.

Report of the Committee on Accidental Poisoning: "Co-operative Kerosine Poisoning Study, Evaluation of Gastric Lavage and Other Factors in the Treatment of Accidental Ingestion of Petroleum Distillate Products," *Pediatrics,* vol. 29, no. 4, April 1962, pp. 648-674.

Roney, J. G., Jr., and M. L. Mall: *Medication Practices in a Community: An Explanatory Study,* Menlo Park, Calif.: Stanford Research Institute, 1966, pp. 12-16.

Rowley, William F., Jr., Eugene Lariviere, and Charles W. Dietrich: "Auto Safety Seats for Children," *The Journal of Pediatrics,* June 1971, p. 1078.

Scherz, Robert G.: "Accidental Childhood Poisoning," *Pediatrics,* vol. 47, June 1971, pp. 1093-1095.

Seddon, J. A.: "Handlebar Injury," *British Medical Journal,* vol. 4, 1969, p. 222.

Seder, Susan: "A New Look at Poisonous Plants," *Family Safety,* Spring 1972, pp. 802-818.

Shulman, B. H., and G. Reddy: "Purse Poisons," *Pediatrics*, vol. 51, January 1973, pp. 126-127.

Smith, E. Ide: "The Epidemiology of Burns," *Childhood Injuries,* 1970, pp. 821-827.

Sobel, Raymond: "Traditional Safety Measures and Accidental Poisoning in Children," *Pediatrics,* vol. 44, November 1969, pp. 811-816.

———: "Safety Measures and Accidental Poisoning," *Pediatrics,* vol. 48, October 1971, pp. 673-674.

Subcommittee on Accidental Poisoning: "Safety Packaging," *AAP Newsletter Supplement,* May 1, 1972.

———: "Safety Packaging," AAP Newsletter Supplement, June 15, 1970.

Thomas, Adrianne, and Sandra Dillard: "Compliance on Sleepwear Labels 'Sporadic, Begrudging,'" *The Denver Post,* August 1, 1973.

Tredgold, R. F.: "Emotional Factors and Accident Causation," *Community Health,* vol. 2, no. 1, July/August 1970, pp. 7-11.

U.S. Department of Health, Education, and Welfare: "Tabulation of 1971 Reports," *National Clearinghouse for Poison Control Centers Bulletin,* September/October 1972, pp. 1-9.

White, W.: "Flammable Fabrics and the Burn Problem," *American Journal of Public Health,* vol. 61, October 1971, pp. 2057-2064.

Wilkinson, A. W.: "Burns," *Community Health,* vol. 2, no. 1, July/August 1970, pp. 23-28.

Wright, Byron W.: "The Control of Child-Environment Interaction: A Conceptual Approach to Accident Occurrence," *Childhood Injuries,* 1970, p. 799.

Pediatric Nutrition

American Academy of Pediatrics: "Absence of Vitamin D in Nonfat Dry Milk," *Pediatrics,* vol. 40, no. 1, July 1967, pp. 130-131.

———: "Correspondence Regarding Iron Fortified Formulas," *Pediatrics,* vol. 48, no. 1, July 1971, pp. 152-156.

———: "Filled Milks, Imitation Milks, and Coffee Whiteners," *Pediatrics,* vol. 49, no. 5, May 1972, pp. 770-775.

———: "Safety of Baby Foods Purchased in Glass Jars," Committee on Nutrition—Statement for Parents, January 1963.

———: "Selected References on Feeding and Nutrition by the Committee on Nutrition," List for Physicians, September 1963.

———: "The Use and Abuse of Vitamin A," Joint Committee Statement on Drugs and on Nutrition," *Pediatrics,* vol. 42, no. 4, October 1971, pp. 655-656.

———: Committee Statement, Committee on Nutrition, "Misuse of Vitamin A," 1973.

———: "Vitamin E in Human Nutrition," *Pediatrics,* vol. 31, no. 2, February 1963, pp. 324-328.

———: "Vitamin K Compounds and the Water-soluble Analogues," *Pediatrics,* vol. 28, no. 3, September 1961, pp. 501-507.

———: "Vitamin K Supplementation for Infants Receiving Milk Substitute Infant Formulas and for Those with Fat Malabsorption," *Pediatrics,* vol. 48, no. 3, September 1971, pp. 483-487.

American Academy of Pediatrics Committee on Nutrition: "Vitamin D Intake and the Hypercalcemia Syndrome," *Pediatrics,* vol. 35, no. 6, June 1965, p. 1022.

———: "The Relation between Infantile Hypercalcemia and Vitamin D: Public Health Implications in North America," *Pediatrics,* vol. 40, no. 6, December 1967, pp. 1050-1061.

Anderson, Thomas A., and Samuel J. Fomon: "Commercially Prepared Strained and Junior Foods for Infants," *Journal of the American Dietetic Association,* vol. 58, June 1971, pp. 520-527.

Asher, Patricia: "Fat Babies and Fat Children," *Archives of Disease in Childhood,* vol. 41, 1966, p. 672.

Beal, Virginia A., and Aldula J. Meyers: "Iron Nutriture from Infancy to Adolescence," *American Journal of Public Health,* vol. 60, no. 4, April 1970, pp. 666-678.

Burman, David: "Iron Requirements in Infancy," *British Journal of Haematology,* vol. 20, 1971, pp. 243-247.

Caffey, J.: *Pediatric X-Ray Diagnosis,* 4th ed., Chicago: Year Book, 1961.

Canadian Pediatric Society: "The Use and Abuse of Vitamin A," *Canadian Medical Association Journal,* vol. 104, Mar. 20, 1971, pp. 521-522.

Clark, F.: "A Scorecard on How We Americans Are Eating," in *The Yearbook of Agriculture: Food for Us All,* Washington, D. C.: U. S. Government Printing Office, 1969, pp. 320-321.

Committee on Nutrition: "Appraisal of Nutritional Adequacy of Infant Formulas Used as Cow Milk Substitute," *Pediatrics,* vol. 31, no. 2, February 1963, pp. 329-338.

———: "Appraisals of the Use of Vitamins B_1 and B_{12} as Supplements Promoted for the Stimulation of Growth and Appetite in Children," *Pediatrics,* vol. 21, May 1958, pp. 860-864.

———: "Childhood Diet and Coronary Heart Disease," *Pediatrics,* vol. 49, no. 2, February 1972, pp. 305-307.

———: "Composition of Milks," *Pediatrics,* vol. 26, no. 6, December 1966, pp. 1039-1049.

———: "Estrogenic and Androgenic Agents in Meats and Poultry," *Pediatrics,* vol. 25, no. 5, part I, May 1960, pp. 896-899.

———: "Expiration Dates on Infant Formulas," American Academy of Pediatrics, Apr. 1, 1972.

———: "Factors Affecting Food Intake," *Pediatrics,* vol. 33, no. 1, January 1964, pp. 135-143.

———: "Fluoride as a Nutrient," *Pediatrics,* vol. 49, no. 3, March 1972, pp. 456-460.

———: "Infant Methenoglobinemia: The Role of Dietary Nitrate," *Pediatrics,* vol. 46, no. 3, September 1970, pp. 475-478.

———: "Iron Balance and Requirements in Infancy," *Pediatrics,* vol. 43, no. 1, January 1969, pp. 134-142.

———: "Iron-fortified Formulas," *Pediatrics,* vol. 47, no. 4, April 1971, p. 786.

———: "Obesity in Childhood," *Pediatrics,* vol. 40, no. 1, part I, September 1967, pp. 455-467.

———"Prepared Infant Formulas and Commercial Formula Services," *Pediatrics,* vol. 36, no. 2, August 1965, pp. 282-291.

———: "Proteolytic Enzymes in Milk in Relation to Infant Feeding," *Pediatrics,* vol. 23, no. 2, February 1959, pp. 408-412.

———: "Trace Elements in Infant Nutrition," *Pediatrics,* vol. 26, no. 4, October 1960, pp. 715-721.

———: "Vitamin B_6 Requirements in Man," *Pediatrics,* vol. 38, no. 6, part I, December 1966, pp. 1068-1076.

Dees, S. C.: "Allergy to Cow's Milk," *Pediatric Clinics of North America,* vol. 6, 1959, p. 881.

Dunning, J. M.: "Current Status of Fluoridation," *New England Journal of Medicine,* vol. 272, no. 30, 1965, p. 272.

Einstein, M. A., and I. Hornstein: "Food Preferences of College Students and Nutritional Implications," *Journal of Food Sciences,* vol. 35, 1970, p. 429.

Finch, Clement A., and Elaine R. Monson: "Iron Nutrition and the Fortification of Food with Iron," *Journal of the American Medical Association,* vol. 219, no. 11, Mar. 13, 1972, pp. 1462-1465.

Foman, S. J., M. K. Younoszai, and L. N. Thomas: "Influence of Vitamin D on Linear Growth of Normal Full-Term Infants," *Journal of Nutrition,* vol. 88, 1966, p. 345.

———: *Infant Nutrition,* Philadelphia and London: Saunders, 1974.

———, Lorn N. Thomas, L. J. Filer, Jr., Edhard E. Ziegler, and Michael Leonard: "Food Consumption and Growth of Normal Infants Fed Milk-based Formulas," *Acta Paediatricia Scandinavica,* Supplement, vol. 223, 1971, pp. 1-36.

Greward, D.: "Infantile Scurvy," *Clinical Pediatrics,* vol. 4, 1965, p. 82.

Hampton, M. C., R. L. Huenemann, L. R. Shapiro, and B. N. Mitchell: "Caloric and Nutrient Intakes of Teen-agers," *Journal of American Dietetics,* vol. 50, 1967, p. 385.

Hartmann, A. F.: "Studies of Amino Acid Administration," *Journal of Pediatrics,* vol. 20, 1942, p. 308.

Hennon, D. K., G. K. Stookey, and J. C. Muhler: "The Clinical Anticariogenic Effectiveness of Supplementary Fluoride-Vitamin Preparations: Results at the End of Three Years," *Journal of Dentistry of Children,* vol. 33, 1966, p. 3.

Hill, L. W.: "Soybean as a Milk Substitute for Potentially Allergic Infants," *Journal of Allergies,* vol. 24, 1953, p. 474.

Holland, N. H., R. Hong, N. C. Davis, and C. D. West: "Significance of Precipitating Antibodies to Milk Proteins in the Serum of Infants and Children," *Journal of Pediatrics,* Vol. 61, p. 181, 1962.

———, ———, ———, and ———: "Infantile Scurvy and Nutritional Rickets in the United States," *Pediatrics,* vol. 29, April 1962, pp. 646-647.

———, ———, ———, and ———: "Iron in Enriched Wheat, Flour, Farina, Bread, Buns and Rolls," *Journal of the American Medical Association,* vol. 220, no. 6, May 8, 1972, pp. 855-859.

Kane, S.: "Nutritional Management of Allergic Reactions to Cow's Milk," *American Practitioner Digest Treatment,* vol. 8, 1957, p. 65.

Kay, J. L., C. W. Daeschner, and M. M. Desmond, "Evaluation of Infants Fed Soybean and Evaporated Milk Formulae from Birth to Three Months. A Comparison of Weight, Length, Hemoglobin, Hematocrit and Plasma Biochemical Values," *American Journal of Diseases of Children,* vol. 100, 1959, p. 264.

Kennedy, B. M.: "Food Preferences of Pre-Army Age California Boys," *Food Technology,* vol. 6, 1952, p. 93.

Kraus, B. S.: "Calcification of the Human Deciduous Teeth," *Journal of the American Dental Association,* vol. 59, 1959, p. 1128.

MacKetith, Ronald and Christopher Wood: *Infant Feeding and Feeding Difficulties,* London: Churchill, 1971.

Meyer, Herman: *Infant Foods and Feeding Practices,* Springfield, Ill.: Charles C. Thomas, 1960.

Omans, W. B., W. Leuterer, and P. Gyorgy: "Feeding Value of Soy Milks for Premature Infants, *Journal of Pediatrics,* vol. 62, 1963, p. 98.

Persson, B., R. Tunell, and K. Ekengren: "Chronic Vitamin A Intoxication during the First Half Year of Life: Description of Five Cases," *Acta Paediatrica Scandinvica,* vol. 54, 1965, p. 49.

Pikering, E. E., D. A. Fisher, A. Perley, et al.: "Influence of Dietary Fatty Acids on Serum Lipids: Studies of the Immature Rhesus Monkey," *American Journal of Diseases of Children,* vol. 102, 1961, p. 42.

Report of the Committee on Nutrition: "The Prophylactic Requirement and the Toxicity of Vitamin D," *Pediatrics,* vol. 31, no. 3, March 1963, pp. 512-525.

Schorr, B. C., Diva Sanjur, and Eugene D. Erickson, "Teen Age Food Habits," *Journal of the American Dietetic Association,* vol. 61, October 1972, pp. 415-420.

Schuck, C.: "Food Preferences of South Dakota College Students," *Journal of the American Dietetic Association,* vol. 39, 1961, p. 595.

Schulman, Irving: "Iron Needs in Infancy," *Journal of the American Medical Association,* vol. 175, 1961, p. 118.

Seeling, Mildred S.: "Are American Children Still Getting an Excess of Vitamin D?" *Clinical Pediatrics,* vol. 9, no. 7, pp. 380-383.

Van de Mark, Mildred S. and Audrey Wright: "Hemoglobin and Folate Levels of Pregnant Teen-Agers," *Research,* vol. 61, November 1972, pp. 511-516.

Walker, Alexander: "The Human Requirement of Calcium: Should Low Intake Be Supplemented?" *The American Journal of Clinical Nutrition,* vol. 25, May 1972, pp. 518-530.

Wharton, M. A.: "Nutritive Intake of Adolescence," *Journal of the American Dietetic Association,* vol. 42, 1963, p. 306.

Willians, Thomas E., Milton H. Donaldson, and Frank Sheppard: "Vitamin K Requirement of Normal Infants on Soy Protein Formula," *Clinical Pediatrics,* vol. 9, no. 2, February 1970, pp. 79-82.

Willis, Norman H.: *Infant Nutrition,* Philadelphia: Lippincott, 1964.

Woodruff, C. W.: "Ascorbic Acid," in G. H. Beaton and E. W. McHenry (eds.), *Nutrition,* New York: Academic, 1964, vol. II, p. 265.

The Working Group on Nutrition and Pregnancy in Adolescence, Committee on Maternal Nutrition, Food and Nutrition Board, National Research Council, National Academy of Sciences: "Relation of Nutrition to Pregnancy in Adolescence," *Nutrition and Pregnancy* (reprinted from *Maternal Nutrition and the Course of Pregnancy,* Washington, D.C.: *National Academy of Sciences,* 1970), pp. 367-392.

Chapter 4

Screening and Diagnostic Tests

In ambulatory pediatrics the nurse will be involved with a multitude of tests, some she will perform herself, some she will train others to perform, some she will simply order performed and interpret the results, and some she will neither order nor interpret, but should be familiar with. This chapter will look closely at some of the more common tests encountered in the outpatient setting and discuss the nurse's role with regard to them.

Tests can generally be divided into screening and diagnostic tests, both of which the nurse will be using frequently. The general purpose of screening tests is to provide a quick, inexpensive measure which can be used with a large population to discover who of that population is most likely to have a certain condition. Only those found to be most likely to have the condition need be tested by the more expensive and time-consuming diagnostic test. For instance, all children should have vision screening tests, but only the few who fail such tests need to see a specialist for more extensive testing. Screening tests can have both false positive and false negative results; in other words, some children will pass a screening test even though they have the condition being tested for, and some will fail the test even though they do not have the condition being tested for. In the case of vision screening, for instance, some children will fail the test, but when referred to the ophthalmologist, they will be found to have no real vision problem; other children may have a vision problem but be able to pass the screening test and hence not get the visual correction which they need; False positive tests cause overreferral; false negative tests cause underreferral. In general, it is better to overrefer than to underrefer, since, in this way, few children with problems will be missed. A large degree of overreferral may be detrimental, however, since it is wasteful of time and money and may be disturbing to the parents.

Diagnostic tests are employed when there is enough evidence to indicate that a child is very likely to suffer from a certain condition; this evidence may be provided by a screening test or may be directly available from the signs and symptoms presented by the child.

Of the many screening and diagnostic tests available, only the more common are discussed in this chapter; the nurse is referred to complete laboratory guides for explanation of the less common tests. This chapter will be concerned with common measurements and with vision, hearing, speech, blood, and urine tests.

COMMON MEASUREMENTS

Taking measurements is a routine procedure which is frequently underrated. This chapter will discuss the importance of some of these measurements and how they are taken and recorded; it will include height, weight, head circumference, temperature, pulse, respiration, blood pressure, and some special measurements.

It is usually the job of the nurse to see that these measurements are taken as well as to interpret them, i.e., decide whether they are normal or need further investigation. One important difference between children and adults is that children grow and change, and this change must be constantly evaluated. Physical measurements of a child reflect his rate of growth; a failure in growth, an acceleration in growth, or any change in growth pattern may be the first clue to serious problems. Taking measurements is easy but extremely important, and measurements must be taken correctly and accurately. Sloppy procedures, lack of recording, or inaccurate interpretation may cause serious problems to be neglected.

RECORDING

Keeping records of measurements is of extreme importance. Isolated heights and weights are useless; it is the rate of growth and change that is important. Measurements must, therefore, be taken periodically and plotted on a graph to be useful. There are many ways to record measurements, and some clinics will record them at the top of the chart page for each visit as well as plot them on a graph kept elsewhere in the chart. The best graphs are set up to show percentages, with the mean and standard deviations above and below the mean. Thus a child's measurements are both plotted and recorded as being at the 90th percentile, 50th percentile, or 3d percentile. Measurements can be taken in pounds and ounces or kilograms and grams or inches and feet or centimeters and meters; many clinics are revising their procedures to include measuring equipment in the metric system and metric graphs for plotting (see Appendix G).

SPECIFIC MEASUREMENTS

Height

Height is an extremely important measure of skeletal and muscular growth and should be followed carefully from birth to adulthood. Height is usually measured at every well-child visit.

The method of measurement varies with age. Some authorities feel that it is so difficult to get an accurate measurement during the first year that they omit that measurement or take it only a few times during the first year. However, most clinics require that the height be measured at every well-child visit. Measuring the height of a young child is best done by two people with the child lying down. One person secures the head, and the other secures the feet; a mark is made at head and heel. Then the child is removed and the distance measured with a metal tape measure. Some clinics have a sliding measuring stick in which the child's head is placed at the headboard and the moveable end stretched to touch the child's heel (see Fig. 4-1). Other clinics have a tape measure fastened to a wooden board, and the child is placed on the board and measured from head to foot. The older children are more easily measured, since they can stand, in their stocking feet, on a standard, balanced adult scale with a built-in tape measure. If one of these scales is not available, a tape measure can be attached to a wall and the child instructed to stand straight against the wall. Make certain that the tape measure begins at the child's heels and is not displaced by a baseboard. When measuring, always use a flat, hard surface to reach from the top of the child's head to the wall so that you are not guessing or adding height because of the hair (see Fig. 4-2).

Once the measurement is taken, it must be plotted on a graph. Height is generally a familial trait, and if parents and grandparents are tall, the child is likely to be tall also. If a child is born with a height at the 25th percentile, he will usually continue to fall at the 25th percentile most of his life. The value of the graph is that it enables the examiner to detect sudden changes in percentile. If that child's height increased to the 50th percentile or dropped below the 3d percentile, further investigation would be indicated. Unusually

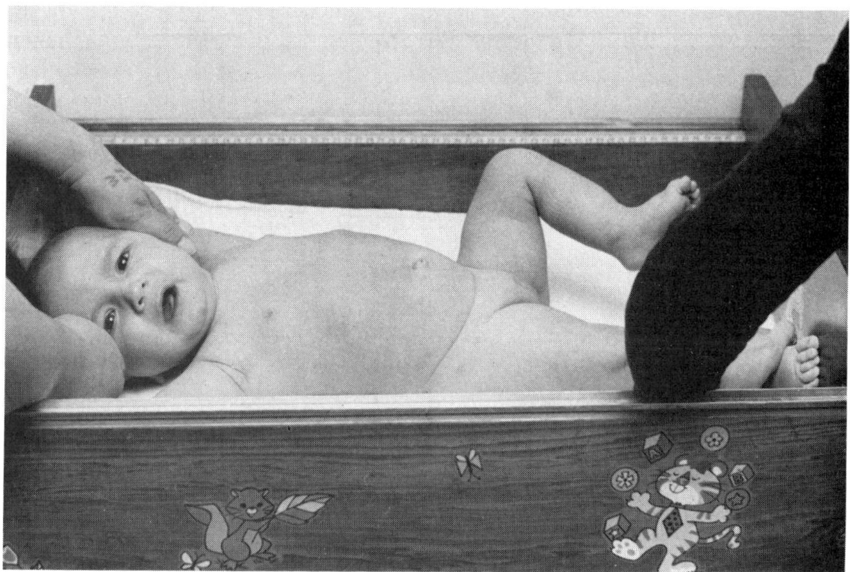

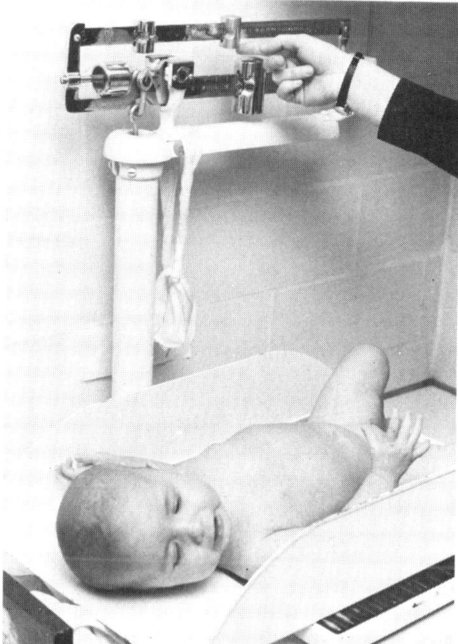

Figure 4-1 Infant being measured for height and weight.

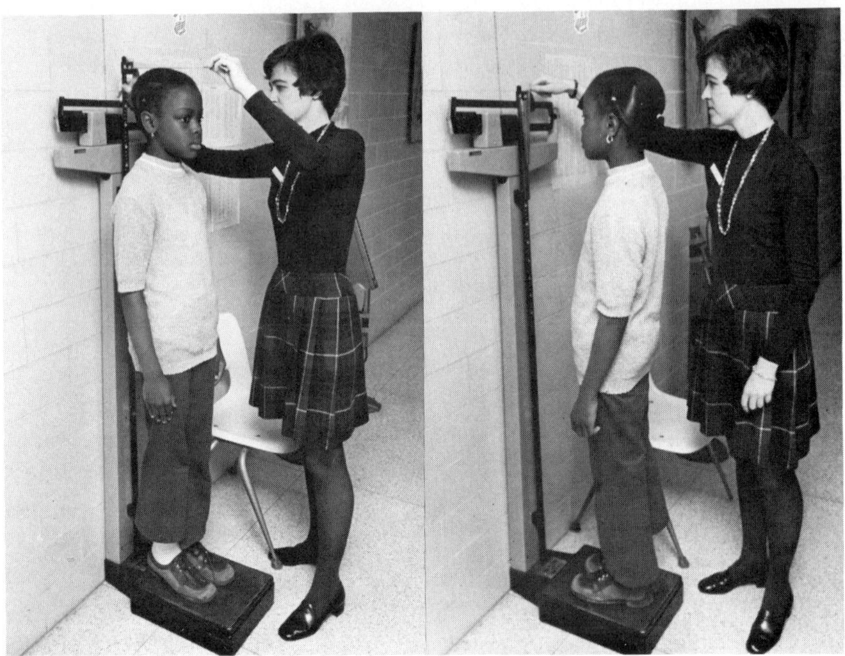

Figure 4-2 Older child being measured for height and weight.

tall stature may be due to heredity, overnutrition, mental retardation, or occasionally overstimulated growth hormones. Abnormally short stature can be due to malnutrition, growth hormone deficiencies, chronic infections, allergies, or distinct diseases such as kidney or heart problems. Short stature may also be inherited.

Weight

Weight is another extremely important index of the child's general growth and nutritional status. The child should be weighed at every visit from birth to adulthood. Since weight can fluctuate suddenly and drastically, it is usually measured at both well-child and sick-child visits.

The method and equipment for weighing varies with age. Infants should have all their clothing removed, including diapers, and are placed in a lying position on a regular baby scale. Remember to balance the scale first with the scale paper. By the time children are walking they can usually be weighed on the adult standing scale. Depending on the situation, all clothing except underpants or just heavy outer clothing and shoes may be removed.

As with height, once the measurement is taken, it is plotted on a graph to show the child's continual weight status. Weight should generally follow the same percentile, and sudden drops or increases warrant further investigation. Percentile increases may indicate overnutrition or, rarely, endocrine disorders. Drops in weight percentile can indicate chronic disease, acute infection, dehydration, emotional problems, or malnutrition.

There are some general rules concerning weight measurements. An average infant is born weighing 3,500 gm (7½ lbs) and is expected to lose 10 percent of this weight during the first few days of life. This means an infant could lose up to 350 gm (or 12 oz.) during this time. Normally infants will regain their birthweight by the 10th to 14th day. Infants generally gain 1 oz./day for the first 6 months. After that, growth is slower, and from age 2 to 10 the child will gain an average of about 5 lbs per year.

Head Circumference

The brain demonstrates growth very rapidly during the 1st year of life, and the best way to evaluate this growth is to plot periodic measurements of the circumference of the skull. Since brain growth is most rapid during the 1st year, most clinics include head circumference measurements at every well-baby visit during the 1st year and some clinics continue into the 2d and 3d year. The most reliable method of measuring is to use a metal or paper tape measure since cloth tapes have a tendency to stretch and give an inaccurate reading. The tape is placed around the broadest part of the head, which is usually over the forehead and occipital protuberance. For greatest accuracy, the tape is placed three times, with a reading taken at the right side, at the left side, and at mid-forehead, and the greatest circumference is plotted (see Fig. 4-3).

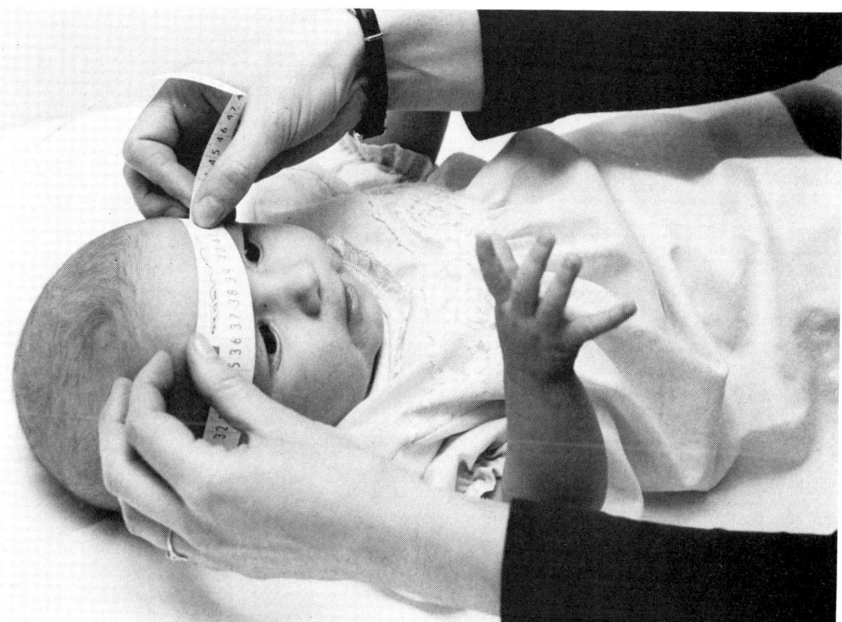

Figure 4-3 Measuring head circumference.

An infant's brain is one-fourth the adult size and will grow to nine-tenths of its final size by the age of 6. In general, a newborn's head circumference is equal to or slightly larger than the chest circumference, and this ratio will continue until the child is 2 years old, when the chest circumference becomes greater than the head size.

As with height and weight, the head circumference measurements must be plotted on a graph. Most clinics use a centimeter graph because it is more accurate. A child with a weight and height in the 50th percentile will usually have a head circumference in the 50th percentile. Marked differences should be investigated. A circumference which increases more rapidly than is expected according to the graph should be further investigated for hydrocephaly, while a graph showing no growth or little growth may indicate microcephaly.

Temperature

Temperatures are not routinely taken on all children. For well-child visits, they are usually omitted, but they must be part of the work-up of every sick child. Since younger children cannot use oral thermometers, most pediatric clinics have a supply of both oral and rectal thermometers. Oral thermometers are usually long and slender, and rectal thermometers are short with a stubby bulb end. Some clinics are beginning to use electronic thermometers because they are accurate and take less time to register. These have a small box which is the measuring device with a probe and disposable cover. The probe may be placed either orally or rectally, and some can be taped into place in the rectum or axilla for constant monitoring, as in the newborn nursery (see Fig. 4-4). Thermometers may be Fahrenheit or Centigrade, with a range of 94 to 110°F and 32 to 43°C (see Table 4-1).

Table 4-1 Temperature Conversions

Centrigrade	Fahrenheit
35.0	95.0
35.5	95.9
36.0	96.8
36.5	97.7
37.0	98.6
37.5	99.5
38.0	100.4
38.5	101.3
39.0	102.2
39.5	103.1
40.0	104.0
40.5	104.9
41.0	105.8
41.5	106.7

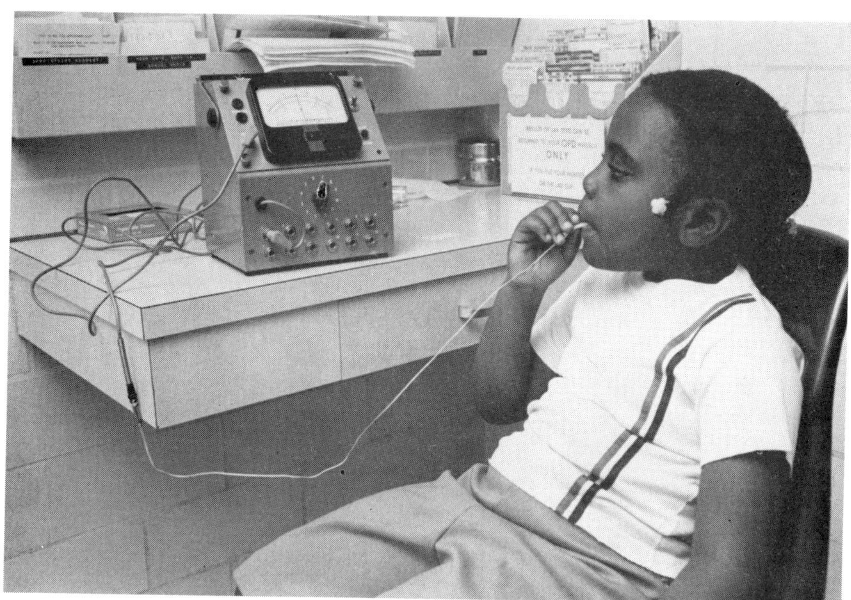

Figure 4-4 Child's temperature being recorded by electronic thermometer.

The choice of thermometer depends on the child's age. If there is any possibility that they will bite the thermometer, young children must have their temperature taken rectally. Children with a stuffy nose must also have their temperature taken rectally since an oral thermometer may interfere with breathing. The child is generally placed across the mother's lap with the child's head hanging on one side and the legs dangling on the other. The diaper or panties are removed, and if necessary, the mother can restrain the child with one arm across the shoulders and one hand firmly on the buttocks. The well-lubricated rectal thermometer is inserted 1 in. into the rectum (see Fig. 4-5). A recent study by Nichols (1972) indicates that the thermometer must stay in place for 4 minutes to obtain an accurate reading. If the room temperature is at least 72°F, the time may be cut to 2 to 3 minutes.

In the newborn nursery the first temperature is usually taken rectally; after that, axillary readings are taken. An oral thermometer is placed under the infant's arm in the axillary area, and the arm is held securely against the body for 4 to 5 minutes. This method is not as reliable with older children because they are more difficult to restrain.

Older children can have their temperature taken orally as long as they are not suffering from some respiratory illness which forces them to breathe through the mouth. Generally by the time children are 6 years old they can understand the instructions for the oral procedure. Some younger children can understand and be trusted, but it is important to be sure that the child

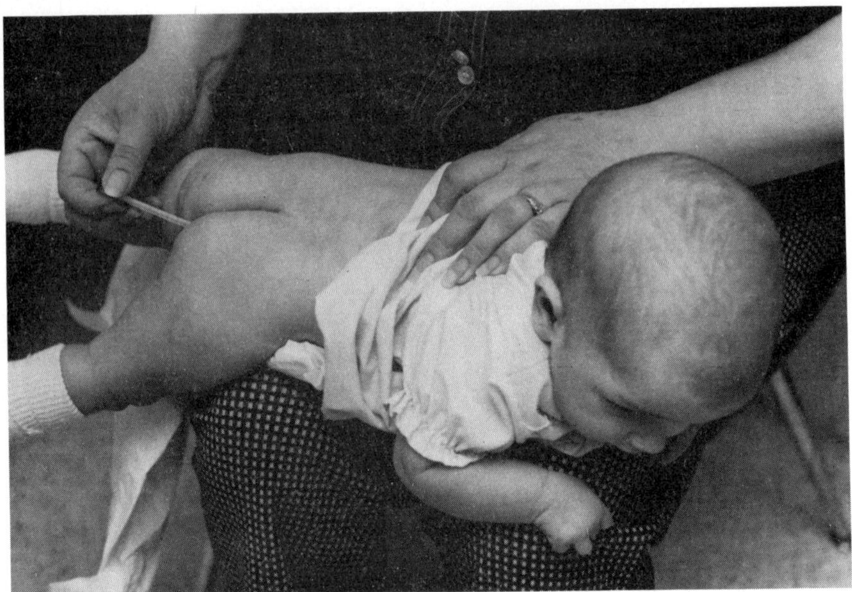

Figure 4-5 Infant's temperature being taken rectally.

will not bite the thermometer. The child should be seated and given an explanation of what is expected before the thermometer is placed under the tongue. Nichols (1972) reported in her study that it took 8 minutes in a room of 65 to 75°F to obtain a stabilized oral temperature.

For ambulatory care, the temperature is usually charted on the top of the day's sheet, but not usually graphed. The normal oral temperature is 95 to 99°F (or 36 to 37°C). Rectal temperatures are normally 1° higher than oral, and axillary temperatures are normally 1° lower than oral. Thus it is important to record both the temperature and the method of obtaining it. Fever in children may be produced by excitement, eating, vigorous exercise, bacterial or viral infections, dehydration, tumors, poisoning, convulsions, and some chronic conditions. A low temperature is seen if the child is in shock or has been chilled or in some infants with infections.

Pulse

Since it directly reflects the heartbeat, the pulse rate is one way of evaluating the state of the circulatory system. The pulse rate should be taken at every visit to the clinic.

In infants the pulse rate is so rapid that it is usually felt for in the dorsal pedalis, femoral, and radial areas, but palpated and auscultated for in the apical area. In the older child the pulse is counted at the radial area. The pulse is checked for rate, rhythm, and quality of beat. A more detailed description of these terms is discussed in the chapter on heart examination in *Physical Diagnosis for Nurses.*

The pulse is usually recorded at the top of the day's chart page. For ambulatory care it is not usually graphed.

Respiration

Observation of the rate, rhythm, and depth of a child's inspiration and expiration is important. Respirations should be checked at every clinic visit and especially at sick-child visits. Newborn infants have very irregular breathing, and their respiration is best obtained while they are resting or asleep. Sometimes palpation and auscultation of the chest make the counting easier. Because of the irregularity of respirations in an infant, it is important to count the rate for a full minute. Older children can be observed as they sit quietly on the examining table, or the respirations can be counted as the examiner listens to the lungs during the examination. For observations the upper clothing must be removed. Children should be unaware of your observations since knowledge of what you are doing may cause them to alter their respirations.

Respiration rates are recorded at the top of the chart for the day's use but are not generally graphed in the pediatric clinic. An increased respiration rate is sometimes found with an increased pulse rate, fever, fulminating infection, or respiratory distress.

Blood Pressure

Blood pressure is the indirect measurement of pressure exerted against the arterial walls during ventricular contractions and relaxations. It should be measured at every well-child visit; however, accurate measurements of infant's blood pressure are difficult to obtain, and the American Academy of Pediatrics recommends beginning the procedure when the child is around 3 years of age. Some pediatricians disagree, and think it should be done on every child at every visit. In this way, the examiner learns to become proficient at the procedure and also knows her limitations with the equipment and age of the child.

Three basic pieces of equipment are needed to measure blood pressure accurately: a sphygmomanometer, a cuff, and a stethoscope. The sphygmomanometer may be mercurial, showing a tube filled with mercury that rises and falls with the pressure changes, or aneroid, showing a spring dial with an indicator that moves with pressure changes. Some practitioners feel the mercurial sphygmomanometer is superior and more likely to give accurate readings. The cuff is an inflatable tube surrounded by a cloth covering that extends beyond the rubberized portion. The cloth portion should be long enough to wrap around the arm several times. Some of the newer cuffs are held together with Velcro at the ends. The last piece of standard equipment is a good stethoscope. If the examiner has trouble hearing through the standard stethoscope, an electronic stethoscope which intensifies the sounds can be obtained. A new apparatus being introduced on the market may replace the three standard pieces of equipment; it is called the Doppler instrument and consists of a small, battery-operated box and a flat probe. It has been shown (Kirkland, 1972) that this instrument overcomes the difficulty of measuring blood pressures in a noisy room. Another useful device is an oscillometer, which transmits the arterial pressures into electrical impulses and can give both systolic and diastolic readings. It is most useful with infants.

The method used to obtain a blood pressure reading varies with the age of the child. For infants under 1 year auscultation is difficult or impossible because the sounds are so faint. A Doppler instrument or oscillometer will overcome this problem. If only the standard three pieces of equipment are available, the flush technique must be used. This is a poor method since it depends on observation and gives only a mean blood pressure. The child's arm is raised above the level of the head, and the blood is "milked" toward the heart. Sometimes an Ace bandage is applied in this position. The cuff is applied and inflated and the arm is lowered to the level of the heart. At this point, the examiner unwraps the Ace bandage and deflates the cuff slowly. The unwrapped part of the arm is observed carefully for the pink flush indicating return of blood to the arm. The reading on the sphygmomanometer at this time is the median between systole and diastole (see Fig. 4-6).

By 3 years of age the usual method of measuring blood pressure can be used. The child is seated with the arm relaxed and slightly flexed on a surface level with the heart. A cuff is selected that covers two-thirds of the child's upper arm, since too large or too small a cuff will give an inaccurate reading. The deflated cuff is wrapped snugly around the arm, leaving enough space to place the stethoscope over the brachial artery in the antecubital area. The stethoscope should be held firmly in place. Once the stetho-

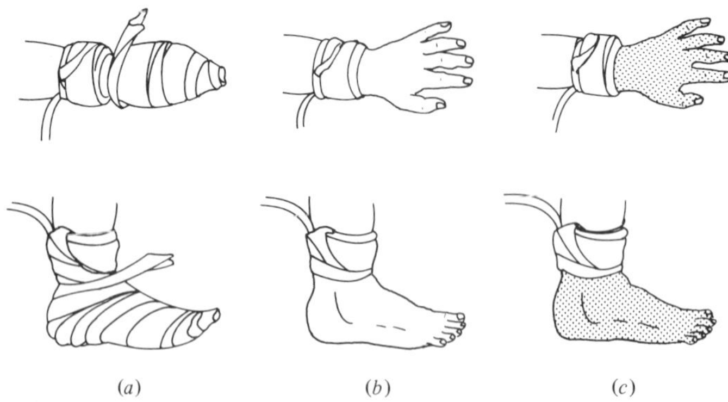

Figure 4-6 Diagrams of the technique of blood pressure measurement by the flush method. *(Source: Printed by permission of Charles C Thomas Publisher, Problems of Blood Pressure in Childhood, by Arthur J. Moss and Forrest H. Adams, 1963, p. 28.)*

scope and cuff are in place, the pressure can be increased to 30 mm of mercury above the disappearance of pulse and then slowly decreased. As the mercury drops, the examiner should listen for five distinct sounds, known as *Korotkoff sounds.*

Phase I: The beginning of gentle, distinct sounds. This is the point of systolic pressure.

Phase II: The gentle sounds of the first phase become longer, producing the sound of a murmur.

Phase III: The sounds become more intense and distinct.

Phase IV: The sounds become faint and muffled.

Phase V: The sounds disappear completely.

In pediatrics it is important to have the correct cuff size. Cuff sizes run from 5 to 14 cm, and it is generally recommended that the child from infancy to 5 years use the 5-cm cuff, the child from 6 to 8 years use the 7-cm cuff, the child from 9 to 14 years use the 9-cm cuff, and the child over 15 use the standard 12 to 14-cm cuff.

Special Measurements

Occasionally there is a need for special measurements, such as sitting height and chest circumference. In children with growth problems it may be useful to compare their sitting height with their standing height. The child should be seated on a firm surface against a wall; the distance from the level of the head to the level of the buttocks is measured with a metal tape measure. By adulthood, sitting height equals one-half of standing height; these adult proportions should be reached around 10 years of age. At birth, the sitting height is 70 percent of standing height; this decreases to 60 percent by the time the child is 2 years old.

The chest circumference is usually measured at birth only, unless the child is showing signs of growth problems. To measure the chest circumference, the tape measure is placed around the chest and across the nipple line. At birth, the chest circumference should be 32 to 35 cm, or 2 cm less than the head circumference. The chest circumference then increases quickly and equals the head circumference until the age of 2; after that, the normal chest will be larger than the head.

It is important to have the average childhood norms available for comparison (see Tables 4-2 and 4-3).

DEVELOPMENTAL TESTING

Some of the most useful of the screening tests available to the nurse working in ambulatory pediatrics are those designed to assess the developmental skills of children. This chapter will discuss three popular screening tests used

Table 4-2 Some General Standard Skeletal Measurements

Percentiles (Boys)								Percentiles (Girls)						
3	10	25	50	75	90	97		3	10	25	50	75	90	97
							Birth							
5.8	6.3	6.9	7.5	8.3	9.1	10.1	Weight, lbs	5.8	6.2	6.9	7.4	8.1	8.6	9.4
18.2	18.9	19.4	19.9	20.5	21.0	21.5	Length, in.	18.5	18.8	19.3	19.8	20.1	20.4	21.1
13.0	13.2	13.5	13.9	14.2	14.6	14.8	Head, in.	12.8	13.1	13.3	13.7	13.9	14.2	14.4
2.8	2.9	3.0	3.2	3.3	3.4	3.5	Hips, in.	2.7	2.8	2.9	3.0	3.2	3.3	3.5
11.7	12.0	12.5	13.1	13.5	14.0	14.5	Chest, in.	11.8	12.1	12.5	12.9	13.4	13.8	14.2
2.6	2.9	3.1	3.4	3.8	4.1	4.6	Weight, kg	2.6	2.8	3.1	3.4	3.7	3.9	4.3
46.3	48.1	49.3	50.6	52.0	53.3	54.6	Length, cm	47.1	47.8	49.0	50.2	51.0	51.9	53.6
33.0	33.5	34.4	35.3	36.2	37.0	37.5	Head, cm	32.5	33.4	33.9	34.7	35.4	36.0	36.6
7.1	7.4	7.7	8.1	8.4	8.7	9.0	Hips, cm	7.0	7.2	7.4	7.7	8.2	8.5	8.9
29.8	30.6	31.8	33.2	34.4	35.7	36.8	Chest, cm	30.0	30.8	31.8	32.9	34.0	35.0	36.0
							3 Months							
10.6	11.1	11.8	12.6	13.6	14.5	16.4	Weight, lbs	9.8	10.7	11.4	12.4	13.2	14.0	14.9
22.4	22.8	23.3	23.8	24.3	24.7	25.1	Length, in.	22.0	22.4	22.8	23.4	23.9	24.3	24.8
15.2	15.4	15.7	16.1	16.3	16.6	17.0	Head, in.	14.9	15.1	15.4	15.7	16.1	16.4	16.6
3.8	3.9	4.0	4.2	4.4	4.5	4.8	Hips, in.	3.7	3.8	3.9	4.1	4.3	4.5	4.8
14.8	15.1	15.5	16.0	16.4	16.9	17.4	Chest, in.	14.4	14.8	15.3	15.7	16.1	16.5	16.9
4.8	5.0	5.3	5.7	6.2	6.6	7.4	Weight, kg	4.4	4.8	5.2	5.6	6.0	6.3	6.8
56.8	57.8	59.3	60.4	61.8	62.8	63.7	Length, cm	55.8	56.9	57.9	59.5	60.7	61.7	63.1
38.7	39.2	40.0	40.9	41.5	42.1	43.2	Head, cm	37.9	38.5	39.2	40.0	40.8	41.7	42.3
9.8	10.0	10.2	10.6	11.2	11.5	12.1	Hips, cm	9.4	9.6	9.9	10.4	10.9	11.4	12.2
37.6	38.3	39.3	40.6	41.6	42.9	44.1	Chest, cm	36.5	37.6	38.8	39.8	40.9	42.0	43.0
							6 Months							
14.0	14.8	15.6	16.7	18.0	19.2	20.8	Weight, lbs	12.7	14.1	15.0	16.0	17.5	18.6	20.0
24.8	25.2	25.7	26.1	26.7	27.3	27.7	Length, in.	24.0	24.6	25.1	25.7	26.2	26.7	27.1
16.6	16.8	17.0	17.3	17.6	17.9	18.1	Head, in.	16.1	16.3	16.5	16.8	17.2	17.5	17.9
4.1	4.2	4.4	4.6	4.7	4.9	5.1	Hips, in.	4.0	4.1	4.2	4.4	4.6	4.9	5.2
15.8	16.4	16.7	17.2	17.7	18.2	18.6	Chest, in.	15.5	16.0	16.4	16.9	17.4	17.9	18.3
6.3	6.7	7.1	7.6	8.2	8.7	9.4	Weight, kg	5.8	6.4	6.8	7.3	7.9	8.4	9.1
63.0	63.9	65.2	66.4	67.8	69.3	70.4	Length, cm	61.1	62.5	63.7	65.2	66.6	67.8	68.8
42.1	42.7	43.3	43.9	44.8	45.4	45.9	Head, cm	40.9	41.4	42.0	42.8	43.6	44.5	45.4
10.5	10.8	11.2	11.6	12.0	12.4	13.1	Hips, cm	10.3	10.5	10.8	11.3	11.8	12.4	13.2
40.1	41.6	42.5	43.7	45.0	46.3	47.2	Chest, cm	39.4	40.6	41.8	43.0	44.2	45.4	46.6
							9 Months							
16.6	17.8	18.7	20.0	21.5	22.9	24.4	Weight, lbs	15.1	16.6	17.8	19.2	20.8	22.4	24.2
26.6	27.0	27.5	28.0	28.7	29.2	29.9	Length, in.	25.7	26.4	26.9	27.6	28.2	28.7	29.2
17.2	17.5	17.7	18.1	18.3	18.5	18.8	Head, in.	16.8	17.0	17.2	17.5	17.9	18.2	18.6
4.3	4.5	4.7	4.8	5.0	5.1	5.4	Hips, in.	4.3	4.4	4.5	4.7	4.9	5.1	5.4
16.5	17.2	17.6	18.1	18.7	19.3	19.6	Chest, in.	16.4	16.8	17.3	17.9	18.3	18.8	19.4
7.5	8.1	8.5	9.1	9.7	10.4	11.1	Weight, kg	6.8	7.5	8.0	8.7	9.4	10.2	11.0
67.7	68.6	69.8	71.2	72.9	74.2	75.9	Length, cm	65.4	67.0	68.4	70.1	71.7	72.9	74.1
43.8	44.5	45.1	46.0	46.5	47.1	47.8	Head, cm	42.6	43.2	43.8	44.6	45.4	46.3	47.2
11.0	11.5	11.9	12.3	12.7	13.1	13.7	Hips, cm	11.0	11.3	11.5	12.0	12.5	13.1	13.8
42.0	43.7	44.8	46.0	47.5	48.9	49.9	Chest, cm	41.7	42.7	44.0	45.4	46.6	47.9	49.2

Table 4-2 *(Cont'd)*

Percentiles (Boys)								Percentiles (Girls)						
3	10	25	50	75	90	97		3	10	25	50	75	90	97
							12 Months							
18.5	19.6	20.9	22.2	23.8	25.4	27.3	Weight, lbs	16.8	18.4	19.8	21.5	23.0	24.8	27.1
28.1	28.5	29.0	29.6	30.3	30.7	31.6	Length, in.	27.1	27.8	28.5	29.2	29.9	30.3	31.0
17.7	17.9	18.3	18.6	18.8	19.0	19.2	Head, in.	17.2	17.4	17.7	18.0	18.4	18.8	19.0
4.5	4.7	4.9	5.0	5.2	5.4	5.6	Hips, in.	4.5	4.6	4.7	4.9	5.1	5.3	5.7
17.1	17.7	18.2	18.7	19.4	20.0	20.4	Chest, in.	17.0	17.4	17.9	18.5	19.0	19.5	20.0
8.4	8.9	9.5	10.1	10.8	11.5	12.4	Weight, kg	7.6	8.3	9.0	9.7	10.4	11.2	12.3
71.3	72.4	73.7	75.2	76.9	78.1	80.3	Length, cm	68.9	70.6	72.3	74.2	75.9	77.1	78.8
44.9	45.5	46.5	47.3	47.8	48.4	48.9	Head, cm	43.6	44.3	45.0	45.8	46.7	47.7	48.4
11.4	11.9	12.4	12.8	13.2	13.7	14.2	Hips, cm	11.4	11.7	12.0	12.4	13.0	13.6	14.4
43.5	45.1	46.3	47.6	49.3	50.7	51.9	Chest, cm	43.1	44.2	45.6	47.0	48.2	49.5	50.9
							15 Months							
19.8	21.0	22.4	23.7	25.4	27.2	29.4	Weight, lbs	18.1	19.8	21.3	23.0	24.6	26.6	29.0
29.3	29.8	30.3	30.9	31.6	32.1	33.1	Length, in.	28.3	29.0	29.8	30.5	31.3	31.8	32.6
17.9	18.2	18.5	18.9	19.1	19.4	19.6	Head, in.	17.4	17.7	17.9	18.3	18.7	19.0	19.3
4.6	4.9	5.0	5.2	5.4	5.6	5.8	Hips, in.	4.6	4.8	4.9	5.1	5.3	5.5	5.8
17.6	18.1	18.6	19.1	19.7	20.3	20.8	Chest, in.	17.4	17.7	18.3	18.8	19.4	19.9	20.4
9.0	9.5	10.2	10.7	11.5	12.3	13.3	Weight, kg	8.2	9.0	9.7	10.4	11.2	12.1	13.1
74.4	75.6	77.0	78.5	80.3	81.5	84.2	Length, cm	71.9	73.7	75.6	77.6	79.4	80.8	82.8
45.6	46.3	47.1	48.0	48.5	49.2	49.8	Head, cm	44.3	44.9	45.6	46.5	47.4	48.4	49.1
11.8	12.4	12.8	13.3	13.7	14.2	14.7	Hips, cm	11.6	12.1	12.4	12.9	13.5	14.1	14.8
44.7	46.1	47.3	48.6	50.1	51.7	52.8	Chest, cm	44.1	45.1	46.5	47.9	49.2	50.5	51.9
							18 Months							
21.1	22.3	23.8	25.2	26.9	29.0	31.5	Weight, lbs	19.4	21.2	22.7	24.5	26.2	28.3	30.9
30.5	31.0	31.6	32.2	32.9	33.5	34.7	Length, in.	29.5	30.2	31.1	31.8	32.6	33.3	34.1
18.2	18.5	18.8	19.2	19.4	19.6	19.9	Head, in.	17.7	17.9	18.2	18.5	18.9	19.3	19.6
4.8	5.0	5.2	5.4	5.6	5.8	6.0	Hips, in.	4.6	4.9	5.0	5.2	5.5	5.7	6.0
18.1	18.5	19.0	19.5	20.0	20.7	21.1	Chest, in.	17.7	18.1	18.6	19.2	19.8	20.2	20.8
9.6	10.1	10.8	11.4	12.2	13.1	14.3	Weight, kg	8.8	9.6	10.3	11.1	11.9	12.8	14.0
77.5	78.8	80.3	81.8	83.7	85.0	88.2	Length, cm	74.9	76.8	79.0	80.9	82.9	84.5	86.7
46.2	47.0	47.7	48.7	49.2	49.9	50.6	Head, cm	44.9	45.5	46.2	47.1	48.0	49.0	49.8
12.1	12.8	13.2	13.7	14.2	14.7	15.2	Hips, cm	11.8	12.4	12.8	13.3	13.9	14.5	15.2
45.9	47.0	48.2	49.5	50.9	52.6	53.7	Chest, cm	45.0	46.0	47.3	48.8	50.2	51.4	52.9
							2 Years							
23.3	24.7	26.3	27.7	29.7	31.9	34.9	Weight, lbs	21.6	23.5	25.3	27.1	29.2	31.7	34.4
32.6	33.1	33.8	34.4	35.2	35.9	37.2	Length, in.	31.5	32.3	33.3	34.1	35.0	35.8	36.7
18.5	18.9	19.0	19.6	19.8	20.1	20.3	Head, in.	18.0	18.3	18.6	18.9	19.3	19.7	20.0
5.0	5.3	5.5	5.7	5.9	6.1	6.3	Hips, in.	4.9	5.1	5.3	5.5	5.8	6.0	6.3
18.7	19.0	19.5	20.0	20.5	21.2	21.6	Chest, in.	18.2	18.7	19.1	19.7	20.4	20.9	21.3
10.6	11.2	11.9	12.6	13.5	14.5	15.8	Weight, kg	9.8	10.7	11.5	12.3	13.2	14.4	15.6
82.7	84.2	85.8	87.5	89.4	91.1	94.6	Length, cm	80.1	82.0	84.7	86.6	88.9	91.0	93.3
47.0	48.0	48.2	49.7	50.2	51.0	51.7	Head, cm	45.8	46.4	47.2	48.1	49.1	50.1	50.9
12.8	13.5	13.9	14.4	15.0	15.5	16.1	Hips, cm	12.5	13.1	13.5	14.1	14.7	15.3	16.1
47.4	48.4	49.5	50.8	52.2	53.9	54.9	Chest, cm	46.3	47.4	48.6	50.1	51.8	53.0	54.2

Table 4-2 ***(Cont'd)***

Percentiles (Boys)								Percentiles (Girls)						
3	**10**	**25**	**50**	**75**	**90**	**97**		**3**	**10**	**25**	**50**	**75**	**90**	**97**
							2½ Years							
25.2	26.6	28.4	30.0	32.2	34.5	37.0	Weight, lbs	23.6	25.5	27.4	29.6	31.9	34.6	38.2
34.2	34.8	35.5	36.3	37.0	37.9	39.2	Length, in.	33.3	34.0	35.2	36.0	36.9	37.9	38.9
18.7	19.1	19.4	19.8	20.0	20.3	20.6	Head, in.	18.2	18.5	18.8	19.2	19.6	20.0	20.3
5.3	5.6	5.7	5.9	6.2	6.4	6.6	Hips, in.	5.2	5.4	5.6	5.8	6.1	6.3	6.6
19.0	19.4	19.8	20.3	20.9	21.6	22.0	Chest, in.	18.6	19.0	19.6	20.1	20.8	21.4	21.8
11.4	12.1	12.9	13.6	14.6	15.6	16.8	Weight, kg	10.7	11.6	12.4	13.4	14.5	15.7	17.3
86.9	88.5	90.2	92.1	94.1	96.2	99.5	Length, cm	84.5	86.3	89.3	91.4	93.8	96.4	98.7
47.5	48.5	49.2	50.2	50.9	51.6	52.3	Head, cm	46.3	47.0	47.8	48.8	49.8	50.8	51.5
13.6	14.2	14.6	15.1	15.7	16.2	16.7	Hips, cm	13.2	13.7	14.2	14.8	15.4	16.1	16.9
48.2	49.3	50.3	51.7	53.2	54.9	55.8	Chest, cm	47.3	48.4	49.7	51.2	52.8	54.3	55.5
							3 Years							
27.0	28.7	30.3	32.2	34.5	36.8	39.2	Weight, lbs	25.6	27.6	29.6	31.8	34.6	37.4	41.8
35.7	36.3	37.0	37.9	38.8	39.6	40.5	Length, in.	34.8	35.6	36.8	37.7	38.6	39.8	40.7
18.8	19.2	19.5	19.8	20.2	20.4	20.7	Head, in.	18.4	18.7	19.0	19.4	19.8	20.1	20.5
5.6	5.8	6.0	6.2	6.4	6.6	6.8	Hips, in.	5.4	5.6	5.8	6.1	6.3	6.6	7.0
19.2	19.6	20.1	20.6	21.3	22.0	22.4	Chest, in.	18.8	19.4	19.9	20.4	21.1	21.7	22.3
12.2	13.0	13.7	14.6	15.6	16.7	17.8	Weight, kg	11.6	12.5	13.4	14.4	15.7	17.0	19.0
90.6	92.3	93.9	96.2	98.5	100.5	102.8	Length, cm	88.4	90.5	93.4	95.7	98.1	101.1	103.5
47.9	48.9	49.6	50.4	51.3	51.9	52.7	Head, cm	46.8	47.5	48.4	49.3	50.3	51.1	52.0
14.2	14.8	15.2	15.8	16.4	16.9	17.4	Hips, cm	13.8	14.3	14.8	15.4	16.1	16.8	17.7
48.9	49.9	51.0	52.4	54.1	55.8	57.0	Chest, cm	47.9	49.3	50.5	51.9	53.5	55.1	56.7
							3½ Years							
28.5	30.4	32.3	34.3	36.7	39.1	41.5	Weight, lbs	27.5	29.5	31.5	33.9	37.0	40.4	45.3
37.1	37.8	38.4	39.3	40.3	41.1	41.9	Length, in.	36.2	37.1	38.1	39.2	40.2	41.5	42.5
5.8	6.0	6.2	6.4	6.6	6.8	7.0	Hips, in.	5.7	5.9	6.1	6.3	6.6	6.8	7.2
19.5	19.9	20.3	20.9	21.6	22.3	22.8	Chest, in.	19.1	19.7	20.1	20.7	21.3	22.0	22.9
12.9	13.8	14.6	15.6	16.6	17.7	18.8	Weight, kg	12.5	13.4	14.3	15.4	16.8	18.3	20.5
94.3	96.0	97.5	99.8	102.5	104.5	106.5	Length, cm	92.0	94.2	96.9	99.5	102.0	105.4	108.0
14.7	15.3	15.7	16.3	16.9	17.4	17.9	Hips, cm	14.4	14.9	15.4	16.0	16.7	17.4	18.3
49.6	50.5	51.6	53.1	54.9	56.6	58.0	Chest, cm	48.5	50.1	51.2	52.5	54.1	55.8	58.1
							4 Years							
30.1	32.1	34.0	36.4	39.0	41.4	44.3	Weight, lbs	29.2	31.2	33.5	36.2	39.6	43.5	48.2
38.4	39.1	39.7	40.7	41.9	42.7	43.5	Length, in.	37.5	38.4	39.5	40.6	41.6	43.1	44.2
	19.5	19.8	20.1	20.4	20.7		Head, in.		18.9	19.3	19.6	20.1	20.4	
6.0	6.2	6.4	6.6	6.9	7.1	7.3	Hips, in.	5.9	6.1	6.3	6.5	6.8	7.0	7.4
19.7	20.1	20.5	21.1	21.8	22.5	23.2	Chest, in.	19.4	20.0	20.3	20.9	21.5	22.2	23.2
13.6	14.6	15.4	16.5	17.7	18.8	20.1	Weight, kg	13.2	14.1	15.2	16.4	18.0	19.7	21.9
97.5	99.3	100.8	103.4	106.5	108.5	110.4	Length, cm	95.2	97.6	100.3	103.2	105.8	109.6	112.3
	49.5	50.3	51.1	51.9	52.6		Head, cm		47.9	49.1	49.9	51.0	51.7	
15.2	15.8	16.2	16.9	17.5	18.0	18.5	Hips, cm	15.0	15.4	15.9	16.5	17.2	17.9	18.9
50.1	51.1	52.2	53.7	55.5	57.2	58.9	Chest, cm	49.2	50.7	51.7	53.1	54.7	56.5	59.0

Table 4-2 ***(Cont'd)***

Percentiles (Boys)								Percentiles (Girls)						
3	10	25	50	75	90	97		3	10	25	50	75	90	97
							4½ Years							
31.6	33.8	35.7	38.4	41.4	43.9	47.4	Weight, lbs	30.7	32.9	35.3	38.5	42.1	46.7	50.9
39.6	40.3	40.9	42.0	43.3	44.2	45.0	Length, in.	38.6	39.7	40.8	42.0	43.0	44.7	45.7
6.2	6.4	6.5	6.8	7.1	7.3	7.5	Hips, in.	6.1	6.2	6.4	6.7	7.0	7.3	7.6
20.0	20.3	20.8	21.4	22.2	22.8	23.3	Chest, in.	19.6	20.2	20.6	21.1	21.8	22.5	23.5
14.3	15.3	16.2	17.4	18.8	19.9	21.5	Weight, kg	13.9	14.9	16.0	17.5	19.1	21.2	23.1
100.6	102.4	104.0	106.7	109.9	112.3	114.3	Length, cm	98.1	100.9	103.6	106.8	109.3	113.5	116.2
15.7	16.2	16.6	17.3	18.0	18.5	19.1	Hips, cm	15.5	15.9	16.4	17.0	17.7	18.5	19.4
50.7	51.7	52.9	54.4	56.3	58.0	59.3	Chest, cm	49.8	51.3	52.3	53.7	55.4	57.3	59.6
							5 Years							
34.5	36.6	39.6	42.8	46.5	49.7	53.2	Weight, lbs	33.7	36.1	38.6	41.4	44.2	48.2	51.8
40.2	41.5	42.6	43.8	45.0	45.9	47.0	Height, in.	40.4	41.3	42.2	43.2	44.4	45.4	46.5
	19.6	19.9	20.2	20.5	20.7		Head, in.		19.0	19.5	19.8	20.2	20.6	
	6.7	6.9	7.2	7.4	7.7		Hips, in.		6.7	6.8	7.1	7.4	7.6	
	20.3	20.8	21.4	22.1	22.6		Chest, in.		19.8	20.2	20.8	21.5	22.2	
15.6	16.6	18.0	19.4	21.1	22.5	24.1	Weight, kg	15.3	16.4	17.5	18.8	20.0	21.9	23.5
102.1	105.3	108.3	111.3	114.2	116.7	119.5	Height, cm	102.6	105.0	107.2	109.7	112.9	115.4	118.0
	49.9	50.6	51.2	52.1	52.6		Head, cm		48.3	49.5	50.4	51.3	52.2	
	17.0	17.6	18.3	18.9	19.6		Hips, cm		17.0	17.4	18.0	18.7	19.4	
	51.6	52.8	54.5	56.2	57.5		Chest, cm		50.2	51.4	52.9	54.6	56.5	
							5½ Years							
	38.8	42.0	45.6	49.3	53.1		Weight, lbs		38.0	40.8	44.0	47.2	51.2	
	42.6	43.8	45.0	46.3	47.3		Height, in.		42.4	43.4	44.4	45.7	46.8	
	6.8	7.1	7.4	7.6	7.9		Hips, in.		6.8	7.0	7.2	7.5	7.9	
	20.6	21.1	21.8	22.5	23.0		Chest, in.		20.0	20.5	21.1	21.8	22.6	
	17.6	19.0	20.7	22.4	24.1		Weight, kg		17.2	18.5	20.0	21.4	23.2	
	108.3	111.2	114.4	117.5	120.1		Height, cm		107.8	110.2	112.8	116.1	118.9	
	17.4	18.0	18.7	19.4	20.1		Hips, cm		17.4	17.8	18.4	19.1	20.0	
	52.4	53.6	55.3	57.1	58.5		Chest, cm		50.9	52.2	53.7	55.5	57.4	
							6 Years							
38.5	40.9	44.4	48.3	52.1	56.4	61.1	Weight, lbs	37.2	39.6	42.9	46.5	50.2	54.2	58.7
42.7	43.8	44.9	46.3	47.6	48.6	49.7	Height, in.	42.5	43.5	44.6	45.6	47.0	48.1	49.4
	19.8	20.0	20.2	20.7	20.9		Head, in.		19.3	19.5	19.8	20.3	20.7	
	7.0	7.2	7.5	7.8	8.1		Hips, in.		7.0	7.2	7.4	7.7	8.1	
	20.9	21.4	22.1	22.8	23.4		Chest, in.		20.3	20.8	21.4	22.2	22.9	
17.5	18.5	20.1	21.9	23.6	25.6	27.7	Weight, kg	16.9	18.0	19.5	21.1	22.8	24.6	26.6
108.5	111.2	114.1	117.5	120.8	123.5	126.2	Height, cm	108.0	110.6	113.2	115.9	119.3	123.3	125.4
	50.2	50.7	51.3	52.5	53.2		Head, cm		48.9	49.5	50.4	51.6	52.6	
	17.7	18.4	19.1	19.8	20.5		Hips, cm		17.7	18.2	18.8	19.5	20.5	
	53.2	54.4	56.1	57.9	59.5		Chest, cm		51.5	52.9	54.5	56.3	58.2	

Table 4-2 ***(Cont'd)***

Percentiles (Boys)								Percentiles (Girls)						
3	10	25	50	75	90	97		3	10	25	50	75	90	97
							6½ Years							
	43.4	47.1	51.2	55.4	60.4		Weight, lbs		42.2	45.5	49.4	53.3	57.7	
	44.9	46.1	47.6	48.9	50.0		Height, in.		44.8	45.7	46.9	48.3	49.4	
	7.1	7.4	7.7	7.9	8.3		Hips, in.		7.1	7.3	7.5	7.9	8.3	
	21.3	21.8	22.4	23.2	23.8		Chest, in.		20.5	21.1	21.8	22.5	23.3	
	19.7	21.4	23.2	25.1	27.4		Weight, kg		19.1	20.6	22.4	24.2	26.2	
	114.1	117.2	120.8	124.2	127.0		Height, cm		113.7	116.2	119.1	122.6	125.6	
	18.1	18.8	19.5	20.2	21.0		Hips, cm		18.1	18.6	19.2	20.0	21.6	
	54.1	55.3	57.0	58.9	60.6		Chest, cm		52.2	53.7	55.3	57.2	59.2	
							7 Years							
43.0	45.8	49.7	54.1	58.7	64.4	69.9	Weight, lbs	41.3	44.5	48.1	52.2	56.3	61.2	67.3
44.9	46.0	47.4	48.9	50.2	51.4	52.5	Height, in.	44.9	46.0	46.9	48.1	49.6	50.7	51.9
	7.3	7.5	7.8	8.1	8.4		Hips, in.		7.2	7.4	7.7	8.0	8.5	
	21.6	22.1	22.7	23.5	24.2		Chest, in.		20.8	21.4	22.1	22.8	23.7	
19.5	20.8	22.5	24.5	26.6	29.2	31.7	Weight, kg	18.7	20.2	21.8	23.7	25.5	27.8	30.5
114.0	116.9	120.3	124.1	127.6	130.5	133.4	Height, cm	114.0	116.8	119.2	122.3	125.9	128.9	131.7
	18.5	19.2	19.9	20.6	21.4		Hips, cm		18.4	18.9	19.6	20.4	21.1	
	54.9	56.1	57.8	59.8	61.6		Chest, cm		52.8	54.4	56.1	58.0	60.1	
							7½ Years							
	48.5	52.6	57.1	62.1	68.7		Weight, lbs		46.6	50.6	55.2	59.8	65.6	
	47.2	48.6	50.0	51.5	52.7		Height, in.		47.0	48.0	49.3	50.7	51.9	
	7.4	7.7	8.0	8.3	8.6		Hips, in.		7.4	7.6	7.9	8.2	8.7	
	22.0	22.5	23.1	24.0	24.8		Chest, in.		21.1	21.7	22.4	23.2	24.1	
	22.0	23.9	25.9	28.2	31.2		Weight, kg		21.1	22.9	25.0	27.1	29.8	
	120.0	123.5	127.1	130.9	133.9		Height, cm		119.5	122.0	125.2	128.8	131.8	
	18.9	19.6	20.3	21.0	21.9		Hips, cm		18.8	19.3	20.1	20.9	22.1	
	55.8	57.1	58.8	61.0	62.9		Chest, cm		53.5	55.1	57.0	59.0	61.2	
							8 Years							
48.0	51.2	55.5	60.1	65.5	73.0	79.4	Weight, lbs	45.3	48.6	53.1	58.1	63.3	69.9	78.9
47.1	48.5	49.8	51.2	52.8	54.0	55.2	Height, in.	46.9	48.1	49.1	50.4	51.8	53.0	54.1
	7.5	7.8	8.1	8.4	8.8		Hips, in.		7.5	7.7	8.1	8.4	8.9	
	22.3	22.8	23.5	24.4	25.2		Chest, in.		21.3	22.0	22.7	23.6	24.5	
21.8	23.2	25.2	27.3	29.7	33.1	36.0	Weight, kg	20.5	22.0	24.1	26.3	28.7	31.7	35.8
119.6	123.1	126.6	130.0	134.2	137.3	140.2	Height, cm	119.1	122.1	124.8	128.0	131.6	134.6	137.4
	19.2	19.9	20.7	21.4	23.3		Hips, cm		19.1	19.7	20.5	21.3	22.6	
	56.7	58.0	59.8	62.1	64.1		Chest, cm		54.2	55.8	57.8	59.9	62.3	

Table 4-2 ***(Cont'd)***

Percentiles (Boys)								Percentiles (Girls)						
3	10	25	50	75	90	97		3	10	25	50	75	90	97
							8½ Years							
	53.8	58.3	63.1	68.9	77.0		Weight, lbs		50.6	55.5	61.0	66.9	74.5	
	49.5	50.8	52.3	53.9	55.1		Height, in.		49.0	50.1	51.4	52.9	54.1	
	7.7	8.0	8.3	8.6	8.9		Hips, in.		7.6	7.9	8.2	8.6	9.1	
	22.7	23.2	23.9	24.9	25.7		Chest, in.		21.6	22.2	23.1	24.0	25.0	
	24.4	26.4	28.6	31.2	34.9		Weight, kg		22.9	25.2	27.7	30.3	33.8	
	125.7	129.1	132.8	137.0	140.0		Height, cm		124.6	127.3	130.5	134.4	137.5	
	19.6	20.3	21.1	21.8	22.7		Hips, cm		19.4	20.1	20.9	21.8	23.1	
	57.6	59.0	60.8	63.3	65.4		Chest, cm		54.9	56.5	58.7	60.9	63.5	
							9 Years							
52.5	56.3	61.1	66.0	72.3	81.0	89.8	Weight, lbs	49.1	52.6	57.9	63.8	70.5	79.1	89.9
48.9	50.5	51.8	53.3	55.0	56.1	57.2	Height, in.	48.7	50.0	51.1	52.3	54.0	55.3	56.5
	7.8	8.1	8.4	8.7	9.0		Hips, in.		7.7	8.1	8.4	8.7	9.2	
	23.0	23.6	24.3	25.3	26.2		Chest, in.		21.8	22.5	23.5	24.4	25.5	
23.8	25.5	27.7	29.9	32.8	36.7	40.7	Weight, kg	22.3	23.9	26.3	28.9	32.0	35.9	40.8
124.2	128.3	131.6	135.5	139.8	142.6	145.3	Height, cm	123.6	127.0	129.7	132.9	137.1	140.4	143.4
	19.9	20.6	21.4	22.2	23.0		Hips, cm		19.7	20.5	21.3	22.2	23.5	
	58.4	59.9	61.8	64.4	66.7		Chest, cm		55.5	57.2	59.6	61.9	64.7	
							9½ Years							
	58.7	63.7	69.0	76.0	85.5		Weight, lbs		54.9	60.4	67.1	74.8	84.4	
	51.4	52.7	54.3	55.9	57.1		Height, in.		50.9	52.0	53.5	55.1	56.4	
	7.9	8.3	8.5	8.9	9.2		Hips, in.		7.9	8.2	8.6	9.0	9.5	
	23.3	24.0	24.8	25.8	26.8		Chest, in.		22.1	22.8	23.8	24.9	26.0	
	26.6	28.9	31.3	34.5	38.8		Weight, kg		24.9	27.4	30.4	33.9	38.3	
	130.6	134.0	137.9	142.1	145.1		Height, cm		129.4	132.2	135.8	139.9	143.2	
	20.2	21.0	21.7	22.6	23.5		Hips, cm		20.1	20.9	21.8	22.8	24.1	
	59.3	60.9	62.9	65.5	68.1		Chest, cm		56.2	58.0	60.5	63.2	66.1	
							10 Years							
56.8	61.1	66.3	71.9	79.6	89.9	100.0	Weight, lbs	53.2	57.1	62.8	70.3	79.1	89.7	101.9
50.7	52.3	53.7	55.2	56.8	58.1	59.2	Height, in.	50.3	51.8	53.0	54.6	56.1	57.5	58.8
	8.0	8.4	8.7	9.0	9.4		Hips, in.		8.1	8.3	8.7	9.2	9.7	
	23.7	24.3	25.1	26.2	27.3		Chest, in.		22.4	23.1	24.2	25.3	26.5	
25.8	27.7	30.1	32.6	36.1	40.8	45.4	Weight, kg	24.1	25.9	28.5	31.9	35.9	40.7	46.2
128.7	132.8	136.3	140.3	144.4	147.5	150.3	Height, cm	127.7	131.7	134.6	138.6	142.6	146.0	149.3
	20.4	21.3	22.0	22.9	23.9		Hips, cm		20.5	21.2	22.2	23.3	24.6	
	60.1	61.8	63.9	66.6	69.4		Chest, cm		56.9	58.7	61.4	64.4	67.4	

Table 4-2 ***(Cont'd)***

Percentiles (Boys)								Percentiles (Girls)						
3	10	25	50	75	90	97		3	10	25	50	75	90	97
							10½ Years							
	63.7	69.0	74.8	83.4	94.6		Weight, lbs		59.9	66.4	74.6	84.1	95.1	
	53.2	54.5	56.0	57.8	58.9		Height, in.		52.9	54.1	55.8	57.4	58.9	
	8.2	8.5	8.8	9.1	9.6		Hips, in.		8.3	8.5	9.0	9.4	10.0	
	24.0	24.7	25.5	26.6	27.8		Chest, in.		22.7	23.6	24.7	25.9	27.2	
	28.9	31.3	33.9	37.8	42.9		Weight, kg		27.2	30.1	33.8	38.1	43.1	
	135.1	138.4	142.3	146.8	149.7		Height, cm		134.4	137.5	141.7	145.9	149.7	
	20.8	21.6	22.3	23.2	24.4		Hips, cm		21.0	21.7	22.9	24.0	25.3	
	60.9	62.8	64.9	67.7	70.0		Chest, cm		57.8	59.9	62.8	65.8	69.0	
							11 Years							
61.8	66.3	71.6	77.6	87.2	99.3	111.7	Weight, lbs	57.9	62.6	69.9	78.8	89.1	100.4	112.9
52.5	54.0	55.3	56.8	58.7	59.8	60.8	Height, in.	52.1	53.9	55.2	57.0	58.7	60.4	62.0
	8.3	8.6	8.9	9.2	9.8		Hips, in.		8.4	8.7	9.2	9.7	10.2	
	24.3	25.1	25.9	27.1	28.3		Chest, in.		23.1	24.0	25.3	26.4	27.7	
28.0	30.1	32.5	35.2	39.5	45.0	50.7	Weight, kg	26.3	28.4	31.7	35.7	40.4	45.5	51.2
133.4	137.3	140.5	144.2	149.2	151.8	154.4	Height, cm	132.3	137.0	140.3	144.7	149.2	153.4	157.4
	21.1	21.8	22.6	23.5	24.8		Hips, cm		21.4	22.2	23.5	24.6	26.0	
	61.7	63.7	65.9	68.8	71.9		Chest, cm		58.6	61.1	64.2	67.2	70.5	
							11½ Years							
	69.2	74.6	81.0	91.6	104.5		Weight, lbs		66.1	74.0	83.2	94.0	106.0	
	55.0	56.3	57.8	59.6	60.9		Height, in.		55.0	56.3	58.3	60.3	61.8	
	8.5	8.7	9.1	9.4	10.0		Hips, in.		8.6	9.0	9.5	10.0	10.5	
	24.6	25.4	26.3	27.5	28.8		Chest, in.		23.5	24.6	25.8	27.0	28.4	
	31.4	33.8	36.7	41.5	47.4		Weight, kg		30.0	33.6	37.7	42.6	48.1	
	139.8	142.9	146.9	151.4	154.8		Height, cm		139.8	143.1	148.1	152.9	157.0	
	21.5	22.2	23.1	24.0	25.3		Hips, cm		21.9	22.8	24.2	25.4	26.8	
	62.5	64.6	66.9	69.9	73.1		Chest, cm		59.6	62.5	65.5	68.5	72.2	
							12 Years							
67.2	72.0	77.5	84.4	96.0	109.6	124.2	Weight, lbs	63.6	69.5	78.0	87.6	98.8	111.5	127.7
54.4	56.1	57.2	58.9	60.4	62.2	63.7	Height, in.	54.3	56.1	57.4	59.8	61.6	63.2	64.8
	8.6	8.9	9.2	9.6	10.1		Hips, in.		8.8	9.2	9.8	10.3	10.9	
	24.9	25.8	26.7	27.9	29.2		Chest, in.		23.8	25.1	26.2	27.4	29.0	
30.5	32.7	35.1	38.3	43.5	49.7	56.3	Weight, kg	28.8	31.5	35.4	39.7	44.8	50.6	57.9
138.1	142.4	145.2	149.6	153.5	157.9	161.9	Height, cm	137.8	142.6	145.9	151.9	156.6	160.6	164.6
	21.9	22.6	23.5	24.5	25.8		Hips, cm		22.4	23.4	24.9	26.2	27.6	
	63.3	65.5	67.8	70.9	74.2		Chest, cm		60.6	63.8	66.7	69.7	73.8	

Table 4-2 ***(Cont'd)***

Percentiles (Boys)								Percentiles (Girls)						
3	10	25	50	75	90	97		3	10	25	50	75	90	97
							12½ Years							
	74.6	80.6	88.7	102.0	116.4		Weight, lbs		74.7	83.7	93.4	104.9	118.0	
	56.9	58.1	60.0	61.9	63.6		Height, in.		57.4	58.8	60.7	62.6	64.0	
	8.8	9.1	9.5	9.9	10.4		Hips, in.		9.0	9.4	10.0	10.5	11.1	
	25.3	26.2	27.2	28.5	29.8		Chest, in.		24.3	25.5	26.6	27.9	29.6	
	33.8	36.6	40.2	46.3	52.8		Weight, kg		33.9	38.0	42.4	47.6	53.5	
	144.5	147.5	152.3	157.2	161.6		Height, cm		145.9	149.3	154.3	159.1	162.7	
	22.3	23.1	24.1	25.1	26.5		Hips, cm		23.0	24.0	25.5	26.8	28.3	
	64.2	66.5	69.1	72.4	75.8		Chest, cm		61.8	64.9	67.7	70.9	75.3	
							13 Years							
72.0	77.1	83.7	93.0	107.9	123.2	138.0	Weight, lbs	72.2	79.9	89.4	99.1	111.0	124.5	142.3
56.0	57.7	58.9	61.0	63.3	65.1	66.7	Height, in.	56.6	58.7	60.1	61.8	63.6	64.9	66.3
	8.9	9.3	9.7	10.1	10.7		Hips, in.		9.3	9.7	10.2	10.8	11.4	
	25.6	26.5	27.7	29.0	30.5		Chest, in.		24.8	25.9	27.0	28.3	30.2	
32.7	35.0	38.0	42.2	48.9	55.9	62.6	Weight, kg	32.7	36.2	40.5	44.9	50.3	56.5	64.5
142.2	146.6	149.7	155.0	160.8	165.3	169.5	Height, cm	143.7	149.1	152.6	157.1	161.5	164.8	168.4
	22.7	23.6	24.6	25.6	27.2		Hips, cm		23.6	24.6	26.0	27.4	29.0	
	65.0	67.4	70.3	73.8	77.4		Chest, cm		62.9	65.9	68.6	72.0	76.7	
							13½ Years							
	82.2	89.6	100.3	115.5	130.1		Weight, lbs		85.5	94.6	103.7	115.4	128.9	
	58.8	60.3	62.6	64.8	66.5		Height, in.		59.5	60.8	62.4	64.0	65.3	
	9.1	9.5	9.9	10.4	10.9		Hips, in.		9.5	9.9	10.4	10.9	11.6	
	26.1	27.1	28.5	29.8	31.2		Chest, in.		25.1	26.2	27.3	28.7	30.6	
	37.3	40.6	45.5	52.4	59.0		Weight, kg		38.8	42.9	47.0	52.3	58.5	
	149.4	153.1	158.9	164.6	168.9		Height, cm		151.1	154.4	158.4	162.6	165.9	
	23.2	24.1	25.2	26.4	27.8		Hips, cm		24.2	25.2	26.5	27.8	29.5	
	66.3	68.8	72.4	75.8	79.4		Chest, cm		63.8	66.6	69.3	72.9	77.7	
							14 Years							
79.8	87.2	95.5	107.6	123.1	136.9	150.6	Weight, lbs	83.1	91.0	99.8	108.4	119.7	133.3	150.8
57.6	59.9	61.6	64.0	66.3	67.9	69.7	Height, in.	58.3	60.2	61.5	62.8	64.4	65.7	67.2
	9.3	9.7	10.1	10.7	11.1		Hips, in.		9.8	10.1	10.6	11.1	11.8	
	26.6	27.6	29.3	30.6	32.0		Chest, in.		25.4	26.4	27.5	29.0	30.9	
36.2	39.5	43.3	48.8	55.8	62.1	68.3	Weight, kg	37.7	41.3	45.3	49.2	54.3	60.5	68.4
146.4	152.1	156.5	162.7	168.4	172.4	177.1	Height, cm	148.2	153.0	156.1	159.6	163.7	167.0	170.7
	23.6	24.6	25.8	27.1	28.3		Hips, cm		24.8	25.8	26.9	28.1	29.9	
	67.6	70.2	74.5	77.8	81.4		Chest, cm		64.6	67.2	69.9	73.7	78.6	

Table 4-2 *(Cont'd)*

Percentiles (Boys)								Percentiles (Girls)						
3	10	25	50	75	90	97		3	10	25	50	75	90	97
							14½ Years							
	93.3	101.9	113.9	129.1	142.4		Weight, lbs		94.2	102.5	111.0	121.8	135.7	
	61.0	62.7	65.1	67.2	68.7		Height, in.		60.7	61.8	63.1	64.7	66.0	
	9.5	9.9	10.3	10.8	11.3		Hips, in.		9.9	10.3	10.7	11.2	11.9	
	27.3	28.5	30.0	31.3	32.7		Chest, in.		25.6	26.6	27.7	29.2	31.2	
	42.3	46.2	51.7	58.6	64.6		Weight, kg		42.7	46.5	50.3	55.2	61.5	
	155.0	159.4	165.3	170.7	174.6		Height, cm		154.1	156.9	160.4	164.3	167.6	
	24.1	25.1	26.3	27.5	28.7		Hips, cm		25.2	26.2	27.2	28.4	30.3	
	69.4	72.3	76.3	79.6	83.1		Chest, cm		65.1	67.7	70.4	74.2	79.2	
							15 Years							
91.3	99.4	108.2	120.1	135.0	147.8	161.6	Weight, lbs	89.0	97.4	105.1	113.5	123.9	138.1	155.2
59.7	62.1	63.9	66.1	68.1	69.6	71.6	Height, in.	59.1	61.1	62.1	63.4	64.9	66.2	67.6
	9.7	10.1	10.5	11.0	11.4		Hips, in.		10.1	10.4	10.8	11.3	12.0	
	28.0	29.3	30.7	32.0	33.4		Chest, in.		25.8	26.8	27.9	29.4	31.4	
41.4	45.1	49.1	54.5	61.2	67.0	73.3	Weight, kg	40.4	44.2	47.7	51.5	56.2	62.6	70.4
151.7	157.8	162.3	167.8	173.0	176.7	181.8	Height, cm	150.2	155.2	157.7	161.1	164.9	168.1	171.6
	24.6	25.6	26.7	27.9	29.1		Hips, cm		25.6	26.5	27.5	28.7	30.6	
	71.1	74.4	78.0	81.3	84.8		Chest, cm		65.5	68.1	70.9	74.7	79.8	
							15½ Years							
	105.2	113.5	124.9	139.7	152.6		Weight, lbs		99.2	106.8	115.3	125.6	139.6	
	63.1	64.8	66.8	68.8	70.2		Height, in.		61.3	62.3	63.7	65.1	66.4	
	9.9	10.2	10.7	11.1	11.6		Hips, in.		10.2	10.5	10.9	11.4	12.1	
	28.7	29.8	31.2	32.6	34.0		Chest, in.		25.9	26.9	28.1	29.6	31.6	
	47.7	51.5	56.6	63.4	69.2		Weight, kg		45.0	48.4	52.3	57.0	63.3	
	160.3	164.7	169.7	174.8	178.2		Height, cm		155.7	158.2	161.7	165.3	168.6	
	25.1	26.0	27.1	28.2	29.4		Hips, cm		25.9	26.7	27.8	29.0	30.8	
	72.8	75.8	79.4	82.9	86.3		Chest, cm		65.8	68.4	71.3	75.1	80.2	
							16 Years							
103.4	111.0	118.7	129.7	144.4	157.3	170.5	Weight, lbs	91.8	100.9	108.4	117.0	127.2	141.1	157.7
61.6	64.1	65.8	67.8	69.5	70.7	73.1	Height, in.	59.4	61.5	62.4	63.9	65.2	66.5	67.7
	10.1	10.4	10.8	11.2	11.6		Hips, in.		10.3	10.6	11.0	11.5	12.2	
	29.3	30.4	31.8	33.3	34.6		Chest, in.		26.0	27.0	28.2	29.7	31.7	
46.9	50.3	53.8	58.8	65.5	71.3	77.3	Weight, kg	41.6	45.8	49.2	53.1	57.7	64.0	71.5
156.5	162.8	167.1	171.6	176.6	179.7	185.6	Height, cm	150.8	156.1	158.6	162.2	165.7	169.0	172.0
	25.6	26.4	27.4	28.4	29.6		Hips, cm		26.1	26.9	28.0	29.2	31.0	
	74.4	77.2	80.7	84.5	87.8		Chest, cm		66.1	68.7	71.6	75.4	80.5	

Table 4-2 ***(Cont'd)***

Percentiles (Boys)								Percentiles (Girls)						
3	10	25	50	75	90	97		3	10	25	50	75	90	97
							16½ Years							
	114.3	121.6	133.0	147.9	161.0		Weight, lbs		101.9	109.4	118.1	128.4	142.2	
	64.6	66.3	68.0	69.8	71.1		Height, in.		61.5	62.5	63.9	65.3	66.6	
	10.2	10.5	10.9	11.2	11.7		Hips, in.		10.3	10.6	11.1	11.5	12.2	
	29.7	30.7	32.1	33.6	35.0		Chest, in.		26.1	27.2	28.3	29.8	31.8	
	51.8	55.2	60.3	67.1	73.0		Weight, kg		46.2	49.6	53.6	58.2	64.5	
	164.2	168.4	172.7	177.4	180.7		Height, cm		156.2	158.8	162.4	165.9	169.2	
	25.9	26.7	27.6	28.6	29.8		Hips, cm		26.2	27.0	28.2	29.3	31.1	
	75.4	78.1	81.6	85.4	88.8		Chest, cm		66.3	69.0	71.9	75.7	80.7	
							17 Years							
110.5	117.5	124.5	136.2	151.4	164.6	175.6	Weight, lbs	93.9	102.8	110.4	119.1	129.6	143.3	159.5
62.6	65.2	66.8	68.4	70.1	71.5	73.5	Height, in.	59.4	61.5	62.6	64.0	65.4	66.7	67.8
	10.3	10.6	10.9	11.3	11.8		Hips, in.		10.4	10.7	11.1	11.6	12.3	
	30.1	31.1	32.5	33.9	35.3		Chest, in.		26.1	27.2	28.4	29.9	31.8	
50.1	53.3	56.5	61.8	68.7	74.7	79.6	Weight, kg	42.6	46.6	50.1	54.0	58.8	65.0	72.3
159.0	165.5	169.7	173.7	178.1	181.6	186.6	Height, cm	151.0	156.3	159.0	162.5	166.1	169.4	172.2
	26.1	26.9	27.8	28.7	29.9		Hips, cm		26.3	27.1	28.3	29.4	31.2	
	76.4	78.9	82.5	86.2	89.7		Chest, cm		66.4	69.2	72.1	75.9	80.9	
							17½ Years							
	118.8	125.8	137.6	153.6	166.8		Weight, lbs		103.2	110.8	119.5	130.2	143.9	
	65.3	67.0	68.5	70.3	71.6		Height, in.		61.5	62.6	64.0	65.4	66.7	
	10.3	10.6	11.0	11.3	11.8		Hips, in.		10.4	10.7	11.2	11.6	12.3	
	30.3	31.2	32.7	34.1	35.5		Chest, in.		26.2	27.3	28.4	29.9	31.9	
	53.9	57.1	62.4	69.7	75.7		Weight, kg		46.8	50.3	54.2	59.1	65.3	
	165.9	170.1	174.1	178.5	182.0		Height, cm		156.3	159.0	162.5	166.1	169.4	
	26.3	27.0	27.9	28.8	30.0		Hips, cm		26.4	27.2	28.4	29.5	31.3	
	77.0	79.4	83.0	86.7	90.2		Chest, cm		66.5	69.3	72.2	76.0	81.0	
							18 Years							
113.0	120.0	127.1	139.0	155.7	169.0	179.0	Weight, lbs	94.5	103.5	111.2	119.9	130.8	144.5	160.7
62.8	65.5	67.0	68.7	70.4	71.8	73.9	Height, in.	59.4	61.5	62.6	64.0	65.4	66.7	67.8
	10.4	10.7	11.0	11.4	11.8		Hips, in.		10.4	10.7	11.2	11.6	12.3	
	30.5	31.4	32.8	34.3	35.7		Chest, in.		26.2	27.3	28.5	30.0	31.9	
51.3	54.4	57.6	63.0	70.6	76.7	81.2	Weight, kg	42.9	46.9	50.4	54.4	59.3	65.5	72.9
159.6	166.3	170.5	174.5	178.9	182.4	187.6	Height, cm	151.0	156.3	159.0	162.5	166.1	169.4	172.2
	26.5	27.1	28.0	28.9	30.1		Hips, cm		26.4	27.2	28.4	29.5	31.3	
	77.5	79.8	83.4	87.1	90.7		Chest, cm		66.6	69.4	72.3	76.1	81.1	

Printed by permission of Paul A. Harper, *Preventive Pediatrics: Child Health and Development,* New York: Appleton-Century-Crofts, 1962, pp. 81–94.

Table 4-3 Normal Blood Pressure for Various Ages (Adapted from data in the literature)*

Age	Mean systolic ± 2 S.D.	Mean diastolic ± 2 S.D.
Newborn	80 ± 16	46 ± 16
6 months to 1 year	89 ± 29	60 ± 10†
1 year	96 ± 30	66 ± 25†
2 years	99 ± 25	64 ± 25†
3 years	100 ± 25	67 ± 23†
4 years	99 ± 20	65 ± 20†
5-6 years	94 ± 14	55 ± 9
6-7 years	100 ± 15	56 ± 8
7-8 years	102 ± 15	56 ± 8
8-9 years	105 ± 16	57 ± 9
9-10 years	107 ± 16	57 ± 9
10-11 years	111 ± 17	58 ± 10
11-12 years	113 ± 18	59 ± 10
12-13 years	115 ± 19	59 ± 10
13-14 years	118 ± 19	60 ± 10

* Figures have been rounded off to nearest decimal place.

† In this study the point of muffling was taken as the diastolic pressure.

Source: R. J. Haggerty, M. N. Maroney, and A. S. Nadas, "Essential Hypertension in Infancy and Childhood," *American Journal of Diseases of Children,* **92:** 535, 1956. With permission of the American Medical Association and W. B. Saunders.

in pediatrics as well as a wide variety of diagnostic tests used for evaluating children's development.

It is important to remember the limitations of screening tests. For example, the Denver Developmental Screening Test does not tell the examiner that the child has cerebral palsy, mental retardation, minimal brain damage, or any other syndrome, only that the child is slow in one of the four large areas sampled. Once this slowness is discovered, the examiner should take a more careful history; perform a more detailed physical examination, including a complete neurological examination; make special arrangements for any additional indicated tests; and get consultation for the child.

Selected Screening Devices

Several developmental tests are popular in pediatrics because they are simple to administer, inexpensive, easily scored, accurate, and reliable in isolating children who need further evaluation. The *Denver Developmental Screening Test* (DDST) was developed to screen young children for early detection of lags in developmental levels. Originally the test was standardized on 1,036 Denver children, and in 1971 it was restandardized on another 236 children (Frankenberg, 1971). A good correlation between specific sections of the DDST and related psychological tests has been shown. As a result of extensive research, the test forms and scoring have been revised several times.

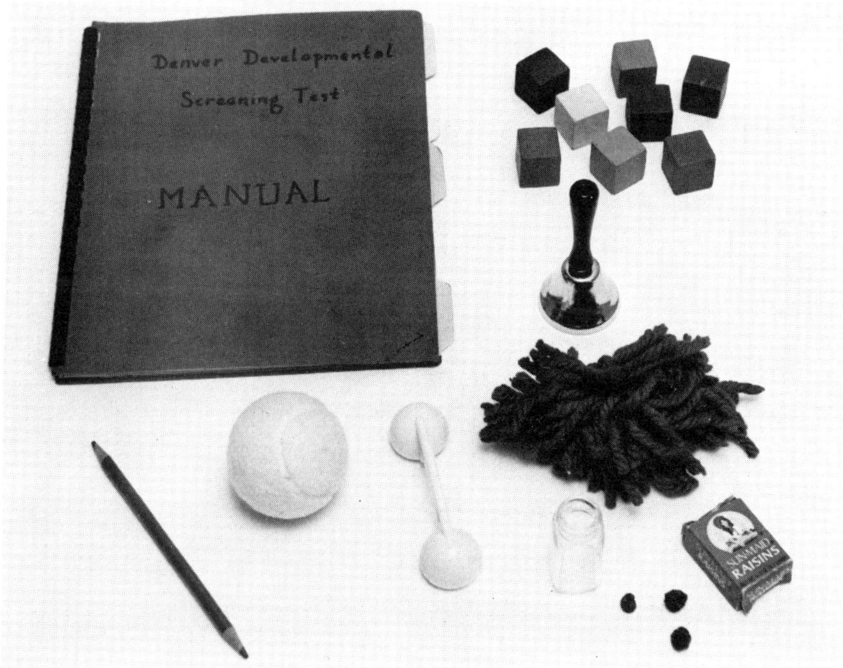

Figure 4-7 Materials used in the Denver Developmental Screening Test.

The original kit includes a tennis ball, eight colored blocks, a rattle, a bell, a pencil, a bottle, raisins, red wool, a pad of test forms, and a manual (see Fig. 4-7).

The test is divided into four large areas: personal-social, fine motor development, language, and gross motor development. Appropriate age levels from birth to 6 years are placed across the top and bottom of the score sheet, and the specific items to be tested are represented by horizontal bars below these age levels. Various points on the bar represent the ages at which 25, 50, 75, and 90 percent of the children pass that item. The area between the 75 and 90 percent is colored a solid blue to emphasize the skills which are particularly relevant to each age. All the bars are labeled with the item to be checked, e.g., "sits, looks for yarn," "hops on one foot," "walks well." If more explanation is needed to perform an activity, a small number appears to the left of the bar and the examiner can turn the form over for additional information. Since the test relies solely on the examiner's observations of the child and the mother's report, activities must be performed exactly as the instructional booklet describes. The examiner may not improvise by substituting a beach ball for the tennis ball or make up new prepositions or definitions. This kind of improvisation invalidates the test.

Before administering the test, it is important that the examiner explain to the mother than the DDST is not an IQ test, but only a developmental screening device to estimate the child's level of maturation in his use of muscles, language, and some social activities. The mother should also be warned that the examiner will be asking the child to perform some activities which are too advanced for his or her age and that the child will probably be unable to accomplish certain tasks.

The examiner, mother, and child should be seated comfortably at a desk or table. To help make the testing more pleasant, the DDST should be

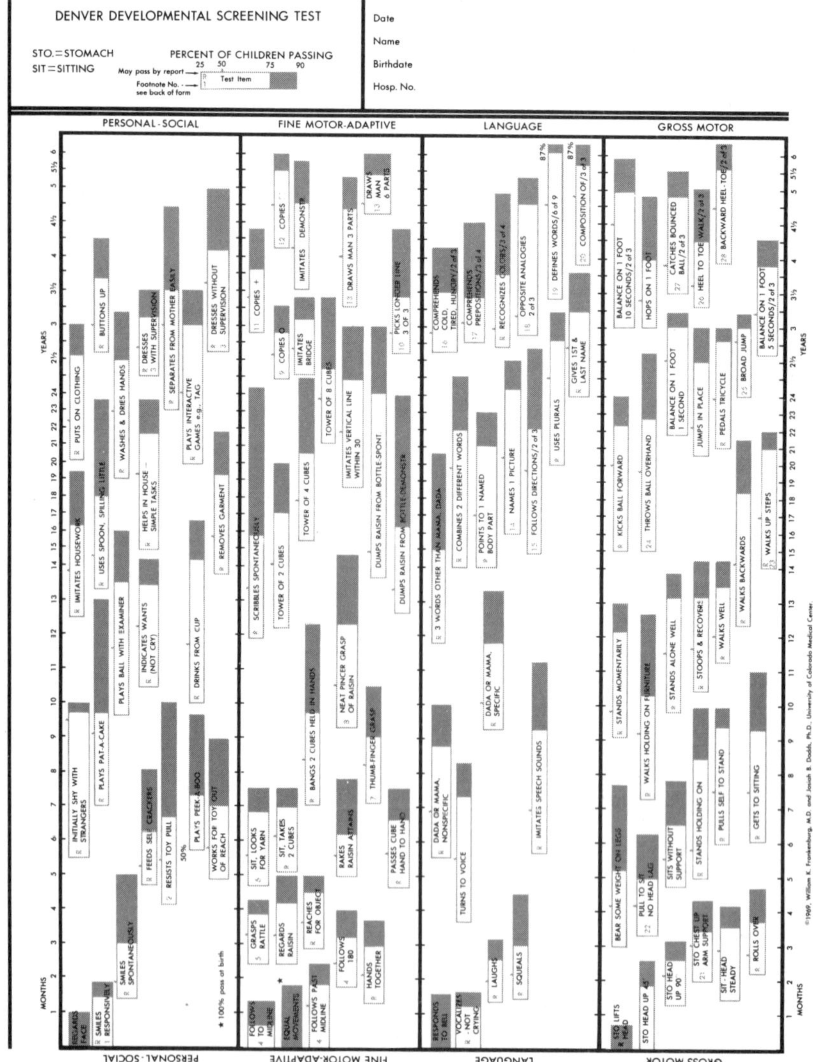

Figure 4-8 The Denver Developmental Screening Test. *(Source: Printed by permission of Dr. William Frankenburg.)*

administered before any painful procedures, such as shots or curetting. It is important to allow time for the child to relax in the examining room and grow accustomed to the examiner before the beginning of the exam. The examiner should start with some easy items so that the child begins with a feeling of success.

The examiner should begin by asking the child's birthday and calculating the age in months, days, and years. If the child was premature, the age is adjusted accordingly. The examiner locates the age across the top and bottom of the score sheet and draws a vertical line from top to bottom to represent the child's chronological age. All items crossing that line are ad-

1. Try to get child to smile by smiling, talking or waving to him. Do not touch him.
2. When child is playing with toy, pull it away from him. Pass if he resists.
3. Child does not have to be able to tie shoes or button in the back.
4. Move yarn slowly in an arc from one side to the other, about 6" above child's face. Pass if eyes follow 90° to midline. (Past midline; 180°)
5. Pass if child grasps rattle when it is touched to the backs or tips of fingers.
6. Pass if child continues to look where yarn disappeared or tries to see where it went. Yarn should be dropped quickly from sight from tester's hand without arm movement.
7. Pass if child picks up raisin with any part of thumb and a finger.
8. Pass if child picks up raisin with the ends of thumb and index finger using an over hand approach.

9. Pass any enclosed form. Fail continuous round motions.
10. Which line is longer? (Not bigger.) Turn paper upside down and repeat. (3/3 or 5/6)
11. Pass any crossing lines.
12. Have child copy first. If failed, demonstrate

When giving items 9, 11 and 12, do not name the forms. Do not demonstrate 9 and 11.

13. When scoring, each pair (2 arms, 2 legs, etc.) counts as one part.
14. Point to picture and have child name it. (No credit is given for sounds only.)

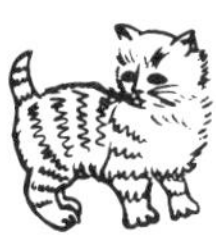
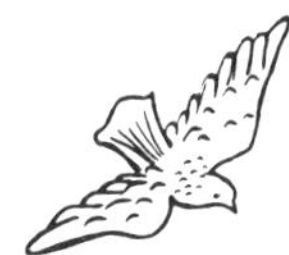
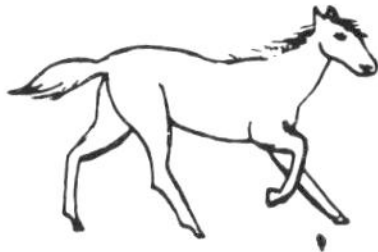
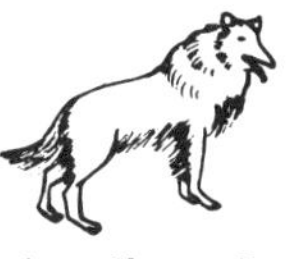
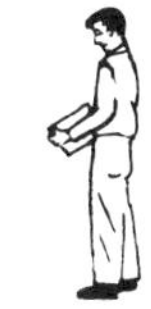

15. Tell child to: Give block to Mommie; put block on table; put block on floor. Pass 2 of 3. (Do not help child by pointing, moving head or eyes.)
16. Ask child: What do you do when you are cold? ..hungry? ..tired? Pass 2 of 3.
17. Tell child to: Put block <u>on</u> table; <u>under</u> table; <u>in front</u> of chair, <u>behind</u> chair. Pass 3 of 4. (Do not help child by pointing, moving head or eyes.)
18. Ask child: If fire is hot, ice is ?; Mother is a woman, Dad is a ?; a horse is big, a mouse is ?. Pass 2 of 3.
19. Ask child: What is a ball? ..lake? ..desk? ..house? ..banana? ..curtain? ..ceiling? ..hedge? ..pavement? Pass if defined in terms of use, shape, what it is made of or general category (such as banana is fruit, not just yellow). Pass 6 of 9.
20. Ask child: What is a spoon made of? ..a shoe made of? ..a door made of? (No other objects may be substituted.) Pass 3 of 3.
21. When placed on stomach, child lifts chest off table with support of forearms and/or hands.
22. When child is on back, grasp his hands and pull him to sitting. Pass if head does not hang back.
23. Child may use wall or rail only, not person. May not crawl.
24. Child must throw ball overhand 3 feet to within arm's reach of tester.
25. Child must perform standing broad jump over width of test sheet. (8-1/2 inches)
26. Tell child to walk forward, heel within 1 inch of toe. Tester may demonstrate. Child must walk 4 consecutive steps, 2 out of 3 trials.
27. Bounce ball to child who should stand 3 feet away from tester. Child must catch ball with hands, not arms, 2 out of 3 trials.
28. Tell child to walk backward, toe within 1 inch of heel. Tester may demonstrate. Child must walk 4 consecutive steps, 2 out of 3 trials.

<u>DATE AND BEHAVIORAL OBSERVATIONS</u> (how child feels at time of test, relation to tester, attention span, verbal behavior, self-confidence, etc,):

Figure 4-8 ***(Cont'd)***

ministered to the child. Items that do not have an R before them must be performed to the examiner's satisfaction. If the child refuses to do an activity, the examiner may request help from the mother by instructing her on the proper way to administer the test. If neither the examiner nor the mother can encourage the child to perform the activity, the examiner places an R (for "refuse") on the bar. As each item is administered, the examiner marks the bar with P (for "pass"), R, or F (for "fail") (see Fig. 4-8).

Once all the items have been administered, the examiner must interpret the results and give some explanation to the mother. There is some controversy over how much or how little to tell the mother. Some feel it is enough to say, "Your child has done well on the DDST." However, many mothers are more curious, and the DDST can provide an opportunity for helping the mother understand what tasks her child can or cannot perform at this age. For example, a 10-month-old who shows no thumb-finger grasp might benefit if the mother understood the child's readiness and began placing in front of him or her some small items (dry cereal, raisins, or small blocks) for practice in reaching and grasping.

With each standardization of the DDST the scoring and interpretation have been modified and redefined, and it is important that the examiner follow the directions found in the manual carefully.

The examiner must remember that the DDST is a standardized screening test and that if the results are to have any validity, the items must be done exactly as the test booklet dictates. For instance, it is not permissible to ask the child, "Which line is bigger?" instead of "Which line is longer?" or to substitute larger, plastic blocks for the set of small, wooden blocks. As the examiner becomes familiar with one age group, the test moves more smoothly and rapidly. However, when in doubt about administering the item or scoring a certain response, the examiner should consult the instruction booklet and follow the directions exactly.

The DDST can take from 5 minutes for an infant to 20 minutes for a 5-year-old, and if used properly, can give valuable information about the child's developmental level. It is well worth the examiner's time to become familiar with the test and proficient in administering it.

Another valuable screening tool for verbal intelligence is the *Peabody Picture Vocabulary Test.* It is to be used on individuals from 2½ years old to adulthood.

The test was standardized on 4,000 children ranging in age from 2½ to 18 years, and reliability was shown not only for children with normal intelligence but also for children with mental retardation, language difficulties, emotional problems, and motor disabilities. Validity was tested by comparison with the Stanford-Binet and Wechsler scales; correlations with these two tests were .50 and .71, respectively.

The original kit includes a booklet of pictures, manual of directions, and 50 scoring sheets (see Fig. 4-9). The test takes about 15 minutes to administer.

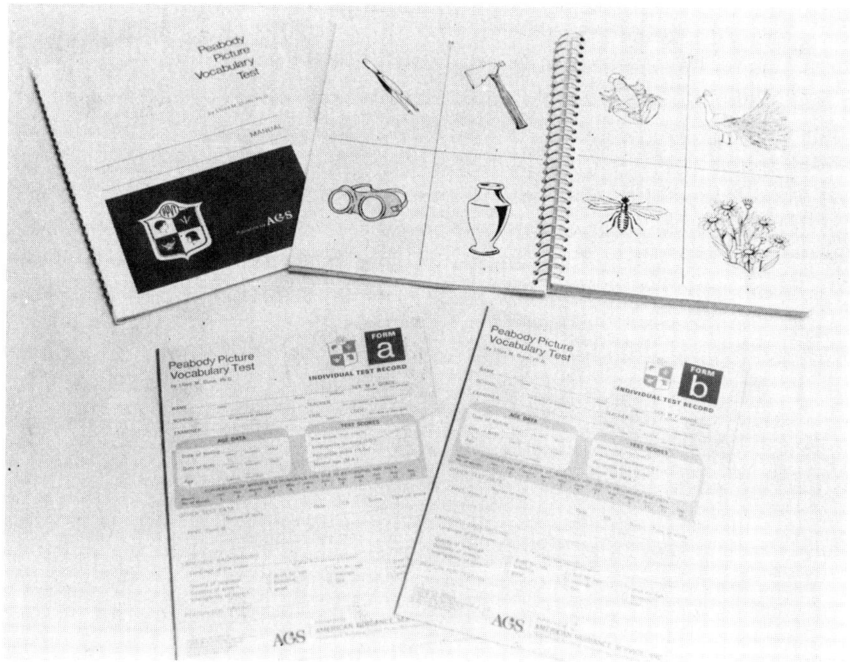

Figure 4-9 Materials used in the Peabody Picture Vocabulary Test.

The Peabody Picture Vocabulary Test is to be given on an individual basis (not to a classroom of children). The examiner and child should have a quiet room with a table and chairs. Past information needed includes the child's name, birthdate, date of testing, age, home language, and the reason for administering the test. The "Series of Plates" booklet is placed in front of the child. The score sheet contains a list of 150 words; however, the top of the score sheet suggests starting points for various age levels. For instance, a 3½-year-old child might be started at picture 15; the examiner would read the stimulus word "pulling," and ask the child to point to the picture best describing that word. The child should point to the picture of the girl pulling the wagon. The word stimulus becomes more difficult and less concrete as the test progresses. It is not a timed test; therefore children may take as long as they like to give an answer. However, after a minute it is wise to offer encouragement by saying, "Try one. Point to one of them." If the child first chooses one picture and then selects a different one, the final response is the one that counts.

The examiner keeps score of the correct and incorrect responses by recording the number of the response picture beside the correct answer and marking through the geometric symbols when an incorrect response is given. Pluses and minuses are not used since the child might interpret the results and thus become discouraged during the testing. The test is terminated when the child gives six incorrect responses to eight consecutive pictures (see Fig. 4-10).

The test manual is needed for the final scoring and interpretation of the examination. Once the child has established a base line for eight consecutive correct answers and a ceiling of six incorrect answers, the raw score is obtained by taking the ceiling item (the last word presented) and subtracting the number of incorrect responses. Thus, if item 49 was the last one presented and the child had 9 incorrect responses, the raw score is 40. The raw score is then located on tables in the manual to obtain the intelligence quotient, percentile score, and mental age. The final scores may then be interpreted according to classifications found in the manual.

Intelligence quotients	Percentage included	Classification
125 and above	5	Very rapid learners
110–124	20	Rapid learners
90–109	50	Average learners
75–89	20	Slow learners
Below 75	5	Very slow learners

Figure 4-10 The Peabody Picture Vocabulary Test. *(Source: Printed by permission of the American Guidance Service, Inc.)*

Plate No.	Word	Key Resp.	Errors*	Plate No.	Word	Key Resp.	Errors*	Plate No.	Word	Key Resp.	Errors*
1	car	(4)___	○	26	teacher	(2)___	♡	51	submarine	(4)___	□
2	cow	(3)___	□	27	building	(3)___	☆	52	thermos	(4)___	△
3	baby	(1)___	△	28	arrow	(3)___	◇	53	projector	(3)___	✙
4	girl	(2)___	✙	29	kangaroo	(2)___	○	54	group	(4)___	♡
5	ball	(1)___	♡	30	accident	(3)___	□	55	tackling	(3)___	☆
6	block	(3)___	☆	31	nest	(3)___	△	56	transportation	(1)___	◇
7	clown	(2)___	◇	32	caboose	(4)___	✙	57	counter	(1)___	○
8	key	(1)___	○	33	envelope	(1)___	♡	58	ceremony	(2)___	□
9	can	(4)___	□	34	picking	(2)___	☆	59	pod	(3)___	△
10	chicken	(2)___	△	35	badge	(1)___	◇	60	bronco	(4)___	✙
11	blowing	(4)___	✙	36	goggles	(3)___	○	61	directing	(3)___	♡
12	fan	(2)___	♡	37	peacock	(2)___	□	62	funnel	(4)___	☆
13	digging	(1)___	☆	38	queen	(3)___	△	63	delight	(2)___	◇
14	skirt	(1)___	◇	39	coach	(4)___	✙	64	lecturer	(3)___	○
15	catching	(4)___	○	40	whip	(1)___	♡	65	communication	(2)___	□
16	drum	(1)___	□	41	net	(4)___	☆	66	archer	(4)___	△
17	leaf	(3)___	△	42	freckle	(4)___	◇	67	stadium	(1)___	✙
18	tying	(4)___	✙	43	eagle	(3)___	○	68	excavate	(1)___	♡
19	fence	(1)___	♡	44	twist	(2)___	□	69	assaulting	(4)___	☆
20	bat	(2)___	☆	45	shining	(4)___	△	70	stunt	(1)___	◇
21	bee	(4)___	◇	46	dial	(2)___	✙	71	meringue	(1)___	○
22	bush	(3)___	○	47	yawning	(2)___	♡	72	appliance	(3)___	□
23	pouring	(1)___	□	48	tumble	(2)___	☆	73	chemist	(4)___	△
24	sewing	(1)___	△	49	signal	(1)___	◇	74	arctic	(3)___	✙
25	wiener	(4)___	✙	50	capsule	(1)___	○	75	destruction	(4)___	♡

The Peabody Picture Vocabulary Test is useful for school nurses evaluating school-age children, as well as for nurses in ambulatory clinics who can incorporate this tool into their routine assessment of children over 2 years of age.

Another popular screening tool is the *Developmental Test of Visual-Motor Integration,* also known as the Beery or VMI, which is designed to assess the visual perception and motor behavior of children between the ages of 2 and 15 years. It is generally given to preschoolers and early schoolagers. The test has been standardized and its validity compared with that of similar tests; correlations with these tests have averaged around .89.

The original kit includes a manual, a package of test booklets, and score sheets; the examiner provides pencils (see Fig. 4-11). The test takes about 20 minutes to administer.

The test booklet consists of nine pages of drawings; each page contains six squares with designs drawn in the top three. Children should be seated comfortably at a table and the test booklet and pencil placed in front of them. They are then directed to copy each of the designs on that page. They may not repeat the form or erase their original work. Only one trial is allowed for each design. Children are asked, "Can you make one like that?" while the examiner points to the first design. The examiner must not trace the design or give it a name. If children understand the task, they are al-

Plate No.	Word	Key	Resp.	Errors*
76	porter	(3)	___	☆
77	coast	(2)	___	◇
78	hoisting	(4)	___	○
79	wailing	(1)	___	□
80	coil	(2)	___	△
81	kayak	(3)	___	✥
82	sentry	(2)	___	♡
83	furrow	(4)	___	☆
84	beam	(1)	___	◇
85	fragment	(3)	___	○
86	hovering	(2)	___	□
87	bereavement	(3)	___	△
88	crag	(4)	___	✥
89	tantrum	(2)	___	♡
90	submerge	(1)	___	☆
91	descend	(3)	___	◇
92	hassock	(2)	___	○
93	canine	(1)	___	□
94	probing	(1)	___	△
95	angling	(1)	___	✥
96	appraising	(3)	___	♡
97	confining	(4)	___	☆
98	precipitation	(4)	___	◇
99	gable	(1)	___	○
100	amphibian	(1)	___	□
101	graduated	(3)	___	△
102	hieroglyphic	(2)	___	✥
103	orate	(1)	___	♡
104	cascade	(3)	___	☆
105	illumination	(4)	___	◇
106	nape	(1)	___	○
107	genealogist	(2)	___	□
108	embossed	(2)	___	△
109	mercantile	(4)	___	✥
110	encumbered	(2)	___	♡
111	entice	(4)	___	☆
112	concentric	(3)	___	◇
113	vitreous	(3)	___	○
114	sibling	(1)	___	□
115	machete	(2)	___	△
116	waif	(4)	___	✥
117	cornice	(1)	___	♡
118	timorous	(3)	___	☆
119	fettered	(1)	___	◇
120	tartan	(2)	___	○
121	sulky	(3)	___	□
122	obelisk	(4)	___	△
123	ellipse	(2)	___	✥
124	entomology	(2)	___	♡
125	bumptious	(4)	___	☆
126	dormer	(2)	___	◇
127	coniferous	(2)	___	○
128	consternation	(4)	___	□
129	obese	(3)	___	△
130	gauntlet	(4)	___	✥
131	inclement	(1)	___	♡
132	cupola	(1)	___	☆
133	obliterate	(2)	___	◇
134	burnishing	(3)	___	○
135	bovine	(1)	___	□
136	eminence	(4)	___	△
137	legume	(3)	___	✥
138	senile	(4)	___	♡
139	deleterious	(2)	___	☆
140	raze	(4)	___	◇
141	ambulation	(2)	___	○
142	cravat	(1)	___	□
143	impale	(2)	___	△
144	marsupial	(4)	___	✥
145	predatory	(3)	___	♡
146	incertitude	(1)	___	☆
147	imbibe	(2)	___	◇
148	homunculus	(3)	___	○
149	cryptogam	(4)	___	□
150	pensile	(3)	___	△

No.	Form	Pass or Fail (P-F)	Observations and Comments	No.	Form	Pass or Fail (P-F)	Observations and Comments
1				13			
2				14			
3				15			
4				16			
5				17			
6				18			
7				19			
8				20			
9				21			
10				22			
11				23			
12				24			

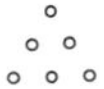

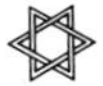

Figure 4-11 The Beery test score sheets. *(Source: Printed by permission of the Follett Educational Corporation.)*

lowed to work on each form until they fail three consecutive designs. If children do not understand the instructions after the first design, the examiner may continue to ask, "Can you make one like that?" and point to each following design. Children should begin with the simple designs and work toward the difficult ones. Although the test is not timed, children should not be allowed to struggle too long over any one design, but should be encouraged to move on.

The test is interpreted by following the criteria set up for each design in the instruction manual. To obtain a valid score, the criteria must be followed exactly; the test booklet should be examined with the individual score criteria and each form passed or failed accordingly. A raw score is calculated by adding all the correct answers up to the three failed designs. The manual provides a table to find the age equivalent score from the raw score. By comparing the child's age equivalent score with his chronological age and by observing the child during the examination, the examiner can assess the child's visual-motor behaviors.

These are three of the most widely used screening tools available today. Additional tools are continually being developed; it is important that the examiner regularly evaluate newer, more refined devices as they become available.

Additional Developmental Tests

While the previously discussed tests can easily be used as screening tests and given in a relatively short period of time, the nurse may need more information about a particular child or may be doing more sophisticated screening on a smaller number of children. The following developmental tests are not screening tools in the usual sense, but within special situations one or two of them might be utilized in such a manner. There are a great many such developmental tests, and the following is only a sampling of some of the more frequently used ones. Only the briefest description is given here. For more detail or for information on the many other tests available, the reader is referred to the bibliography at the end of this chapter. If the nurse needs to become proficient at administering one of these tests, she should seek out the nearest testing center and ask for a demonstration and help in learning the specific test. Scoring will be mentioned, but due to the wide range of interpretation the nurse must be careful in reaching decisions of normality or abnormality.

The *Bender Visual-Motor Gestalt Test* tests perceptual ability and spatial relationships of individuals between the ages of 4 and adulthood. The early standardization included only 474 adults between the ages of 15 and 50 years. Only as recently as 1964 was the test standardized on children. Over the years many modifications of the test have been made. Presently the test consists of a series of nine designs which the child is asked to copy. The test kit includes a design booklet, paper, pencil, manual, and score sheets. Generally it takes 10 to 15 minutes for the child to be shown the designs and copy them. From the nine designs, 105 items are scored, and the score is compared with scales provided in the manual.

The *California First-Year Mental Scale,* also known as the Bayley mental scales, tests infants between the ages of 1 and 18 months. The early standardization was on 54 middle-class children between the ages of 1 and 21 months. The test is divided into several sections: postural development, motor development, perception, attention span to objects and humans, language, object manipulation, understanding commands, and problem solving. Many of the tasks are taken from the Gesell scales. Once a raw score is obtained, the test provides an estimated mental age.

One of the more popular infant tests is the *Cattell Infant Intelligence Scale.* It is used on children between the ages of 3 months and 2½ years to determine their intelligence quotient. Many standardizations have been done, but the original covered 274 children in a longitudinal study with 1,346 actual tests given. It was found to have very high correlations with other tests on children after the 9th month of age. Items were picked from other tests to provide a continuity between tests for very young infants and tests for the older child. All the items are grouped by age, and each age is tested in five areas. The test includes material such as rattles, a toy, a cup, cubes, a spoon, peg board, paper and pencil, picture cards, an instruction manual, and score sheets. The child is placed in a high chair or on the mother's lap or examining table. The examiner places certain objects in front of the child and asks for certain responses, either motor or verbal. Usually the test takes around 20 to 30 minutes. Scoring is done by placing a plus or minus beside each task on the score sheet and adding all pluses to find the raw score, which is applied to a formula to obtain the basal age, mental age, and intelligence quotient of the child.

The *Developmental Screening Inventory for Infants* (DSI) is used on infants between the ages of 4 weeks and 18 months. The test is taken from Gesell and is divided into categories of adaptive behavior, language, personal-social tasks, and gross and fine motor behavior. Materials for the test include a cup, embroidery hoop, bottle, round candies, picture book, crayon, paper, and blocks. The infant is placed on the examining table or sits on the mother's lap while different objects are presented; the examiner observes for specific responses. Scoring is separate for each category tested.

The *Full-Range Picture Vocabulary Test,* or Ammons vocabulary test, tests for daily, used vocabulary. It was set up to test children between the ages of 2 and 17 years and standardized on 589 children within that age range. Validity was tested by a comparison with the Stanford-Binet test. Materials include a series of 16 drawings, an instruction manual, and score sheets. The test comes with two forms, each containing 85 words. As the examiner pronounces the word, the child must point to the drawing best describing the word; the entire test takes from 10 to 15 minutes. Scoring is based on the norms given in the instructional manual.

One of the most familiar tests is the *Gesell Developmental Schedules.* Originally it was standardized on 107 children, and there has been much controversy over the small sample, the economic status of the children (all middle class), and the low correlations with standard IQ tests. Standardization continues, and it is still a widely used and imitated test. There are two forms: the infant schedule and the preschool schedule. The infant schedule tests the child from 4 weeks to 1 year of age and is divided into four large areas: motor, adaptive, language, and personal-social. The preschool schedule tests the child from 15 months to 6 years and has the same categories. Kits for both tests include a baby ring, blocks, bottle and pellet, book, cup, paper, pencil, picture cards, ball, instruction booklet, and score sheets. Much of the examination depends on the observations of the tester. With infants, the examiner simply places the baby on the examining table or mother's lap, presents certain items, and watches the response. With older children, the examiner may show certain items or ask for certain tasks and the child responds or performs appropriately. As each task is completed, the examiner assigns a plus for correct and a minus for incorrect responses. The final raw score is applied to an algebraic formula to obtain percentile and rank.

The *Goodenough-Harris Drawing Test* may be used for children between the ages of 3 and 15 years to assess intelligence and personality traits. In 1950 it was standardized on 2,975 children across the United States. Materials are simple, with only a test booklet, pencil, and instruction manual. The test is not timed, but generally takes around 15 minutes and may be given individually or in groups. Older children may fill in their own background information (name, sex, date, grade, age, birth date, father's occupation). Children are told to draw three pictures in the spaces provided: a man, a woman, and a self-portrait. Younger children may need a rest period between pictures. Using the manual, the examiner scores each individual figure according to specific standards supplied in the manual. Specific items on the figure are given a score of 1 if drawn according to specification; the raw score is applied to a formula to obtain a standard score and percentile.

The *Illinois Test of Psycholinguistic Abilities* (ITPA) was developed to test language development in children between the ages of 2½ and 9 years. It was standardized on 700 children within the age range of the test. The test is divided into nine large areas: automatic auditory-vocal, visual decoding, motor encoding, visual-motor sequencing, auditory-vocal association, vocal encoding, auditory-vocal sequencing, visual-motor association, and auditory decoding. Materials include an instructional manual, test sheets, and certain objects (cup, ball, block, etc.), and a picture book. The ITPA can be given only individually. The examiner follows instructions in showing the child certain objects or pictures and asking for specific responses. The raw scores of each section are converted into profile scores and plotted on a percentile graph.

The *Marianne Frostig Developmental Test of Visual Perception,* called simply Frostig, is used with children between the ages of 3 and 8 years to isolate perceptual problems. Standardization began on 1,800 schoolchildren between the ages of 5 and 9 years and continues today. Studies show a reliability of .80 on a test-and-retest basis. A validity of .44 to .50 is found if the scores are compared with teacher ratings; a somewhat lower validity (.32 to .40) appears when scores are compared with scores from the Goodenough-Draw-a-Man Test. There is still much controversy over the standardization.

The test is divided into six large areas: eye-hand coordination, figure-ground discrimination, constancy, spatial position, spatial relations, and a total score called a *perceptual quotient.* Materials include demonstration cards, instructional manual, score sheets, and administration sheets. The test is not timed, but generally requires 30 to 45 minutes. The child should be comfortably seated at a desk or table and given a pencil and the administration sheets. The examiner introduces each section of the demonstration cards and gives instructions. The child is asked to accomplish certain tasks such as drawing lines between two boundaries or connecting dots on the page. The raw score is obtained by using the booklet, which gives the criteria for each task. The perceptual quotient and perceptual age are obtained from the raw score.

The *Minnesota Preschool Scale* is used to test the nonverbal, verbal, and intelligence quotient of children between the ages of 3 and 6 years. It was standardized on 900 children, and when the two forms of the test were given 1 week apart, the reliability ranged from .68 to .94. Equipment for the test includes test cards, a large doll, a small doll, a cup, a large ball, a small ball, a watch, scissors, pencils, paper, 12 cubes, secured and loose cubes, a key, a penny, cardboard, and a cardboard clock. The child is presented with one of the test items at a time and asked certain questions, such as: "What is this?" A raw score is obtained by adding the number of correct answers in the verbal and nonverbal sections and applying this to a formula to get the percentile placement and intelligent quotient equivalent. This test is not widely used because of the age limitations.

The *Oseretsky Tests of Motor Proficiency* may be used on children between the ages of 5 and 16 years to assess general coordination, hand coordination, speed, voluntary movements and synkinesia. The equipment includes wooden boxes, 20 pennies, paper, wooden spool, 40 match sticks, a rubber ball, a block of wood, a 6-ft-long rope, ruled paper, a wooden hammer, 2 mazes, 36 playing cards, a matchbox, a book, pencils, a wooden sieve, a wooden stick, a stop watch, an instruction booklet, and score forms. It is a timed test. As the child performs the tasks, the examiner puts a plus beside the items correctly done and a minus beside the incorrect responses. If the task requires both hands or feet and the child uses only one, a score of half is given. As with all tests, it is best to begin with tasks that the child can easily do. Items are given until the child fails all the items within one grouping. The raw score is applied to a formula to obtain the mental level and the motor level.

The *Piaget Right-Left Awareness Test* was developed to test handedness of schoolchildren between the ages of 5 and 11 years. It is a simple test in which children are given several verbal commands requiring them to differentiate between their right and left hands. The examiner sits opposite the child and says, "Show me your right hand," or shows the child several objects and asks the child on which side each object is placed. Equipment needed includes a coin, pencil, bracelet, and key. The raw score of the items passed is applied to a grid for appropriate ages for each task.

The *Preschool Inventory* is a simple screening tool to give information on children between the ages of 3 and 6 years and predict that child's probability of success in school. It was standardized on 389 children. Besides the instruction manual and score sheets, the examiner needs three small colored cars, eight large crayons, a box of checkers, and three cardboard boxes. The test is timed. The examiner asks the child to perform certain tasks described in the manual. As the child accomplishes each task, the examiner scores the correct answers. A total raw score of 64 points can be accrued and is converted to a percentile by following instructions in the manual.

The *Preschool Readiness Experimental Screening Scale* (Press) was developed to assess the level of maturation of children between the ages of 4 and 5 years. Although standardization is still inadequate, preliminary findings on 75 children indicate high reliability. Validity has been tested by a comparison with the Slossen Intelligence Test; it, too, appears good. Minimum equipment is needed: the instruction manual, score sheets, tongue blades, paper, and pencil. The test is divided into five large categories (introduction, colors, numbers, general, and drawing), with three questions in each category. The test can be administered during the physical examination of the child or done separately. Either way, it takes about 2 to 3 minutes. The child is simply asked a list of questions, some requiring a verbal response and some a motor response. Scoring is kept simple and ranges from 0 to 10.

A very familiar intelligence quotient test is the *Stanford-Binet Scales.* Originally the Stanford-Binet was standardized on 1,500 school and preschool children. Over the years the standardization has continued, and additional studies now include over 3,000 subjects tested. The test may be used on individuals from 2 years to adulthood. Originally there were two forms, but recently these have been combined into one form. The test is divided into age levels and several categories: visual perception, visual imagery, visual memory, thinking, memory and attention, abstractions, reasoning, vocabulary, and concepts. Materials include a set of toys (doll, car, scissors, utensils, doll chair, etc.), a test booklet, and score sheets. To administer the test to younger children takes between 40 and 50 minutes, while testing older children and adults may take as long as 60 to 70 minutes. Initial items are chosen slightly below the child's expected level to give a feeling of success. All the items in all the areas are given until the child reaches a ceiling level. As the child responds to the requests, the examiner assigns a plus for correct answers and a minus for incorrect items. It is expected that the child will have a scattering of scores in several different areas. The raw score is applied to a formula to obtain the child's mental age and intelligence quotient.

The *Vineland Social Maturity Scale* is used on individuals from 1 year to adulthood; it assesses the person's independence and self-reliance. Originally it was standardized on 620 children. Test items are arranged according to age and fall into eight categories: general self-help, self-help in eating, self-help in dressing, self-direction, occupation, communication, locomotion, and socialization. Test materials include the instruction booklet and score sheets. The individuals being tested do not have to be present as long as representatives who know them well answer the questions being asked. Scoring is a complicated process of graduation from "absolutely can do" to "positively cannot do," including "beginning skill," "no opportunity," etc. Each score is given a credit; the total score is converted into a raw score and finally into percentiles and age value.

The *Wechsler Intelligence Scale for Children* (WISC) includes three scales: the WPPSI scale for children from 4 to 6½ years, the WISC scale for children from 7 to 10 years, and the WAIS scale for anyone over 16 years of age. Earlier forms of the test have been standardized. Test materials include the manual, test items, and test score sheets. Generally the test takes one hour to administer, and it should be given individually. The test is divided into two sections. The verbal section includes information, comprehension, arithmetic, similarities, and vocabulary. The performance section includes block design, picture completion, picture arrangement, object assembly, mazes, and coding. The examiner administers each subtest as quickly as the child can respond. Additional information on items or explanation can be asked for if the examiner does not understand the subject's first answer. Scoring is difficult, since the answers are scored not only for correctness but for surrounding responses, e.g., slowness, compulsiveness, lack of organization. The final score gives the child's intelligence quotient.

There are, of course, many more developmental tests available than those listed in this chapter, but this list should give the reader some idea of the wide range of development that can be tested. This list also skips the many fine guides that have been developed to help the examiner look at the child, such as the Yale Developmental Screening tool or the Washington Guide to Promoting Development in the Young Child. Both of these guides take items from standardized tests, but are not standardized themselves as tests. They can, however, give the observer a good deal more organized, detailed information about a child than unplanned, spontaneous observation. Some of the standardized developmental tests mentioned in the chapter are much better than others, and some are more specific than others; the nurse will soon learn her own preference.

VISION TESTING

Vision screening is an extremely important part of the care of children of all ages. Difficulty with vision is both a common and a serious condition. If a child's vision has always been poor or if it has become poor gradually, the child is likely to be unaware that a problem exists. Unless the defect is rather severe, the parents will probably be unaware of it also. Although it is easy to tell if a child is suffering from a very severe degree of poor vision, it is quite difficult to pick up less incapacitating, yet important losses. Preschoolers who have some lessened degree of visual acuity will miss out on many of the experiences that are important in their perceptual and cognitive development. Their eye-hand coordination may be poor; they may not learn to distinguish important aspects of pictures that should lay the foundation for later reading ability. Schoolchildren who cannot see well are missing important parts of their education that they may never be able to make up. Therefore, detecting visual problems is important because of the significance to the individual child and because of the large numbers of children who have such problems. Vision impairment is the fourth most common disability in the United States; it is the leading cause of handicapping conditions in childhood (Krupke et al., 1970). From 5 to 10 percent of the preschoolers in this country have vision problems, while 20 to 30 percent of the school-age children have such problems (Green and Richmond, 1962). Many of these problems are not being currently detected. This is particularly true of the preschool group, in which only 2 percent receive any type of vision examination (Lippman, 1971). The importance of such screening is clear from the fact that although 7½ million schoolchildren suffer from some type of visual difficulty, only one-fourth of these will manifest symptoms (Lippman, 1971). The other three-fourths would never be found without some type of visual examination. The fact that many of these children never are found is evident from the report of Armed Forces rejections in 1964–1965. Of those individuals who were rejected for eye defects, 75 percent had defects that could have been prevented or treated in childhood (Krupke, 1970). Certainly the most dramatic case is that of the child with a minor degree of crossed eyes; if the defect is caught early, the child can have perfect vision for life, but if it is missed, the child may totally lose the vision in one eye by school age. This is certainly a pressing reason for regular vision screening of preschoolers.

Vision is not only very important but also a very complicated function. It deserves careful evaluation at each well-child visit. A thorough history and careful observation are necessary. Methods of screening the six most important aspects of vision will be discussed in this chapter: visual acuity, farsightedness, nearpoint vision, heterophoria, color vision, and visual fields. These will be discussed with regard to methods now available for evaluation at various age levels. First, however, it is important to be aware of some general eye-related complaints that may indicate visual difficulties. Any child who seems to be either inattentive or excessively attentive to visual clues should be suspected of having visual problems. Such children may contort their face, squint their eyes, close one eye, cock their head or thrust it forward, or hold their body tensely while looking at things in the distance. Children who frequently try to brush things away from their eyes or who rub their eyes excessively (some of these children will have recurrent styes as a result) should be examined carefully. A physical finding or history of permanently or transiently crossed eyes demands ophthalmological consultation. Children should be asked whether they can see the blackboard, and they should be observed while reading from the blackboard as well as reading from books. Sitting very close to the television set may be an indication of visual problems although many children with adequate vision seem to do this from habit. At any rate, a careful physical examination and thorough history should accompany visual testing to discover possible eye problems.

Visual Acuity

Visual acuity is arbitrarily defined as the ability to see a standardized symbol at a standardized distance. Classically, this refers to a Snellen "E" or alphabet chart seen at 20 feet. The Snellen alphabet chart is by far the most accurate and should be used whenever possible. Generally it can be used with children above the third grade. It is important that the test be given accurately. Some charts are available which provide adequate illumination, but most charts come without lighting, and the lighting should be tested with a light meter. The light should fall evenly across the chart without shadows or glare and should measure between 10 and 30 footcandles. If lighting in the area is inadequate, it can be supplied by a 75-watt bulb in a gooseneck lamp, situated 5 ft away at a 45° angle. It is important to test children individually so that they cannot memorize the chart while waiting in line. One examiner should be stationed at the chart and one with the child. The examiner usually begins with the 20/30 or 20/40 line and works either up or down depending on how well the child does. Each child should be tested as far down the chart as he or she is able to read. A passing score on a line consists of reading the *majority* of letters on that line; this will differ from line to line since the lines vary in length. It is important to expose the entire line at once rather than a single letter at a time for this age group, since some authorities feel (e.g., Sheridan, 1970) that exposing one letter at a time may allow certain children with amblyopia to be missed. Vision tested by the single-letter method can be as much as 1½ lines better than that tested by exposure of the whole line. The vision of both eyes together will never be poorer than that of either eye singly; for this reason, most authorities suggest not beginning the test with both eyes (it may be necessary with younger children in order to accustom them to the test). Some (e.g., Lippman, 1970), however, do suggest beginning the test with both eyes uncovered, since this may reveal a tropia. If a near and far cover test is done, however (as it should always be), a tropia will be seen anyway. Children should be able to read the 20/20 line by the fourth grade; any who are unable to read this line with either eye should be referred for further examination. Children from the age of 4 years through the third grade, should be able to read the 20/30 line accurately with both eyes, and children younger than this are expected to read the 20/40 line. These standards differ from those available 10 years ago; it has been shown that children's vision is much better than once believed. Any children who do not read the line appropriate for their age with each eye should be referred; furthermore, any children who show a two-line difference between eyes, even though the worst eye is seeing at a level appropriate for the child's age (for instance, a 3-year-old who has 20/20 vision in one eye and 20/40 in the other), should also be referred, since this difference may result in the child suppressing the vision in the poorer eye and eventually losing it completely. For this reason, all children should be tested as far down the chart as they are able to see.

If the building in which the testing is being done does not have a space long enough to utilize the 20-ft chart, two alternatives exist. The Snellen chart is made in a 10-ft version which, though less desirable since it has been less thoroughly standardized, is generally quite adequate. A second possibility is to use the 20-ft chart with a mirror. In this situation, the examiner sits next to the child with the 20-ft chart between them. Both the examiner and the child look directly into a mirror 10 ft in front of them in which they can see each other and the chart. This arrangement has certain advantages; only one examiner is necessary, and she can remain close to the child, helping to maintain rapport. If an alphabet chart is used, it must be one specially constructed for use with a mirror; that is, the letters are printed backward so that they appear normally oriented to the child looking in the mirror.

For children who are too young to utilize an alphabet chart, the next best standardized chart is the Snellen E, sometimes called the illiterate E since it does not require knowledge of letters (see Fig. 4-12). Some feel that this is slightly less good, since no curves or complicated letters are used which might detect certain forms of astigmatism. Nonetheless in practice it is almost as good as the alphabet chart. Most E charts have the letter E oriented in four directions: up, down, right, and left. This is important since oblique angles are usually too developmentally advanced for the age of the child who must use the E chart. The mechanics of testing with the E chart are basically the same as those for the alphabet chart. There are some problems, however, usually related to the age group with which this chart is used. One is that certain preschool children are still having difficulties with directionality. Children are generally asked to point a finger, hand, or entire arm in the direction which the E is pointing (or in which the "legs of the table" are pointing). This requires them not only to see the letter, but also to comprehend the idea of direction, to match this direction to the direction of their hand, and to be reasonably agile in making their hand or arm conform to the direction in their mind. In other words, this tests not only vision, but several other complicated skills; when children give an incorrect answer, it is difficult to be sure that it is their vision that is at fault. There are several approaches to this problem. One is to paste colorful, easily recognized pictures (e.g., a dog, a rabbit, a boy, and a girl) on the wall above, below, and at each side of the chart and then ask the child to say which picture the E is pointing to. This, at least eliminates the difficulty in motor maneuvering and in mentally matching the direction of the letter to the direction of an arm or hand. It does not eliminate the basic problem with directionality, however. Another very helpful step is to ask mother to practice with the child at home the week before the test. This considerably increases the rate of testability. The National Society for the Prevention of Blindness has printed forms of the E chart for use in testing children at home (see Fig. 4-13) which can be sent home the week before the examination. In a clinic situation, it might be wise to institute a system where such a chart with an explanatory letter is automatically sent to the home of children from about 3 years of age on up. Practice in using the chart can also be given in a classroom setting by the teacher or nurse and is sometimes more effective than individual practice. The other difficulty in testing preschool children is the difficulty of gaining rapport. The mirror method described above is particularly helpful in this

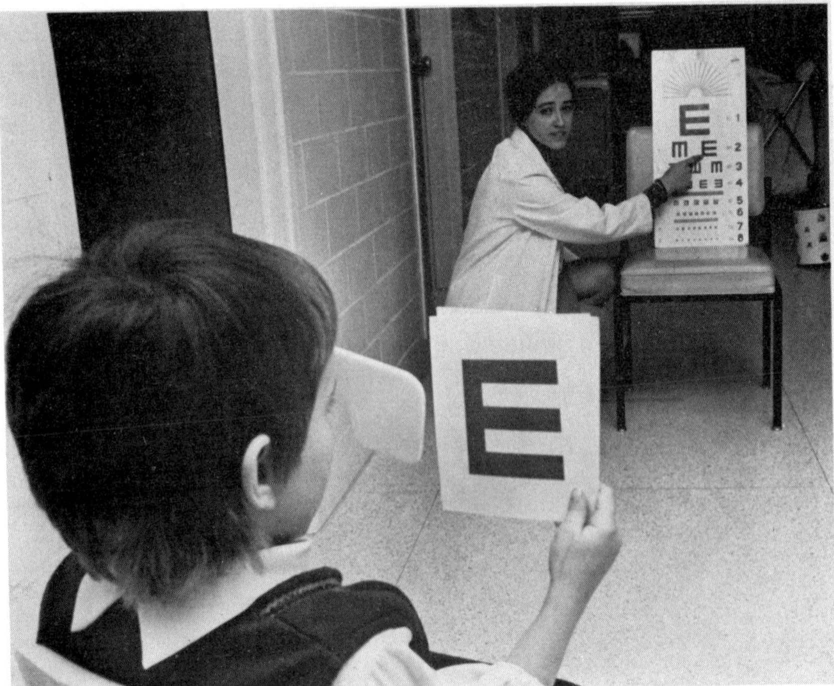

Figure 4-12 Child being tested with the E chart.

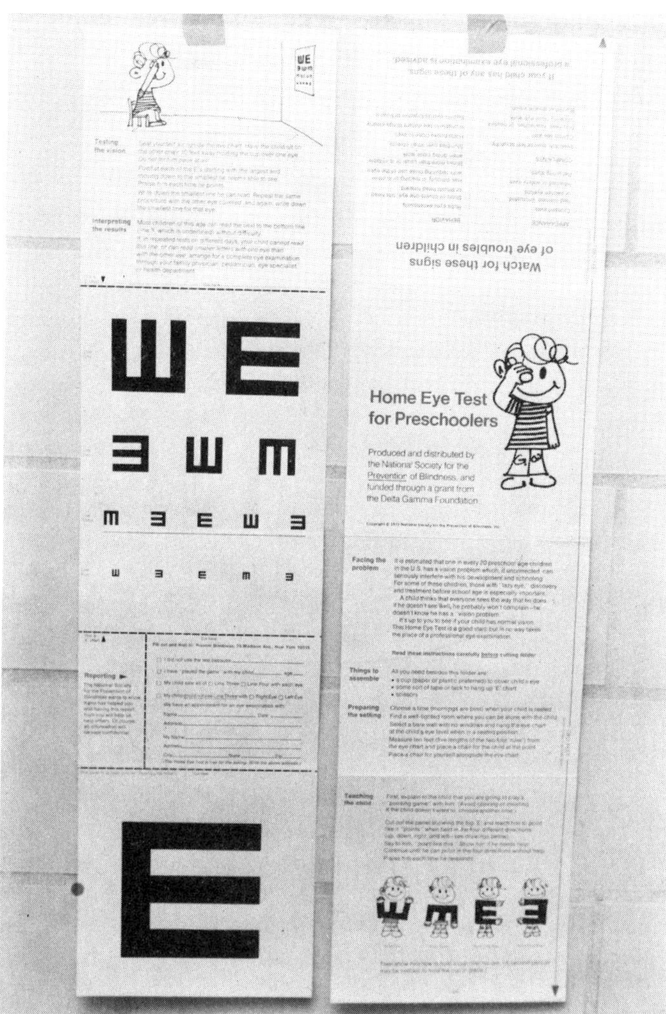

Figure 4-13 E chart for home testing.

situation. Children this age may also have difficulty in looking at one letter at a time. For this reason, the National Society for the Prevention of Blindness suggests that single-letter exposure may be used for children below kindergarten. As note earlier, some authorities disagree, saying this may mask amblyopia. It is important that the nurse record which method was used in testing.

Because the two Snellen charts are the best standardized, it is important to use them if at all possible; the accuracy of the results justify the extra time involved in having the child practice with the mother or in setting up a mirror arrangement or in any other measures that may be useful. If it is impossible to use the Snellen charts, however, the next best tests are those which utilize certain figures from the Snellen. The Landholt rings chart is exactly the same as the illiterate E chart, but uses the letter C instead. The same problems are inherent in it—the problem of directionality and the difficulty in keeping the child's interest and the authors have found no advantage in it. The Ffooks chart is similar but utilizes a square, circle, and triangle (because these figures are developmentally recognized first). Since they are not the exact letters of the Snellen, their standardization is less accurate. By far the best test the authors have found for younger children is the Stycar test. This test is available in several forms. All forms have letters selected from the standardized Snellen which are recognized at a developmentally early stage. After working with several thousand young children, Mary Sheridan isolated V, A, T, C, O, L, H, U, and X as the most easily recognized letters. The Stycar chart is similar to the Snellen alphabet chart but uses only these letters. Since children are not yet able to name the letters, they are given a card with the nine letters on it. They merely point to the letter which matches the letter being pointed to on the chart. For younger children, the test uses fewer letters: for the 4-year-old, seven letters are used; for the 3-year-old, five letters are used; and for the 2-year-old, only four letters are used. Only a single letter is shown at a time to younger children. This, of course, has the disadvantage of single-letter testing discussed above. Sheridan also suggests that the test be given at 10 ft with the use of a mirror. It has been found that 100 percent of the 4-year-olds are testable with the seven-letter method, 80 percent of the 3-year-olds are testable with the five-letter method, and 30 percent of the 2-year-olds can be tested using four letters. These are extraordinarily high rates of testability for these age groups. Lippman (1970), who compared the E test at 20 ft, the E test at 10 ft, the Allen cards (to be discussed later), the Stycar test, and the Starcar test (to be discussed later), determined that children found the Stycar easiest to learn, that it was highly accurate, and that testability became much higher with the Stycar on the second attempt than it did with the test at 10 ft although they were similar on the first attempt. It seems unfortunate that such a useful test as this is not more widely used in the United States.

If none of the more standardized tests (i.e., the Snellen alphabet, E, Landholt rings, or Stycar) can be used with a child, the next choice is one of the picture charts. These are far less standardized, and therefore far less accurate, and it should seldom be necessary to use them. Not only are they less standardized, but most of them are difficult to use because of the child's lack of familiarity with the pictures used. In Lippman's study (1970) it was found that testability rates are one-third lower with children from lower economic groups than rates from higher economic groups; the pictures used are generally of things a middle-class child rather than lower-class child would be familiar with. Some of the tests are also put out in color. Although color may add interest, color charts are even less standardized than black-

and-white ones. Probably the Allen cards are the best of the available picture tests, since greater effort has been put into their standardization (see Fig. 4-14). The tests consist of a series of black-and-white pictures (e.g., a telephone, a birthday cake, a man on a horse, a Christmas tree) which are shown to a child by an examiner as he slowly comes toward the child. The distance at which the child is first able to recognize three of the pictures is used as the numerator over the denominator of 30. A 3-year-old should achieve a score of 15/30; a 4-year-old, a score of 20/30. Any child who misses the appropriate pictures or who shows a 5-ft difference between eyes should be referred. Examples of other picture charts available are the Osterberg chart (see Fig. 4-14), a Danish chart of black-and-white figures such as a swan, house, Christmas tree, man, and key; the Kindergarten chart, with colored pictures of a circle, heart, flag, sailboat, and cross; the A.O. and B&L test, which is similar to the kindergarten chart but has black-and-white pictures; and the California Clown test, in which the clown's hand points in various directions. Other tests which might be considered picture tests are Sjogren's Hand and Withnell's Blocks (see Fig. 4-14). Sjogren's Hand is very much like the illiterate E test. However, in the attempt to turn the E into the more interesting picture of a hand, the standardization has been lost. The child may often determine the correct answer by the thickness of the palm rather than through an ability to distinguish between the fingers. Withnell's Blocks are inexpensive and quite portable. The cards depict one, two, or three rectangles in both horizontal and vertical positions (in order to detect certain types of astigmatism). Although more work has been put into standardizing this particular test, it still lacks the exact standardization of the Snellen, and in addition, it lacks the added interest of picture charts. The

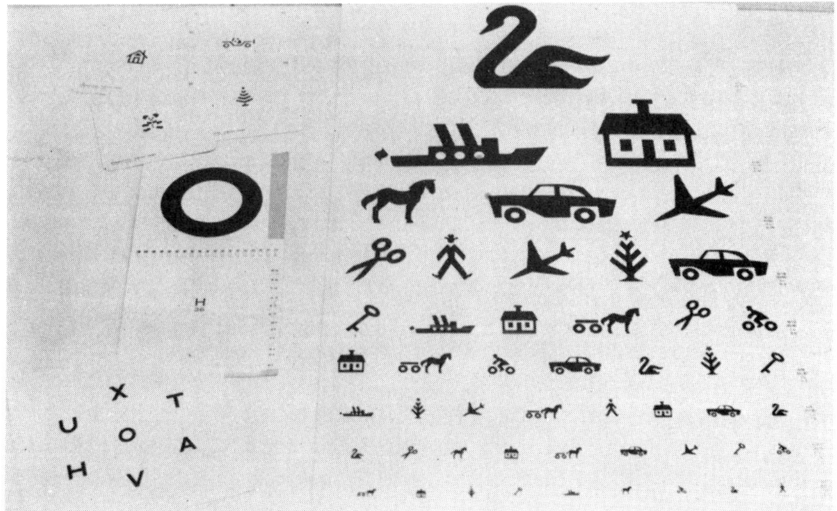

Figure 4-14 Vision testing materials: Allen cards, Osterberg chart, and Stycar test.

child must be able to count up to 3 in order to report how many blocks he sees.

For very young children, not even the picture tests will suffice, and only a rough estimate of their vision can be made. Again the most useful tests for this age group have been popularized by Mary Sheridan. The Starcar is a test devised by her which utilizes two sets of seven small toys—a car, plane, chair, knife, spoon, fork, and doll—one of which the examiner holds at 10 ft against a black background. The child has a similar set of toys (in different colors than the test toys so that the child is unable to match by color) which he holds up to match the one chosen by the examiner. This test cannot be exactly equated with the Snellen standards, but Sheridan advises that the child who can distinguish between the small knife and fork at 10 feet has vision equal to 20/20; a child who cannot distinguish between the large fork and knife should be referred for further evaluation. This is a more difficult test to administer, and the nurse should do it rather than delegating it to ancillary personnel. Sheridan has been able to use this test from about 21 months until the Stycar letters are usable.

For children below 21 months, there is only one rough test available, and again, it is seldom used in this country. This test consists of rolling standard sized balls across a dark background and seeing whether the child can follow them at a distance of 10 ft. Again it is impossible to equate this test exactly to Snellen standards, but Sheridan says that a baby from 6 to 9 months can be expected to follow the ¼-in. ball; a 10-month-old will follow a ⅛-in. ball; and by 12 months, the child should follow all balls. This test is more difficult to do monocularly since babies often object to having one eye closed, but it is sometimes worthwhile trying.

Heterophoria

Next to acuity testing, the most important screening test of vision available is the screening test for heterophoria. This is the most serious visual condition, particularly in preschool children, that the nurse is likely to encounter with any degree of frequency. *Heterotropia* refers to the situation in which a child's eyes do not focus together in such a way as to transmit good coordinated binocular vision; *heterophoria* is a tendency, not always overt, toward the same problem. This results from some type of inequality between the eyes or eye muscles which prevents each eye from focusing on exactly the same point at the same time. Sometimes this is obvious, as in cases of severely crossed eyes, but often it is more subtle and requires careful observation and screening procedures to detect. It is extremely important to detect this condition because in some cases if it is undetected, the child will learn to suppress the vision in one eye completely; if not caught until school years, there is a good chance that this vision will never be regained. Neither the child nor the parents will ordinarily be aware of this problem, and therefore routine screening for it is essential. Hatfield (1966) found that 20.9 percent of the eye problems found in his sample of 3-year-olds were problems of this type. Many babies will exhibit intermittently crossing eyes. If such a muscle imbalance is horizontal rather than vertical, if it is not constant, and if it becomes gradually better, it can be considered normal up until the age of 6 months. After this, it may be normal, but should be referred to an ophthalmologist for careful evaluation. After this age, any history of eyes which cross when the child is tired or sick or occasionally for unknown reasons should also be referred for ophthalmological consultation. When such crossing is overt and constant, it is referred to as *tropia.* Where there is merely a tendency to such crossing, it is called a *phoria,* and must usually be detected by certain screening methods. These screening methods should be incorporated into every well-child examination. The first of these is called the *corneal light reflex* (or Hirschberg's reflex) and should be done in both a near-point (i.e., about 14 in.) and far-point (i.e., about 20 ft) position. The child is asked to look straight ahead at a particular spot designated by the examiner. The examiner then shines a penlight into the child's eyes and notes where the light reflex falls. It should fall on exactly the same position in each eye; any asymetricality should be referred for further consultation. In order to evaluate this carefully, it is important that the child's eyes remain completely still, giving the examiner enough time to determine where the light reflex is falling. This can usually be explained to older children. With young babies, a bright, flashing, moving toy is ideal, since they will generally focus on it long enough for such a determination. It is often wise to turn out the room lights, since overhead lights will also be reflected in the eyes and it may be difficult to tell which light reflex is coming from the room lights and which from the examiner's penlight.

The next test which should also be done at each visit is called the *cover test.* It is another method of making manifest a phoria which cannot usually be seen. This test is also begun by having the child focus on a specified spot, first 14 in. away and then 20 ft away. While the child is focusing on the spot, one eye is covered. It is important that the eye be covered completely so that it is unable to focus. It is also important that neither the eye nor the eyelashes be touched, since this will cause the child to blink when the cover is moved, and the examiner will not be able to see the response of the pupil. The cover should be held over the eye from 5 to 10 seconds and then removed fairly abruptly. The examiner then watches the *previously covered* eye to see if it moves. If there is a phoria, the covered eye will have begun to wander when it was unable to focus on the designated spot (i.e., when it was covered), and when the cover is removed, the eye will attempt to refocus with a sharp jerky movement. It is this movement which will indicate to the examiner that the eye has a phoria. This procedure is repeated for both eyes both at the near point of 14 in. and the far point of 20 ft. Although a very slight movement can be normal, the authors feel that any movement requires a referral to an ophthalmologist. Since the consequences of underreferral are so grave (i.e., amblyopia with possible irreversible loss of sight in one eye), it is better to err on the side of overreferral.

Farsightedness

Although young children are normally slightly farsighted, some authorities feel that it is important to detect an abnormal amount of farsightedness or hyperopia. For preschoolers and schoolchildren through the second grade, this is done by having them read the 20-ft line of the E or alphabet chart at a distance of 20 ft through a +2.25 lens. Normally, a child should be unable to accomodate enough to see this line clearly. If the eyes *do* accomodate, and the child is able to read four of the six symbols correctly, this amount of hyperopia may be an indication that this child is more likely to develop eye fatigue or symptoms of muscle imbalance. Not all ophthalmologists agree that this test is worthwhile for the preschooler, so before initiating this screening it is wise for the nurse to consult with the ophthalmologist in the community to whom children will be referred. The procedure is more commonly accepted for older schoolchildren. Generally it is recommended that a +1.75 lens instead of a +2.25 be used on children in the third grade and older.

Near-Point Vision

Near-point vision refers to the acuity achieved by the eyes at a distance of 13 to 14 in. (reading distance). It is almost always the same as acuity at a distance of 20 ft. The primary condition in which a difference will be seen is presbyopia, a condition of old age. In young children, accomodative powers are great, and even a child who might have difficulty in reading for longer periods of time will usually be able to adapt for the few minutes necessary for the test. For this reason, the National Society for the Prevention of Blindness does not recommend its routine use. It is possible that a phoria may become manifest during its use, but this should be detected when doing the near-point cover test. Again, this test may be more useful with older school-age children. Most of the charts available for testing acuity at 20 ft are also available in sizes standardized for near-point testing at 14 in.

Color Blindness

Not all clinicians agree that testing for color vision is important. The authors, however, feel that every boy should be tested for color blindness, preferably during kindergarten. Since color blindness is so rare in girls, routine testing of them is probably not necessary. Although color blindness is not correctable, it is important to know that it exists. One reason the authors recommend testing during kindergarten is the increasing use of color in educational materials, for instance Sullivan's *Words in Color* and the Cuisenaire rods used so often today. If the teacher is aware that a child is color-blind, much misunderstanding can be eliminated when using these materials. Awareness of this defect is also important in considering occupational choices since certain occupations rely heavily on color vision. Color testing needs to be done only once, since the results will not change. The classic materials for testing color vision are the Ishihara plates, and these are still used with adults and older children. They consist of a series of plates with figures composed of dots hidden in a background of similar dots. The only cue to help the individual distinguish the figure is the color. If the person is color-blind, the figure remains hidden. There are four types of plates: the *vanishing-figure* plate, which contains a figure that a person with color vision can see but a person with either red or green color blindness cannot see; the *diagnostic* plates, which contain two hidden figures, one which can be seen only if a person has normal red vision and the other which can be seen only if normal green sensitivity is present; the *transformation* plates, which also have two hidden figures, one which is seen only with normal vision and one which should be seen only with abnormal color vision; and the *hidden-digit* plate, with figures which persons with abnormal color vision can see but which those with normal color vision cannot see. These last two types are not totally accurate, since some people with normal color vision are able to see the figures which should be seen only by color-blind individuals.

An improvement has been made on the Ishihara plates by adding plates to detect difficulties in yellow-blue color vision. These are the AOHRR polychromatic plates, which, although they have just been discontinued, are still used in most places. They are considered to be more valid than the Ishihara, and are 100 percent effective with red-green difficulties and somewhat less effective with blue-yellow defects. The test consists of 24 plates, including 4 demonstration plates and 20 test plates. A quick screening test can be given by selecting only the high- and low-chroma plates. Individuals missing these can be further tested with the more moderately hued plates. It is important to use the lamp which comes with the test since normal room light completely invalidates the findings. These plates are useful with children who have reasonably good figure-ground skill and who can name the letters, numbers, and geometric figures on the plates. For younger children, tracing the figures can sometimes be useful although this requires considerable eye-hand coordination.

For children too young to be tested by these plates, some researchers have used such tasks as matching colored yarns or putting colored table tennis balls in similarly colored muffin tin compartments. Various forms of color wheel matching tests are also used. None of these are accurate. The only other test known to the authors to be constructed specifically for young children is Guy's color vision test (see Fig. 4-15). This test uses the Ishihara plates but provides matching figures that the child can point to rather than actually naming them (the same principal utilized in the Stycar test). Although no research has been done on this test, the authors have found it quite easy to use with young children. However, since only the high-chroma plates are used, it might be possible to miss children with more minor degrees of color defects. For this reason, if Guy's test is given in kindergarten,

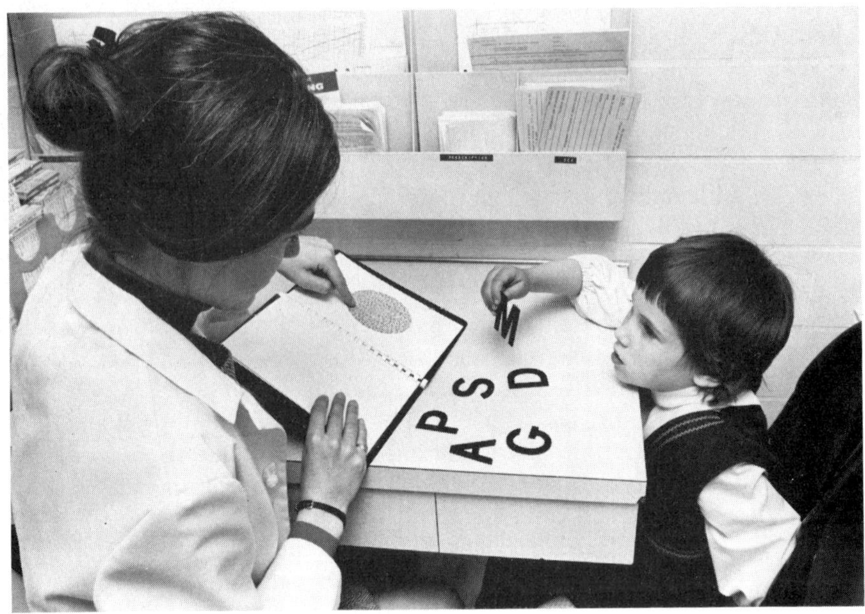

Figure 4-15 Testing for color vision with Guy's color test.

it might be wise to rescreen children when they are old enough to utilize the AOHRR plates.

Visual Fields

Testing for visual fields is usually considered part of the neurological examination, although we are including it under visual screening techniques. The object of this screening is to assess the child's peripheral vision. It is possible to have limited peripheral vision due to ocular, neurological, or pituitary problems (usually a pituitary tumor). The procedure for this test begins with the child facing the examiner, about 3 ft away, with the examiner's arms outstretched halfway between the child and herself. The examiner then moves the fingers of one or both hands at a spot she herself can see and asks the child to tell her which finger is moving. This should be repeated in all four quadrants of vision, first with both eyes and then with each eye individually. When the eyes are tested individually, the examiner must remember to close her own left eye while the child closes his right eye and vice versa. Because there is really no standard, the child's peripheral vision must be compared with that of the examiner. For this reason it is essential to keep the moving finger exactly halfway between the examiner and the child. Roughly, peripheral vision is expected to be 60° on the nasal side, 100° on the temporal side, and 130° in both vertical directions. The only more objective method of measuring peripheral vision is with a machine called a *multiple pattern field screener,* but this is available in very few places.

Testing Infants

When dealing with infants, it is impossible to test specifically all the aspects of vision discussed above. It is important, however, to be sure that they have at least some vision. Historically, there has been a gradual increase in the awareness of how well infants can see. As we devise better and better methods of assessing infants' vision, it becomes clear that infants have an acuity better than we have realized simply because we have not had adequate methods of testing. This is still true. It used to be thought that an infant had an acuity of 20/670; today it is felt that acuity is actually 20/450. Chances are that it is better than that; we are simply still unable to test it well. For clinical purposes, the nurse should at least be certain that every newborn she examines can see. This can be done in three ways: the following response, the turning-to-light response, and the nystagmus response to an optokinetic drum. The following response consists of just that: following. Even a newborn will show the ability to track a light or bright object for limited distances. An infant who does this certainly is not blind; the nurse does not, of course, know how well the infant sees. If an infant is held face up in the examiner's arms with the back of the head toward a source of bright light, such as a window, the eyes of a normally sighted infant will turn toward the source of light. Again, no measurement of vision is possible, but at least the nurse is assured that the baby can see. A third method of testing for presence of some vision is by using an optokinetic drum. Generally the drum has stripes on it although some have various pictures on them. When the drum is twirled slowly in front of the infant's open eyes, nystagmus will be elicited if vision is present (see Fig. 4-16).

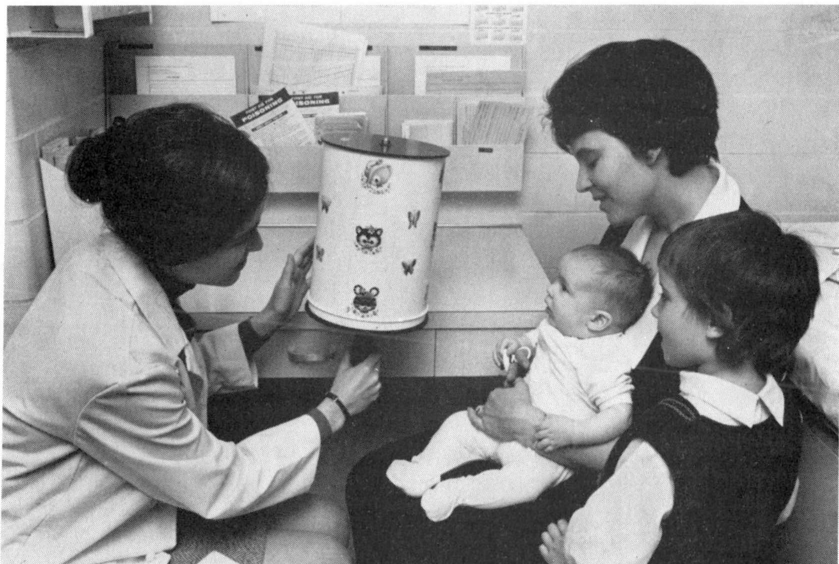

Figure 4-16 Nystagmus test for vision.

When and Where to Do Vision Screening

A child's first visual examination should be performed soon after birth, usually in the nursery. In the normal newborn, testing methods already discussed are sufficient; in premature infants, periodic visual examinations should be done by an ophthalmologist during infancy and later (the effects of retrolental fibroplasia are not always immediately evident). After that the nurse should make some attempt to assess the child's visual abilities at every well-child visit. The appropriate methods for various age groups have been discussed above. It is also important not to overlook the family's assessment of the child's vision. In very serious visual problems, the parents will often be the first to suspect a problem; in more minor problems they may be unaware of the difficulty.

With children over 2½, it may be possible for mother to test the child's eyes with an E chart at home long before it is possible for an unfamiliar examiner to test them. The National Society for the Prevention of Blindness has created a card for such testing which mothers can use at home (Fig. 4-13). Press (1968) found that more visual problems were discovered by mothers than by nurses and that there was only a 4.6 percent rate of overreferrals. Trotter (1966) compared testing by mothers with testing by volunteers and found mothers much more accurate. Home testing can be an extremely important adjunct to the office visits. At this time, 94 percent of the preschool children in this country have never received a vision screening exam; this situation could be greatly improved by teaching mothers to test their own children. Cards for home testing are available at no cost from local chapters of the National Society for Prevention of Blindness.

In addition to testing at every well-child visit, it is usually recommended that schools test children's vision according to the schedule discussed before since many of the children of this age do not sec a physician regularly.

HEARING TESTING

As with vision screening, a careful evaluation of the child's hearing is an essential part of every well-child visit. Estimates of children in this country with some degree of hearing impairment vary from 2 to 12 percent, and of these, 3 to 5 percent have defects serious enough to interfere with schoolwork (Moghadam et al., 1968). This figure is far greater for those living in poorer socioeconomic conditions, either rural or urban; it is estimated that about 19.8 percent of these children suffer from hearing loss (Fay et al., 1970). It is important that all nurses be alert to clues indicating the possibility of future language disorders, since hearing and language are so closely related. Children who should arouse the nurse's suspicion include babies who babble normally until about 6 months and then gradually decrease in sound production (even totally deaf babies will babble the first few months);

who constantly miss high-pitched consonants and fricatives such as "s," "sh," "ch," "f," "th," and sometimes "k"; who pay little attention to the radio or who turn its volume up above the comfort level of others in the house; who are consistently inattentive to speech; who manifest garbled speech; whose voice quality is poor or whose voice is quite loud or a monotone; who consistently drop word endings; who use mostly vowel sounds after 1 year of age; who do not turn to the source of sound by 4 months, who omit initial consonants after age 3; whose speech is highly unintelligible after age 3; who are not talking at all by age of 2; who are inconsistent in responses to speech or environmental sounds during the first 2 years; who do not understand commands or instructions by 18 months; who do not react with a startle to loud noises during the 1st year; or who do not react to name or commands by 6 to 9 months. Although these behaviors may be normal or may indicate other problems, they should make the nurse highly suspicious about the child's hearing or language development.

Types of Hearing Loss

Hearing loss can be of two types: peripheral and central. Peripheral losses can be either conductive or sensorineural. Conductive losses are the most common in young children. They are caused by some physical obstruction which interferes with the sound waves being conducted from the outside air through the middle ear. Most often, the obstruction is in the form of thick fluid such as exists in serous otitis or glue ear. During the acute phase of otitis media, one third of children will have some hearing loss, which will last until the infection is completely healed and probably for 1 or 2 weeks after that. Children with conductive losses lose hearing acuity equally in all frequencies, although it is sometimes more accentuated in the lower frequencies. Air and bone conduction are equally poor.

Sensorineural or cochlear hearing loss refers to a loss caused not because of a problem in the middle or outer ear, as is true for conductive loss, but because of a defect in the inner ear, usually with the cilia or fluid system of the cochlea; sometimes damage to the 8th (acoustic) cranial nerve will result in such a loss. This type of loss is permanent (or at least has always been considered so until the advent of acupuncture as a possible cure for nerve deafness). It affects primarily high frequencies and results in a general loss of clarity in hearing acuity. Air conduction is generally about 10 decibels lower than bone conduction, and recruitment may be present; recruitment is the abnormal increase in sound intensity when nearing the threshold; in other words, a person hears less and less clearly as the sounds become softer and softer until, suddenly, as the lowest hearing threshold is neared, the sounds become disproportionately louder.

Central hearing losses can be either retrocochlear losses, which are uncommon in children, or losses due to brain damage, either generalized throughout the brain or localized to the temporal area.

Causes of Hearing Loss

Hearing loss can appear at birth or later in childhood. It is important to detect hearing loss which is present from birth as soon as possible; many specialists recommend putting hearing aids on children by 6 months of age to achieve the best results. Hearing losses present at birth may be of a hereditary nature, and a careful family history in this regard should always be taken. Some such hereditary diseases will appear at birth, but most will be progressive and become manifest only gradually. Other congenital problems can also result in hearing losses. Cleft palate is frequently associated with frequent serous otitis media and often results in eventual hearing loss. Children with this defect should have their hearing evaluated regularly. Prenatal infections may result in hearing losses of the sensorineural type in infants. Syphilis and rubella during the first 4 months of pregnancy are well-known causes; other viruses are probably implicated as well. Losses resulting from such prenatal infection may be present at birth, but may not become evident until the child is older; therefore these children should be followed carefully even though as newborns they appear to have normal hearing. Metabolic or endocrine problems in the pregnant woman as well as various kinds of poisoning (quinine, salicylates, alcoholic overdoses) may also cause the newborn to suffer hearing losses. Any pregnant woman who has taken such drugs should have her infant carefully evaluated. Obstetric trauma, birth anoxia, Rh or ABO incompatability or kernicterus are other conditions known to be associated with an increased incidence of hearing loss in the newborn. Again, such loss may be present in the newborn, but may not become evident until later.

Other agents can cause hearing loss later in childhood. Most common of these is chronic, frequent otitis media or serous otitis. Any child with such a history should be evaluated very thoroughly. Labyrinthitis of otitic origin, especially in infants, is often implicated, as are infectious diseases which affect the auditory nerve or organ of Corti (examples of these are measles, mumps, viral neuritis of the 8th nerve, and meningitis and encephalitis, particularly when caused by Hemophilus influenza). Drugs may also be etiologic; particularly ototoxic are neomycin, kanamycin, and streptomycin. These drugs may result in immediate loss or may be responsible for a loss which is delayed by 2 to 3 months; it is often characterized by recruitment. A careful history for these drugs should always be taken. Impacted wax is an infrequent but real cause of some conductive loss in older children, as are inflammed adenoids which block the opening to the eustachian tube, often resulting in serous otitis. Progressive inherited deafness may also become evident only in later childhood.

Screening Tests

The nurse working in ambulatory pediatrics must be alert to all such suggestive clues indicating the possibility of hearing loss, but even without such indications, every child deserves a careful hearing evaluation at every well-child visit. The type of evaluation will differ with the age of the child. This chapter will discuss some of the screening tests available for various age groups as well as some of the diagnostic tests which are utilized in the specialist's more thorough evaluation.

Tests used with the school-age child will be discussed first since they are, in general, the easiest to administer and the most clearcut. There are several such tests available, and although the nurse should be aware of them, it is the authors' strong opinion that only an audiometric screening test is adequate for evaluation of school-age children. Certainly some of the commonly used tests are clearly inadequate. Examples of these are coin-click tests, watch-tick tests, and whispered-voice tests. These are all tests in which the examiner roughly compares the patient's hearing with his own. They are not standardized, and in the case of a child, in whom accurate hearing is so vital, they can only be considered insufficient. Tuning forks, also, although useful for certain specific purposes, are not adequate for the hearing evaluation of a child.

Tuning-Fork Tests Three tuning-fork tests are commonly used: the Weber, the Rinne, and the Schwabach. The Weber test is performed by striking the tuning fork to make it vibrate and placing the stem in the midline of the scalp. The child is then asked if it is louder in either ear or if it is the same in both. A normally hearing child will hear it equally well in both ears. If the sound lateralized to one ear, a conductive loss may exist in that ear or a sensorineural loss may exist in the opposite ear. In any case, such a child needs further evaluation by an audiologist. This test is usually impossible with preschoolers, who are unable to comprehend the concept of comparing loudness between the ears.

The Rinne test is performed by striking the tuning fork until it is vibrating, and then placing the stem on the child's mastoid until he no longer hears it. At this point, the fingers of the fork, which are still vibrating, are placed in midair, 1 to 2 in. in front of the concha and the child is asked whether he can hear them. Since air conduction should be about two times better than bone conduction, the child should be able to hear the fingers of the fork vibrating in the air after he can no longer hear the stem of the fork vibrating on his mastoid process. Any child who is unable to do so should be referred for further evaluation.

The Schwabach test is less commonly used. It consists of comparing the patient's bone conduction to that of the examiner's. The stem of the vibrating fork is placed on the child's mastoid until he can no longer hear it; it is then placed on the examiner's mastoid. If the examiner can still hear the vibration after the child has said he can no longer hear it, the child should be referred for further evaluation. The frequencies usually suggested as best for the tuning forks which are to be used in these tests are the 256, 512, and 1,024. These tests give the nurse an idea of the difference between air-conduction level and the bone-conduction level in the child's hearing, but they give no indication of the actual level of hearing which the child has. They should be used only as supplementary to the audiometric screening.

Audiometric Tests Audiometric testing has been used since the early 1900s when the Western Electric Company produced the first multiple mass screening audiometer. It is important that the nurse be familiar with audiometers and certain terminology pertaining to their use although she will generally be responsible only for supervising others in administering the tests. Many types of audiometers are available, and a listing of those which have met the standards of the Subcommittee on Conservation of Hearing of the American Academy of Ophthalmology and Otolaryngology is published regularly in the *Transactions of the American Academy of Ophthalmology and Otolaryngology*. Audiometers are basically similar although there are some differences. They may be either battery-operated or electric, and they may be either the standard type or of special adaptation such as those used only for neonates, those which can be used for automatic screening, and those which can be used for screening with multiple earphones. All will have an on-off button, an output selector which directs the noise to the right or left ear, earphones (red for the right and blue for the left ear), a hearing threshold level to regulate the loudness, a frequency lever, sometimes an air-bone selector, and sometimes a masking device. Machines should be calibrated to the ANSI standards which were adopted in 1969. If old machines are used which are calibrated to the previously used ASA standards, a conversion table should be attached to the machine and the results translated into the new standards.

It is important that the nurse be familiar with certain terms and abbreviations commonly used in testing hearing so that she will be able to record her own findings and to understand the recordings of others. dB is the abbreviation for the term *decibel*, which refers to the degree of loudness or intensity of a sound. Hz and cps are abbreviations for *Hertz* and *cycles per second*, that is, the pitch or frequency of a sound. *Recruitment* refers to the pathological subjective increase of 10 to 20 decibels when nearing the threshold; this symptom is caused by damage to the cochlear portion of the ear. *Threshold* is the faintest tone which can be heard 50 percent of the time. *Air conduction* is the conduction of sound from the air through the outer and middle ear; *bone conduction* refers to the conduction of sound through the bone. *Masking* is a noise introduced into the better ear in a situation in which one ear hears considerably better than the other. It is not used in screening. Abbreviations for recording should also be familiar to the nurse. Findings from air conduction are always indicated by a solid line. This line is interrupted by the symbol O for the right ear and X for the left ear; □ is used as a symbol for the right ear masked during air conduction and △ for the left ear masked in air conduction. When air conduction is performed without earphones, as in the case of very young children who are afraid of earphones, it is done in a soundproof room by a specialist who records a blue S for the findings of the left ear and red S for the findings of the right ear. S stands for *sound field,* the term used for the open, soundproofed room. Bone conduction is indicated by a dotted rather than solid line. In bone conduction, the symbol > indicates the right ear unmasked; < indicates the left ear unmasked; ▶ symbolizes the right ear masked; and ◀ indicates the left ear masked. Although not all these symbols will be used in the type of screening the nurse will usually be involved in, it is important that she be familiar with them since reports from the audiologist will often use them.

The human ear can hear from about 20 to 20,000 Hz, but of these, the most important speech frequencies are 500, 1,000 and 2,000 Hz; 3,000, 4,000, and 6,000 Hz are sometimes considered important for environmental sounds. Sounds over 6,000 Hz are rarely important in human hearing. Many specific audiometric screening tests are available, but all of them specify certain of these important sounds to be tested. Specific directions for the various audiometers come with the machines, but some pointers are important for all of them. Children should always be positioned in such a way that they are unable to see the examiner's hands operating the interrupter switch. The interrupter switch should be used to channel the noise first to one ear and then to the other, always in an irregular pattern so that children are not able to respond to the pattern rather than the actual sound.

Several types of screening tests are used for school-age children. The Massachusetts test uses a multiple-earphone audiometer, and the child is asked to circle yes or no when hearing a sound of 500, 4,000, and 6,000 Hz. As many as 40 children can be tested at one time, and this test is generally rapid and efficient in fourth grade and above. A similar test is the Glorig Automatic Group Screening Test. This test can be used with as many as 40 children with multiple headphones attached to one machine. It is automatic and requires no trained personnel. It is effective only after the level of about third grade. The Reger-Newby Group Screening Test is operated in the same automatic manner, and the child is asked to count the number of sound spurts heard at each frequency. The Johnston Group-Tone is another multiple-earphone audiometric test. It is constructed in such a way that the child can respond by raising a hand rather than recording an answer as is done in the other tests. Not all earphones receive the sound at the same time, so children are prevented from responding solely on the criterion that children next to them are raising their hand. The advantage to this method is that children who are not yet old enough to write can be tested; the disadvantage is that a trained person is necessary since the test is not totally automatic; it is often found that the children below fourth grade are not testable even with this method since they require more individualized attention.

In 1961 the National Conference on Identification Audiometry recommended that whenever possible, individual audiometric tests be given (Fig. 4-17) although it recognized that mass screening was more economical and could be used where economics was the deciding factor. This body suggested that the frequencies of 1,000, 2,000 and 6,000 Hz be tested at the level of 20 dB (ANSI) and that the 4,000-Hz level be tested at 30 dB (ANSI). Referrals were to be made if the child could not hear any of these frequencies at the suggested decibels, but because of the inefficiency of changing the decibel lever twice during each test, this recommendation was later changed to testing all frequencies at the 25-dB level and referring children who failed either the 1,000- or 2,000-Hz level or the combination of both the 4,000- and 6,000-Hz level. Holding the decibel dial constant and changing only the frequency dial is called the *sweep check* method. Other authorities suggest the same

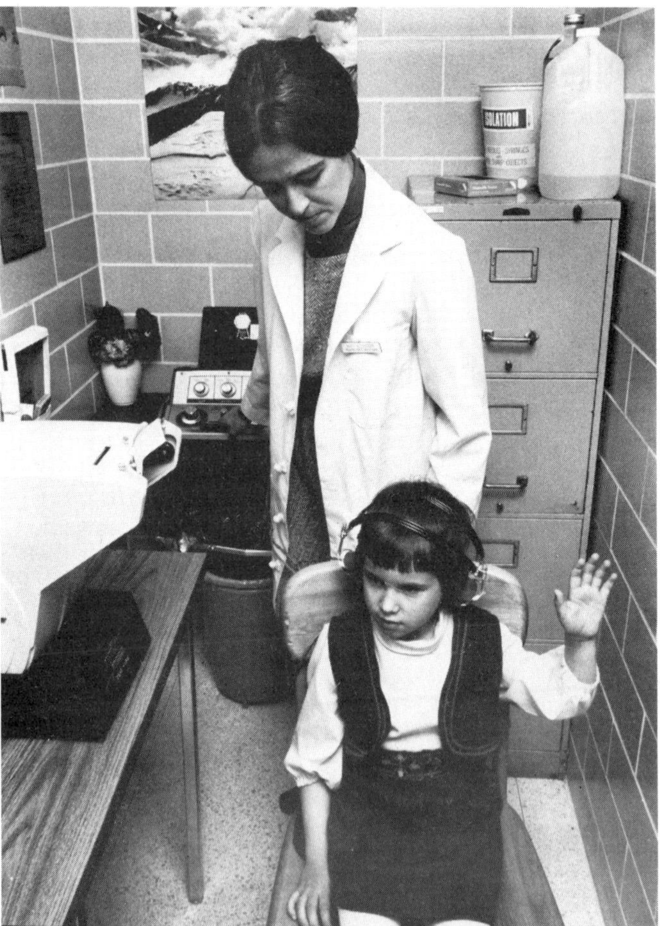

Figure 4-17 Individual audiometric testing.

method but use different decibel or frequency levels. Glorig and House (1957) have suggested modifying this test to only one or two frequencies; they used either the 4,000-Hz frequency or the 2,000- and 4,000-Hz frequencies together. Miller and Polisar (1964), however, have shown that the one-frequency test will find only 39 percent of the hearing defects and the two-frequency test will find only 46.2 percent. Some tests, such as Frankenberg's screening test, include the 500-Hz level as well, but this and the 250-Hz level are particularly prone to interference from ambient noise and are probably not suitable for noisy clinics.

Diagnostic Testing

Children who fail the screening audiometric test should be rescheduled for a second screening after an interval of 2 weeks; if they again fail, they should be referred to an audiologist who will perform a more definitive threshold audiogram. This test uses the same machine and the same basic principles of audiometric screening but differs slightly in technique and purpose. The goal of the threshold audiogram is to find the child's threshold (i.e., the lowest level at which a sound is audible 50 percent of the time) for each frequency. The Committee on Conservation of Hearing of the American Academy of Ophthalmology and Otolaryngology recommends that this be performed by the ascending technique; that is, the tester begins below the level at which he expects the child to hear and proceeds to increase the decibels by 10 until the child can hear; the decibels are then decreased in steps of 5 until the child can no longer hear. This technique, known as the Hughson-Westlake ascending technique, is continued until the child's threshold is discovered for each frequency. This test is much more time-consuming and requires more skill than the screening tests and should probably not be utilized by the nurse if a trained audiologist is available.

Further diagnostic testing may be performed in the form of speech audiometry. In general, speech sounds are not as accurate as pure tones in assessing accurate levels of total hearing ability, but in certain circumstances they may be more accurate since they test the amount of hearing that the child is able to utilize when listening to spoken communication. Usually spondees (i.e., two-syllable words phonetically balanced with random high and low frequencies) are used, although occasionally monosyllables, sentences, and connected discourse are used. Such testing may miss high-frequency losses since the words may be recognized by the frequency vowels, but, as stated before, this may be useful in discovering how well the child has learned to utilize what hearing he has. The audiometer necessary for speech audiometry is different from that used for pure tone audiometry and is generally available only in speech clinics. Although one form of speech audiometry, the fading-numbers test, has been used in the past for screening purposes, this is no longer considered adequate and only pure-tone audiometry should be used in screening.

When and Where to Do Hearing Screening

Generally, it is recommended that audiometric screening be scheduled in the school at the kindergarten, first, third, fifth, and seventh grades every year and that it include all transfers to the school during the preceding year no matter what grade they are in. In the clinic situation, hearing evaluation should be done as part of every physical examination, and as follow-up to any disease known to be potentially ototoxic (e.g., measles, mumps, otitis media, any disease with high fever, and upper respiratory infections even without known ear infections); after administration of ototoxic drugs such as streptomycin, kanamycin, and neomycin; and regularly in high-risk groups as discussed earlier.

Testing Preschoolers Preschoolers and toddlers are somewhat more difficult to test, but it is at least as important and maybe more important to be sure these children are hearing well. They are not old enough to be aware of whether they are developing a hearing loss or not, and hearing is crucial to the important skills they are learning, particularly their language skills. Audiometric testing using pure tones is the most accurate measure available, and some mature preschoolers will be able to cooperate easily with this method. Most younger children, however, will need certain modifications. As in vision testing with the E chart, it is worth taking some extra time to help this age group understand the audiometric test since there is no other test as accurate. Patience is usually the most important component to successful testing with this age group. Inclusion of mother in the testing and asking mother to practice the testing at home using earmuffs and a whistle the week before the examination are extremely helpful. Sometimes open-field audiometry in which no earphones are used is necessary, but this requires a soundproof room and a skilled audiologist; it is impossible to test the ears separately with this method. But for high-risk children who cannot be tested in other ways or for children about whom the nurse has a question, this may be necessary.

In general, audiologists will attempt to use play audiometry to test children of this age, and many of these techniques can be adopted by the nurse in the clinic setting. The underlying assumption of play audiometry is that the child will be much more responsive if meaning is given to the sound. Some elaborate mechanisms, such as the peep show in which the child can push a button when a sound is on and activate a doll or cause some other interesting visual stimuli or the frequently used pedacoumeter in which seven puppets will pop out if the button is pushed in response to a sound, are available in specialized hearing clinics but seldom if ever in outpatient pediatric clinics. The nurse can attempt on a simpler level, however, to create more interest in the test. This is usually done by having the child use a more interesting response than the traditional hand raising. Sometimes children will enjoy putting a ring on a peg or a block in a box. It is usually best to start without earphones on and with very loud sounds to which mother responds by putting a block in a box. Then she and the child respond together, and the mother guides the child's hand with the block in it into the box at the appropriate moment. Gradually the child is allowed to do this alone. Only when the child understands the game completely are the earphones put on. This may require several sessions, sometimes with practice in between visits at home. An excellent example of this is seen in the film "Too Young to Say," available from the John Tracy Clinic. Speech audiometry is sometimes used for this age group because although it lacks some of the accuracy of the pure-tone testing, it is inherently more interesting to the young child. One picture test consists of four phonetically similar words with matching pictures. The words are filtered through known frequencies and the child is asked to point to the appropriate picture (Bennett, 1961). The more widely used Verbal Auditory Screening for Children (VASC) is a similar test consisting of 12 spondees and stimulus pictures.

Experiments have also been done by Downs and the University of Denver in which familiar animal sounds are filtered at specific frequencies and the child is asked to point to the picture of the animal which made such a sound. This test is not commonly available, however.

Mary Sheridan, one of the world's leading authorities on the sensory screening of young children, feels strongly that children of all ages should be tested not only for pure-tone sensitivity, but for hearing of actual speech as well. As discussed previously, it is impossible to standardize speech sounds as accurately as pure tones, particularly without the use of filtered speech monitored by a specialized audiometer. Sheridan, however, has worked extensively with this problem and has devised several spoken tests which are easily administered clinically. These consist of a series of identification tests in which children are asked to point to one of several toys in front of them. For the 3- to 7-year-old, Sheridan devised a seven-toy test, which uses a set of seven toys, the names of which are carefully selected to test an ascending frequency scale of sounds. Starting from the lowest-pitched words, the names are "spoon," "doll," "fork," "car," "knife," "plane," and "ship." The examiner first ensures that the child knows all the appropriate names and then, standing at ear level, 10 ft from the child, names the toys in this order in a moderate tone of voice. The child is asked to point to each toy as it is named. For the younger child, (2 to 3 years old), Sheridan devised a six-toy test consisting of a cup, spoon, ball, car, doll, and brick. Again the sounds used in the words appear in an ascending order of frequency. Finally, Sheridan reports success using the five-toy test (by omitting the spoon) for children as young as 1½ years.

One of the most exciting technological advances in auditory screening has been the recent introduction of impedance tests. These test for conductive loss in a more objective and sensitive way than has ever been possible before. An impedance bridge is an attachment which can be used with specialized audiometric equipment. One end is placed inside the external auditory canal and the other is attached to the machine. A measured amount of force is then emitted and the resistance encountered is registered. The resistance comes from the tympanic membrane; a middle ear which is filled with fluid, as in the case of serous otitis, will cause the tympanic membrane to be stiffer than normal, and more resistance will be measured on the graph; a middle ear in which the ossicles are missing or broken will result in a very loose tympanic membrane, and less-than-normal resistance will be measured on the graph. This test takes only a few seconds to administer and requires no response or even cooperation from the child; for this reason it is suited for infants and young children. Although it cannot pick up sensorineural deafness, it is exquisitely sensitive to the most common type of hearing loss in young children—conductive loss from serous otitis; in this situation it is much more reliable than the commonly used pneumonic otoscopic tests. It is hoped that impedance machines will be widely available in outpatient pediatric clinics in the near future.

If a child is too young or too immature to be tested by the audiometer through either pure-tone or speech audiometry, the nurse must resort to less standardized techniques.

Testing Infants For toddlers, and young infants, the most reliable test available is that devised by Hardy as a modification from the early work of the Ewings. This is a test in which the child is held in the mother's lap and has his attention visually attracted directly in front of him. A noisemaker is then sounded to one side and the examiner observes whether a head or eye turn localizes the sound. This test is best performed with two examiners, one producing the sound to the side. The sounds produced should be of high frequency (a high-pitched rattle, the unvoiced consonants of "S" or "Sh," or the opening of a small ball of crisp tissue paper), medium frequency (a medium-pitched rattle or a metal teaspoon stirring gently against the rim of a cup), and low frequency (a xylophone, a low-pitched rattle, or the examiner's voice saying "baa," "bu," or "ga"). It is important for the examiner making the noise to stay completely out of view on a level with the child's ear, about 2 to 3 feet behind the child. By 3 months of age localization efforts should begin and the child will turn either the entire head or the eye toward the source of the sound if it is localized at ear level. By 6 months the localization response should be reasonably well developed, and a mere eye turn is not enough; a turn of the entire head is required. At 9 months, sharp localization is expected to sounds produced at the level of the ear or below, and by 1 year, the child should be able to localize either above or below the ear level. This is only a rough test since many frequencies are included in all such noisemakers; Clark (1956) analyzed 24 different such noisemakers and found a minimum of five frequencies in each. Testing of this kind is clearly demonstrated in the film "Auditory Screening of Infants," available from the Maryland State Department of Health, 301 Preston St., Baltimore, Maryland. With neonates, testing is even more difficult. Neonatal audiometers such as the Xenith Nemometer and the Vicon Apriton are available. These emit the frequency of 3,000 Hz at 80, 90, and 100 dB. They should be held 10 in. from the ear. The most consistent reliable response indicating that the infant has heard the noise is an eyeblink, sometimes called the *acousticopalpebral reflex.* A *Moro* or *acoustic muscle reflex* (generalized flexing), an *auditory oculogyric reflex* (a horizontal movement of the eyes in infants over 4 months), an *arousal response* (eye opening, stirring, or limb movement), a cessation of movement or vocalization, or a change of expression are also considered evidence that the infant has heard. It is important that infants being tested be in the "drowsy state," that is, not so active that they are responding to many stimuli and not in such a deep sleep that they will not respond to any stimuli. This kind of testing is quite subjective, and even with training, Moncur (1968) found that 39 percent of the "yes" responses recorded by the examiner came at a time when no sound was even emitted. Downs and Hemenway (1969) screened 17,000 infants of whom 500 failed. Of these 500, only 15 had real hearing problems, and 1 child who passed did have a hearing loss. In spite of the high amount of overreferal and the missed child, Downs and Hemenway feel this procedure is justified, since the PKU test which has been instituted by law finds only 1 in 4,000 to 6,000.

Attempts have been made to find more objective response criterion. Bartoshuk (1962) used a change in the heart rate in both newborns and fetuses in utero; Heron and Jacobs (1969) used changes in respiration as the response. A "Papousek cradle" has been especially constructed for this purpose; the child is placed in the cradle and actual head turnings to sound are reported to be quite consistent (Bench, 1970).

A few very specialized, sophisticated techniques are also available for testing infant hearing, but only in a few institutions around the country. The Psychogalvanic Stimulus Response (PGSR), sometimes called electrodermal audiometry, is based on a Pavlovian stimulus-response model. Since children respond to a central nervous system stimulation with mild increase in sweat gland activity, the test is begun by coupling an electric shock with a sound. Each time these two stimuli are emitted, increased sweat results; eventually, the child is conditioned to the sound (if the child can hear it) and the electric shock is discontinued. After that, the child is tested for sweat responses to various frequencies. This test is used only after about 18 months with children who cannot be tested in other ways. It has many disadvantages; some children cannot be conditioned, and these are often the same ones who cannot be conditioned to play audiometry. Psychotics, psychoneurotics, and children with certain endocrine problems cannot be conditioned. The child cannot be too active, but cannot be sleeping or sedated. In spite of these limitations, this test is useful for certain children, but requires a skilled person to administer it.

Electroencephalographic audiometry (EEGA or EAR) has certain advantages over PGSR. It can be used with children under 18 months, and it is done with the child either sleeping or sedated. An EEG is taken while various sound frequencies are emitted, and a skilled person can interpret the changes in the EEG pattern to sound. It is not always accurate since some changes occur spontaneously and to other stimuli and because adaptation will often occur rather rapidly. As of this writing, it is not very standardized and is done in only a few institutions in the country. It does hold promise for future hearing testing of young children, however.

In summary, then, it is important that each child's hearing be tested by the most accurate method available appropriate to his or her age. Children who are high risk because of the situations discussed previously or whose parents are concerned about their hearing deserve particularly careful evaluation. Any child who fails the test or about whom the nurse is uncertain should be referred for more sophisticated evaluation.

SPEECH TESTING

Another very important part of well-child care is the periodic evaluation of speech development. Some specifics of how a child develops the various aspects of speech will be discussed in Chapter 5. In this chapter, more emphasis will be placed upon clinical evaluation of the individual child's speech. It is important to be generally aware of the developmental sequence of vocal sounds from the beginning cry through adultlike speech. This is particularly true of the developmental sequence of the sounds of articulation, which are repeated here for the reader's convenience:

3 to 4 years: lip sounds—"m," "p," "b," "w," "h,"
4 to 5 years: tongue contact sounds—"n," "t," "d," "ng," "k," "g," "y,"
5 to 6 years: "f"
6 to 6½ years: "v," "th" (voiced, as in "then"), "ch," "sh," "l"
6½ to 7 years: "z," "s," "r," "th," (voiceless, as in "this")

Knowledge of normal development in this area will help alert the nurse to early danger signs. Even in infants and toddlers some of these danger signs are already apparent. Some indications that should alert the nurse to evaluate a child carefully are difficulty in sucking, lack of musical inflection in early babbling, not responding with a startle to loud noises during the first year, not looking for the source of moderately loud sounds by eye or head turning by 4 to 8 months, not reacting to one's own name or commands such as "no-no" by 6 to 9 months, inconsistent response to speech or environmental sounds during the first 2 years, excessive drooling, not speaking at all by the age of 2 years, not comprehending commands or instructions by 18 to 24 months, or any expression by the parents that they are concerned about the child's speech or hearing development. Fuller (1970) found a history of abnormal crying in 19 percent of the children with poor speech and only 1 percent of children with normal speech. He also found a higher incidence of prenatal complications in the children with speech problems. An older child may also present certain signs which should alert the nurse to the possibility of hearing or speech problems. The nurse should evaluate very carefully any child who uses mostly vowel sounds in speech after the age of 1 year, any child in whom the amount of verbalizing decreases rather than increases at any time from birth to 7 years, any child who consistently drops word endings, or any child in whom the voice is a monotone, extremely loud, largely inaudible, or of poor quality.

Causes of Speech Problems

The most common cause of speech problems is mental retardation, while the second most common cause is loss of hearing (this is why many of the early danger signs of lost hearing are the same as those indicating the possibility of future speech problems). Fiedler (1971) found a "poor environment" in 45 percent of the children with speech problems, but in only 15 percent of those without speech problems. Certain anatomical problems can cause poor speech also. Cleft palate is a common etiology for speech problems. This refers not only to overt clefts but to submucous clefts as well. For this reason it is important for nurses always to include a check for submucous cleft in their physical examination of the mouth. This is done by palpating the upper hard palate to make sure it is intact. If a submucous cleft exists, a large notch will be felt (see Fig. 4-18); this can frequently be seen as well if the patient is asked to say "ah." It is important to remember that submucous cleft is frequently associated with a bifid uvula, and any child with a bifid

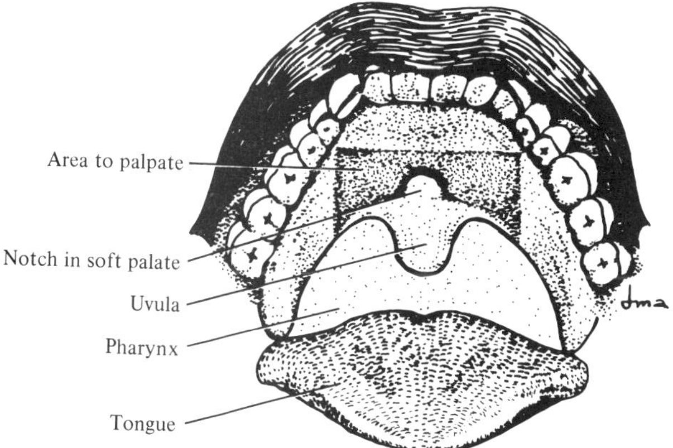

Figure 4-18 Area to be palpated for submucous cleft palate.

uvula should be examined very carefully for the existence of submucous cleft. Children with cranial nerve damage in which they lost control of their uvula or portions of the mouth and throat may also have poor speech, while children with tumors of the larynx may present with persistently hoarse speech. Problems with lip mobility which may be reflected in poor pronunciation of such sounds as "p," "b," "wh," "m," "f," and "v" are seldom organic, but may need a speech specialist to correct them. Difficulties with malocclusion may result in inaccurate articulation of the sounds "s," "z," "sh," "zh," "ch," and "j." Anatomical problems of the tongue are usually problems of either tongue thrust or paralysis of the tongue. Tongue thrust is a controversial subject. Such a condition apparently does exist, but its etiology, normal prognosis, and cure are not clear. This problem is sometimes referred to as *reverse swallowing* and consists of a backward movement of the tongue in the swallowing process, ending with a thrust of the tip of the tongue against the front teeth. Both dental and speech problems may result. This pattern is probably normal in certain very young children, but when it persists into the ages of active speech development, problems can arise: it should always be gone by the time of the eruption of permanent teeth (7 to 9 years) but can cause problems long before this. The nurse can examine for this by placing her fingers over the child's masseters while breaking the lip seal with her thumbs (Fig. 4-19). The child is then asked to swallow, and the nurse feels for a contraction of the muscles of mastication. Normally a significant contraction can be easily palpated; in children with tongue thrust, this contraction is felt either very slightly or not at all. It is interesting to note that this condition is never noted in children who have been breastfed for most of their infancy. This has led many to believe that this is caused by certain types of nipples, particularly very long nonpliable nipples. In fact, one of the commercial nipples, Nuk, is said to prevent tongue thrust because of its similarity to the human breast; this has not been proven, however.

Articulation Testing

Although it is important to be aware of all aspects of a child's speech—articulation, lexicon, syntax, and semantics—by far the most clinically useful screening tests are available for articulation. In general, these tests attempt to test individual sounds within the context of other sounds (that is, within words). Sounds are usually tested in three positions: word initial, word medial, and word final. Some tests test several positions in one word; although this is less time-consuming, it requires very good listening ability on the part of the examiner. Probably the least important position is word medial. It has been found that when this position was not tested, only 1 percent of the children with speech defects were missed.

One of the biggest difficulties in administering such tests is accurately assessing the sound being tested. It takes some concentration to be able to listen only to the sound being tested and not to be influenced by the sur-

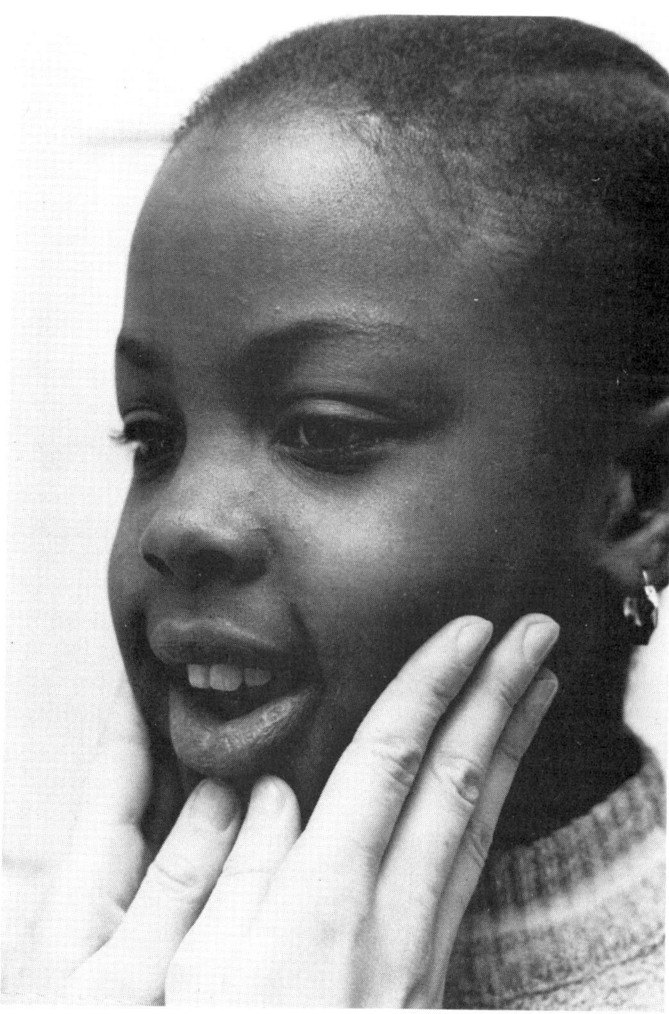

Figure 4-19 Examining a child for tongue thrust.

rounding sounds. Although Irwin (1970) has found a very high correlation between examiners, the examiners in his study were speech pathology majors in college who had had a great deal of practice in this kind of listening. It is important for the nurse to be aware of this problem and to carefully train herself, ideally by working with a speech therapist or by obtaining such films as the one which teaches the Denver Articulation Screening Test, available from Laradon Hall, Denver, Colorado. It is easy to assume that you are hearing correctly when you are in fact not doing so.

The screening tests available for assessing speech are of three types: spontaneous, word imitative, and nonsense imitative. In the spontaneous type, the child speaks a familiar word without having heard it first. The most common technique used in this type of test is to present a picture and ask the child to name it. The word imitative test is one in which the examiner says a word and asks the child to repeat it. The nonsense imitative test is one in which the examiner says a nonsense word (such as "shuk" to test the word initial "sh" sound) and asks the child to repeat it. There is controversy concerning which of these types is best. Carter and Buck (1958) and Snow and Millisen (1954) have shown that there are fewer errors when children repeat nonsense words than when they repeat real words. This seems to indicate that even though children hear the examiner pronounce a word, if it is a well-known word that they have heard pronounced in a different way before, they will proncounce it the way they are used to hearing it rather than the way the examiner pronounces it. An example of this is the use of the word "mother" in the Denver Articulation Screening Test. Many Black children repeat this word as "mothah," according to their own dialect. This certainly does not indicate that the children are incapable of using a word final "r" sound: it indicates merely that they do not think that sound is appropriate in that word, and they repeat the word with their correction. Carter and Buck (1958) and Snow and Millisen (1954) have further shown that there are fewer errors in imitative testing than in spontaneous testing; that is, it is apparently less difficult for children to imitate a word they have just heard than it is for them to pronounce a word which they know but have not just heard.

The most important attribute of a screening test, however, is its ability to predict future problems. The difficulty lies in the fact that articulation errors, even when age-inappropriate, tend to decrease without any kind of therapy from the first through the third grade. In other words, when a child of this age is found with an articulation defect, is it very possible that it will go away with no help at all. However, if the examiner waits until the third grade and the defect persists, it will be much more difficult to correct than if it had been referred in the earlier years. The problem, then, is determing which types of defects will disappear by themselves. This is not entirely known, and when possible the nurse should refer any child with a problem to a speech therapist. However, the question of how to predict which kinds of articulation problems will disappear spontaneously has been studied and some things are known. Intelligence and social maturity do not seem to have any effect on the disappearance of the problem. It is probable that the more consistent the error, the less likely that it will correct itself. There are also specific types of errors (like lateral lisps) which are less likely to disappear without therapy. Carter and Buck (1958) found that when a child made an error on the spontaneous test *which did not correct itself on the nonsense test,* this error was less likely to be outgrown. Steer and Drexler (1960) tested kindergarteners and found that the best predictor of speech errors which would not self-correct were (1) the overall number of errors, (2) the overall numbers of errors in word-final position, (3) the number of errors of omission in word-final position, and (4) errors in the "f" and "l" sounds (these sounds are particularly developmentally relevant at the kindergarten level). In order to avoid excessive overreferral, then, it might seem best, at least from the information available at this time, to use the comparison of a spontaneous and an imitative nonsense test. Unfortunately, the authors know of no commonly used test of this type suited for the clinical situation. Findings from the Steer and Drexler study are also useful in this regard.

Many types of tests are available for both screening and diagnostic purposes. The most complete and most commonly used diagnostic test is the Templin-Darly Diagnostic Test of Articulation, which is composed of 176 items in both picture card version and reading version. The format for this test is a sentence spoken by the examiner with a missing word to be filled in by the child. A picture to prompt the correct word accompanies the sentence. For instance, the examiner may say,"This is Smokey the ______," and show the child a picture of a bear. A comparable Templin-Darly screening test is also available and consists of 50 items.

Fiedler (1971) has devised a home screening examination which asks the child to perform and includes certain articulation skills and includes a survey of certain pertinent historical information such as pregnancy and labor problems. This test is specific for 3-year-olds. The Predictive Screening Test of Articulation (PSTA) was devised by Van Riper (1969) in order to predict which articulation errors would not correct themselves. It consists of some imitation of nonsense words, some imitation of words in sentences, some tests of recognition of misarticulation, and some items of skill in which the child imitates a rhythm by clapping his hands. Van Riper clearly states that this test is not yet fully tested, and one would assume that he does not yet feel it is adequate for clinical use. The Laradon Articulation Scale also attempts to predict which articulatory problems need therapy, but its predictive powers have not yet been proven. The Carter-Buck tests previously discussed also attempt to be predictive and actually consist of three subtests: one which tests spontaneous articulation, one which tests word imitative articulation, and one which tests nonsense syllable imitative abilities. The score is a comparison of the tests. This test is quite lengthy, however, and certainly cannot be considered a screening test. The Picture Articulation Test by Irwin and Musselman (1962) is quite short since it incorporates several of the sounds being tested into one word. Although the shortness is an advantage clinically, the increased skill required to hear several sounds correctly in one word probably makes this test a poor choice for the nurse working in the ambulatory setting. The Developmental Articulation Test is rather lengthy and has been criticized because it does not contain enough blends. The Deep Articulation Test exists in both picture and written forms and tests sounds in many different contexts. It is quite thorough and lengthy, and must be considered a diagnostic rather than a screening test. Many other tests are available, such as the Arizona Articulation Proficiency Scale, the Photo Articulation Test, and the Meacham Language Development Scale, but none of these are suited to clinic use by the nurse. The test with which the authors have had the most success is the Denver Articulation Screening test, which is constructed for use as a screening tool by persons who are not speech therapists. It takes about 10 minutes to administer, and although it comes with pictures to help maintain the child's interest, it is basically a word imitative test; that is, the nurse says the word and the child repeats it. Twenty-two words are used, and only one sound in each word is tested. Again, the authors would like to emphasize that the test may appear deceptively easy, and it is suggested that nurses spend some time comparing their assessment of sounds with that of a speech therapist or with the films available from Laradon Hall. The test is scored according to percentiles of children who have acquired certain sounds at certain ages. Figure 4-20 shows the test itself and the scoring mechanism.

Vocabulary Testing

Lexicon, or vocabulary, is an aspect of speech that is somewhat less understood. The development of a vocabulary seems to be related to both environment and intelligence, and intelligence tests are often heavily weighted with

---

Instructions: Have child repeat each word after you. Circle the underlined sounds that he pronounces correctly. Total of correct sounds is the raw score. Use charts in Fig. 4-20(*b*) to score results.

Name:

Hospital no.:

Address:

Date: _____ Child's age: _____ Examiner: _____

Raw score: _____

Percentile: _____ Intelligibility: _____ Result: _____

1. table	**6.** zipper	**11.** sock	**16.** wagon	**21.** leaf
2. shirt	**7.** grapes	**12.** vacuum	**17.** gum	**22.** carrot
3. door	**8.** flag	**13.** yarn	**18.** house	
4. trunk	**9.** thumb	**14.** mother	**19.** pencil	
5. jumping	**10.** toothbrush	**15.** twinkle	**20.** fish	

Intelligibility: (circle one)
1. Easy to understand
2. Understandable half the time
3. Not understandable
4. Cannot evaulate

Comments:

Figure 4-20(a) Denver Articulation Screening Examination Test Form for children $2\frac{1}{2}$ to 6 years of age. Printed by permission of Amelia F. Drumwright, University of Colorado Medical Center, 1971.

To score DASE words: Note raw score for child's performance. Match raw score line (extreme left of chart) with column representing child's age (to the closest *previous* age group). Where raw score line and age column meet, number in that square denotes percentile rank of child's performance when compared with other children that age. Percentiles above heavy line are *abnormal,* below heavy line are *normal.*

Percentile Rank

Raw score	2.5 yr	3.0 yr	3.5 yr	4.0 yr	4.5 yr	5.0 yr	5.5 yr	6 yr
2	1							
3	2							
4	5							
5	9							
6	16							
7	23							
8	31	2						
9	37	4	1					
10	42	6	2					
11	48	7	4					
12	54	9	6	1	1			
13	58	12	9	2	3	1	1	
14	62	17	11	5	4	2	2	
15	68	23	15	9	5	3	2	
16	75	31	19	12	5	4	3	
17	79	38	25	15	6	6	4	
18	83	46	31	19	8	7	4	
19	86	51	38	24	10	9	5	1
20	89	58	45	30	12	11	7	3
21	92	65	52	36	15	15	9	4
22	94	72	58	43	18	19	12	5
23	96	77	63	50	22	24	15	7
24	97	82	70	58	29	29	20	15
25	99	87	78	66	36	34	26	17
26	99	91	84	75	46	43	34	24
27		94	89	82	57	54	44	34
28		96	94	88	70	68	59	47
29		98	98	94	84	84	77	68
30		100	100	100	100	100	100	100

Figure 4-20(b) Denver Articulation Screening Examination Percentile Ranking.

To score intelligibility:		Normal	Abnormal
	2½ years	Understandable half the time, or "easy"	Not understandable
	3 years and older	Easy to understand	Understandable half the time Not understandable

Test result: 1. Normal on DASE and intelligibility = normal
2. Abnormal on DASE and/or intelligibility = abnormal

If abnormal on initial screening, rescreen within 2 weeks. If abnormal again, child should be referred for complete speech evaluation.

Figure 4-20(b) ***(Cont'd)*** Printed by permission of Amelia F. Drumwright, University of Colorado Medical Center, 1971.

vocabulary subtests. In fact most verbal or written tests presuppose a certain level of vocabulary. Some specific tests do exist for evaluating the lexicon. Examples of these are the Houston Test of Language Development and subtests of the Illinois Test of Psycholinguistic Ability, the Picture Story Test, and the Peabody test (Fig. 4-10). Of these, probably only the Peabody can be considered a screening test applicable for use in a clinical situation. It may be useful for the nurse to keep in mind some of the commonly estimated sizes of vocabulary at various ages. The first word is usually said at about 14 months for boys and 3 to 6 months earlier for girls. Between 8 months and 2 years, most children acquire about 100 words; by 3 years, the estimate is usually about 900 words, and by 4 years, 1,500 words. The older the child, the less exact is the estimate of vocabulary, since it is impossible to discover exactly how many words a child knows and speaks. Smith (1941) found that the average vocabulary of first graders was 23,700; by twelfth grade this had increased to 80,300 words, showing a steady increase all through the school years. This study concerned only recognition vocabulary (that is, words children could recognize when they heard them or saw them), not spoken vocabulary. Smart and Smart (1970) estimates the adult spoken vocabulary to be much less—about 20,000 words.

Syntax Testing

Syntax, that is, the way a child combines words into sentences according to certain grammatical rules that indicate meaning, is much more difficult to test, and few tests are available for this purpose. Most of those which are available have been constructed for research purposes; a very few are available for diagnostic purposes; and only one known to the authors has been specifically made for screening purposes. One difficulty is that there are so many different aspects of syntax, and little is known about the development of these specific aspects. As will be discussed in Chapter 5, we know something about the development of negative and interrogative sentence structures and something about certain morphological tasks like the formation of verb tenses and noun pluralization, but we know almost nothing about the development of the ability to use passive sentence structures, possessives, variations of word order, reflexive pronouns, or many other aspects of English grammar. We know even less about the learning of the grammatical rules by children speaking other languages. Probably the best known tests are the ingenious figures and nonsense words used by Berko (1958) to test for development of pluralization and tense rules. She would show a child a picture of an imaginary amoebalike figure and say to the child, "Here is a wug." Then showing a picture of two such figures, she would ask the child to fill in the missing word in the sentence "These are two ______." In this way, she could tell when a child would pluralize by adding an "s," by adding an "es," by adding an "ez," or by changing the word itself (as in the plural of "goose"—"geese"). In a similar way she would show a picture of a man doing an imaginery activity and say, "This is a man who knows to spow. He is spowing. He did the same thing yesterday. What did he do yesterday? Yesterday he ______." This test discovered much about normal development of certain morphological forms.

Attempts have been made to design other tests of syntactic development. Carrow (1968) constructed such a test although it can be used only in assessing receptive language. The Michigan Picture Language Inventory (Lerea, 1958) tests both expressive and receptive syntactical development by asking the child to supply the missing word in a sentence. In such a way, it is able to test such grammatical constructions as comparative adjectives, demonstratives, adverbs, articles, prepositions, pronouns, verb tenses, and possessives, but is unable to test structures which utilize word order such as passive sentences, negatives, questions, auxiliary verb constructions, and noun phrases. This test is sometimes used in speech clinics. The Imitation, Comprehension, Production Test (ICP) is another available test (Fraser, Bellugi, and Brown, 1963). It also tests both expressive and receptive grammatical abilities by using sentence pairs with pictures. There are no norms available for this test, however. The only test known to the authors to be constructed specifically for screening purposes is the Northwestern Syntax Screening Test (NSST), designed by Lee in 1969. This test also uses sentence pairs and stimulus pictures to elicit both receptive and expressive ability. For instance, four pictures are presented to the child: a picture of two cats playing, a picture of an adult woman holding a little boy, a picture of an adult woman and a cat, and a picture of a cat nursing a litter of kittens. The examiner then says two sentences: "This is a mother cat," and "This is mother's cat," and the child is asked to point to each of these pictures. This tests the receptive ability to understand possessive nouns. Then only two pictures are shown, the mother cat and mother's cat. The examiner again repeats the two sentences. After this each picture is shown separately and the child is asked to repeat the sentence which is appropriate to it. This is considered the test of expressive ability. The test is designed for use with children from 3 to 8 and takes approximately 15 minutes to administer. Norms are available for both receptive and expressive ability for all ages. At present, this test is used primarily in speech clinics. It is probably not worth using routinely in well-child visits, but it might be useful for the nurse to have available for children about whose slow language development she is concerned.

LABORATORY TESTING OF BLOOD

The nurse's role varies with regard to screening and diagnostic tests for blood. With some tests, the nurse should know when to perform them, draw the specimen, test the sample, and interpret the results; with more complicated tests the nurse may be involved only in ordering the procedure and helping in the interpretation.

Normals are given for each test, but these vary widely from laboratory to laboratory, and nurses must be familiar with their particular laboratory's values.

Although this text has not been written as a laboratory manual, some general statements are made about test methods. Some of the methods discussed are the older, more laborious, methods of performing these tests. Many of the newer laboratories in large medical centers are equipped with electronic equipment that allows these tests to be done more accurately, more rapidly, and with less expense. The principle of the tests remains the same, however.

Normal Blood

Blood cells appear very early in the developing embryo. By the 2d month of gestation the fetal liver is producing red blood cells; by the 4th month the spleen makes additional cells; by the 5th gestational month bone marrow begins producing blood cells. Until a child is 7 years of age all his bones contain bone marrow to produce such cells. After that period, besides the spleen and the liver, only the clavicles, ribs, scapula, skull, and sternum produce cells.

Blood is composed of both fluid and solid elements. The fluid portion of blood is called *plasma* and is produced by the liver and lymphoid tissue. Plasma is a clear, watery substance which contains certain proteins: albumin, globulin, and fibrinogen. Albumin is utilized in osmotic pressure stabilization; globulins are needed for immunity; and fibrinogen is necessary for the clotting mechanism. Plasma volume remains fairly stable during health, but can change dramatically during certain diseases. Increased plasma volume is seen in rubeola, rubella, leukemia, infectious mononucleosis, and some allergies. It may decrease after severe burns, dehydration, hemorrhage, or surgery. The solid elements of blood include red blood cells, white blood cells, and platelets.

Red Blood Cells Red blood cells (erythrocytes) are biconcave disks which carry the hemoglobin used in oxygen exchange. Five stages are seen in erythrocytic development: hemocytoblasts (or pronormoblasts) contain a large nucleus and are produced by the red bone marrow; these develop into basophils (or erythroblasts) which begin synthesizing hemoglobin, gradually becoming polychromoatophils (or erythroblasts) and later normoblasts. Normoblasts begin to lose their nuclei and to form reticulocytes (or early erythrocytes), which show only a fragment of a nucleus; gradually the nuclei disappear entirely and the mature erythrocyte appears (see Fig. 4-21).

Normally the biconcave shape of the erythrocyte changes only slightly to allow the cell to slide through the various capillaries. However, in certain diseases the cells assume peculiar shapes and make this gliding action difficult or impossible. Chronic anemias sometimes show bizarre shaped cells, obstructive jaundice shows pear-shaped cells, and the familiar sickle cell is seen in sickle cell disease. Uremia frequently produces cells with spiny projections. The normal erythrocyte lives from 100 to 120 days and then disintegrates within the liver. The normal total count can vary; however, the newborn contains roughly 6 million to 8 million erythrocytes, and this number falls to around 4 million to 5 million by adulthood. After childhood an erythrocytic count over 6 million can be seen in dehydration, anoxemia, cardiac disease, and bone marrow hyperplasia. Any count below 4 million is considered low and is frequently seen in anemia.

White Blood Cells White blood cells (leukocytes) are rounded, nucleated cells which protect the body by a process of phagocytosis (i.e., destruction of foreign bodies). All leukocytes display 3 main stages and around 16 substages of development. The maturation process is (1) myeloblast, (2)

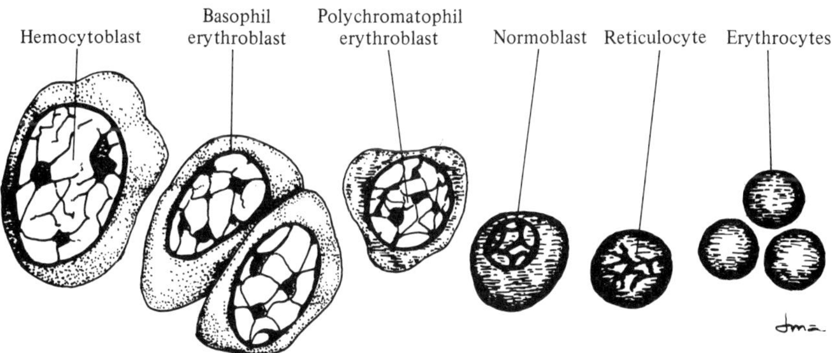

Figure 4-21 Red blood cell development.

promyelocyte, and (3) mature myelocyte with a round, rough nucleus (see Fig. 4-22).

The normal leukocyte lives from 1 to 5 days and is probably destroyed by the liver, spleen, lung, or intestinal tract. The normal leukocytic count varies with age, the newborn showing 10,000 to 20,000 per cubic millimeter and the 8- to 9-year-old showing the adult level of 5,000 to 10,000 per cubic millimeter. There are five varieties of leukocytes: neutrophils, eosinophils, basophils, monocytes, and lymphocytes. While all produce phagocytosis, each functions slightly differently. Neutrophils engulf bacteria and aid in the formation of pus. Eosinophils have less efficiency in phagocytosis but respond primarily against foreign protein, allergic reactions, and parasites. Basophils are present in the storage and release of heparin, and lymphocytes help produce globulins and antibodies. These varied leukocytes all have normal ranges which differ at certain ages (see Table 4-4).

Abnormal leukocyte values often pinpoint specific conditions, and the leukocyte count may be a total of all varieties or individual tallies. Leukocytosis (increased leukocytes) can be physiological or pathological. Physiological leukocytosis occurs at birth, during the 9th month of pregnancy, and after exposure to excessive sunlight. Pathological leukocytosis may be caused by infection, severe hemorrhage, cancer, ingestion of certain drugs (chloroform, quinine), dehydration, or leukemia. Leukopenia (decreased leukocytes) may be seen in some infections, bone marrow defects, malaria, rubeola, mumps, and aplastic anemia.

Platelets Platelets (thrombocytes) are smaller than erythrocytes, circular with rough edges and a definite nucleus, and utilized in blood coagulation. Bone marrow produces the thrombocyte, which begins as a megakaryocyte and develops through several stages to a mature cell. The normal thrombocyte lives from 3 to 5 days and is destroyed by the spleen. The normal platelet count is around 200,000 to 400,000 per cubic millimeter. There is a physiological increase in platelets during pregnancy and normal menstruation and with excessive exercise. Low platelet counts are seen in thrombocytopenia, aplastic anemia, infectious mononucleosis, and mega-

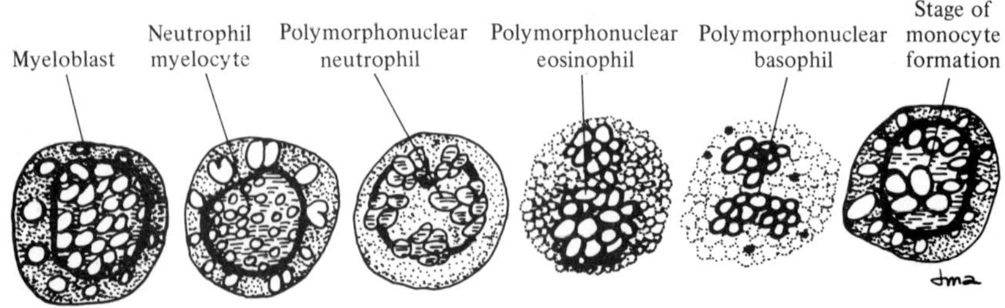

Figure 4-22 White blood cell development.

karyocytic thrombocytopenia. High platelet counts occur in thrombocytosis, trauma, and hemorrhage and post splenectomy.

Obtaining the Specimen

Most blood samples for screening or routine diagnostic testing come from capillary or venous blood.

Capillary blood is sufficient for a good many blood tests, and it is easily obtained. Included in the needed equipment are (1) dry cotton balls, (2) alcohol sponges, (3) lancets (or hemolets), (4) two capillary tubes or pipettes (capillary tubes are usually heparinized), (5) clay for closing one end of capillary tube, and (6) a bandage for the younger child. The choice of site varies with age. Infants usually have sufficient surface area on the large toe or lateral heel, while older children and adults usually have capillary blood drawn from the end and lateral side of the middle or index finger or sometimes from the earlobe. Blood flow is increased if the finger or toe is warm; running the extremity under warm water or asking older children to open and close the hand several times sometimes makes it easier to obtain sufficient blood.

Table 4-4 Normal Values for Leukocytes

Age	Neutrophils, %	Eosinophils, %	Basophils, %	Monocytes, %	Lymphocytes, %
Premature infant					
0–24 hours	15.49	1.22		3.24	14.62
3 weeks	8.67	1.22			15.17
Full-term infant					
24 hours	23.3	1.32	0.08	5.28	6.10
1–7 days	22.05	2.92	0.057	5.18	14.45
7–30 days	5.8	6.0	2.5	6.8	12.1
3 months	8.1	3.9	0.1	5.0	51.0
6 months	10.6	3.2	0.2	8.0	37.2
12 months	29.25	1.9	0.0	3.4	27.6
Preschool					
2 years		2.9	0.2	6.1	21.98
4 years	13.98	5.9	0.2	7.4	24.3
6 years	14.1	3.15	0.2	6.31	24.5
School					
10 years	31.0	2.9	0.2	6.1	14.4
12 years	12.2	2.9	1.8	3.8	16.0
Adult					
18–20 years	13.9	6.5	2.2	2.9	16.1

Printed by permission of Ross Laboratory, *Children are Different*, Columbus, Ohio: Ross Laboratories, 1970, pp. 104–105.

The position of the child's extremity and the examiner's hand can make the difference between a good puncture and a nonproducing puncture. The child's hand and finger should be at a lower level than the elbow with the arm and hand firmly on a table or the examiner's knee. The examiner's hand should rest on her own knee or the table for support (see Fig. 4-23).

The area should be scrubbed with cotton and alcohol and either allowed to dry or wiped dry with a dry cotton ball. The child's finger is grasped firmly between the examiner's fingers (since the pressure reduces the pain slightly), and with a swift, firm swing, the lancet is plunged through the skin. A good puncture requires that the lancet point fully penetrate the skin; a slight nick will not do. The first drops of blood are removed and the capillary tube held to the site for drawing up the specimen. Two tubes are drawn for comparison and in case one tube breaks. The finger should not be "milked," since this damages the red blood cells and may give false readings. Once the specimen is drawn, a dry cotton ball is applied to the site and the child instructed to hold the cotton tightly over the site for a few minutes. Some children like a bandage to show off their bravery. This is not a painless test, and the child should be allowed to cry and should be comforted after the procedure. Before transporting, the capillary tubes must be stoppered on one end with a plug of clay. This need be done at only one end.

If more than a few drops of blood are needed, venous blood must be withdrawn. This is a more complicated procedure, but a necessity for some screening and diagnostic tests.

The equipment needed for venous samples includes (1) a blood pressure cuff or tourniquet, (2) cotton balls, dry and with alcohol, (3) a large (#20 to #23) needle and syringe or a Vacutainer, and (4) the proper collecting

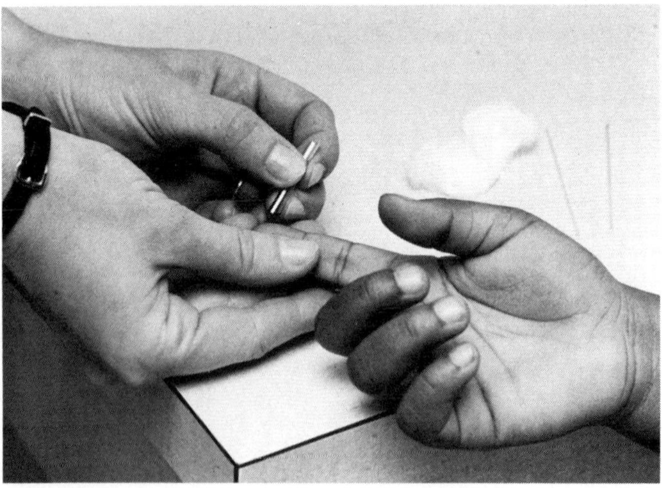

Figure 4-23 Capillary blood being drawn from a child's finger.

tubes. The choice of site for venous blood varies with age. For older children and adults the median basilic and/or median cephalic veins at the inner elbow are good sites. Newborns can have venous blood withdrawn from the jugular vein, femoral vein, or longitudinal sinus (running near the angle of the anterior fontanel). However, nurses may wish to confine their venous blood punctures to the older child at the elbow area and let someone else withdraw the samples at the other sites.

The position of the child's extremity and the examiner's hand is important. Since this is a painful procedure, the child will have to be firmly restrained. The arm of the child should be relaxed and resting on a firm surface. The examiner may brace her fingers and hand against the child's arm (see Fig. 4-24).

The blood pressure cuff is inflated to a point below systolic and above diastolic, or the tourniquet is applied between the shoulder and elbow. The child can be instructed to open and close the fingers vigorously several times. It is wise to palpate the veins for location and firmness before scrubbing the area firmly with an alcohol sponge and allowing it to dry. With one hand holding the skin taut, the other hand slides the needle into the vein with the bevel facing upward and the plunger slightly withdrawn. If blood is to be drawn into the syringe, the plunger can be slowly withdrawn to the level needed. If blood is to be drawn into special collecting tubes and a Vacutainer is used, the blood will appear in the Vacutainer; the first tube can be pushed into the needle and following tubes connected carefully so as not to

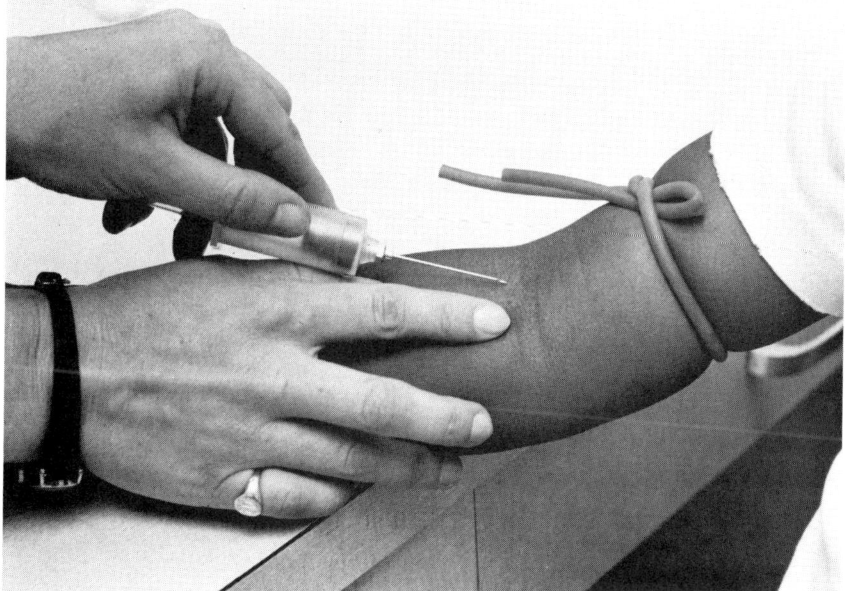

Figure 4-24 Venous blood being drawn from a child's arm.

disturb the needle point in the vein. When a sufficient sample has been withdrawn, the tourniquet is removed, a dry cotton ball is placed over the puncture site, a slight pressure is applied, and the needle is withdrawn. Then firm pressure is put on the site to help coagulation.

Knowing how to perform these two procedures should enable the nurse to obtain specimens for all screening blood work and a good many diagnostic blood tests.

Screening Tests

Several procedures that can be considered screening tests will be described here: colorimetric G6PD, colormetric lead, Dextrostix, galoctosemia, hematocrit, hemoglobin, Sickledex, serum hexosaminidase assay, and tests for venereal disease. Each examiner must choose which of the listed tests are appropriate and needed and must ensure that follow-up can be provided for children with positive findings. Thus an area containing many Black children might need routine Sickledex; the community with many Jewish descendants might benefit from the serum hexosaminidase assay; and a community filled with old, dilapidated homes might warrant the colorimetric lead screening test, etc. While all these tests are considered screening, not all are simple, easily performed tests, and the nurse may have to find a laboratory that is equipped and knowledgeable enough to run some of the tests.

Colorimetric Test for G6PD Glucose-6-phosphate dehydrogenase (G6PD) is a deficiency of glucose metabolism within the red blood cell causing hemolytic anemia; it is present in 10 percent of the Black male population. It is also found in some Caucasians, especially from the Middle Eastern countries, and in some Chinese children.

Although some laboratories are equipped to run this test on capillary blood, most require 4 ml of venous blood. The blood must be drawn into heparinized, citrated, or oxalated tubes for transporting to the laboratory. This is not a simple test, and the nurse will not generally run it. Generally the procedure requires that the blood be centrifuged and the red packed cells watered, buffered, and mixed with several chemicals, including a brilliant cresyl blue dye. The mixture is sealed in the test tube with a layer of mineral oil and placed in the water bath. Readings are taken at specific times (at 50, 75, and 100 minutes and at 2 and 6 hours). A normal reading shows complete decolorization at 100 minutes, and an abnormal reading shows partial or no decolorization after 100 minutes. Any abnormal readings mean the specimen should be sent for the diagnostic test.

Colorimetric Lead Screening Children who eat old paint or inhale fumes from lead-containing substances have an increase in the lead levels of their blood which causes increased erythrocyte destruction and delayed hemoglobin synthesis leading to anemia. Many of these children are suspect from their living conditions—old houses which were painted many decades ago or houses situated near high-speed roadways where there are many fumes and exhausts. Some children become suspect with a history of pica—eating nonfood substances such as paint, dirt, and cigarette butts. This test is not easy to run, and the nurse will need the assistance of a laboratory and laboratory technicians.

Only capillary blood is needed, and the specimen can be drawn up in heparinized capillary tubes. The equipment needed by the laboratory includes a test tube with rubber plug, scale, burner, special filter paper, and some specific chemicals such as sulfuric acid and ammonium citrate. A 40-ml test tube is weighed, the blood sample added, and the tube reweighed. Chemicals are added and the tube is left standing for 30 minutes; then it is heated and additional chemicals added. The tube is shaken for 30 seconds, and the special filter paper is then inserted into the mixture and a reading taken. The reading is then applied to a formula to obtain the standard.

Interpretation is based on a microgram percent, and there is much controversy over the normal range. Some feel that any level between 60 and 100 microgram percent may be toxic with no symptoms and that any level over the 100 microgram percent will show symptoms. Others feel that a lead level below 40 microgram percent is normal, a level between 40 and 80 microgram percent is suspect and needs referral, and any level over 80 microgram percent needs immediate care. The nurse must check with the laboratory to know how to interpret results.

Dextrostix Some children, especially newborns, are prone to changes in blood glucose, and any large changes can be damaging to the child. Dextrostix reagent strips are simple dipsticks that can be used to measure hyper- or hypoglycemia.

Because only a drop of capillary blood is needed, the heel, finger, or earlobe can be punctured with a lancet and the special filter paper held to the wound for absorption. The only equipment needed besides the puncture apparatus is a watch, running water, the special filter paper, and the standardized color chart. After placing one large drop of blood on the special filter paper, wait exactly 60 seconds, quickly wash the filter paper with running water (from tap or wash bottle) for 1 or 2 seconds and hold the filter paper against the color chart for interpretation.

Only a gross estimate of the amount of glucose present is possible with a range of 0, 25, 45, 90, 130, 175, and 250 mg/100 ml of blood. No color or a creamy yellow color is a negative normal reading; dark purple is a positive or abnormal reading and indicates that the child should be referred for more diagnostic testing.

Galactosemia Screening Galactosemia is an autosomal recessive trait causing a deficiency of galactose-1-phosphate uridyl transferase which causes the galactose to increase, resulting in galactosemia and galactosuria. If it is allowed to continue, the infant will develop cataracts, mental retardation, and hepatic failure; without treatment the disease is fatal. The only treatment is restriction of galactose intake; in order to be effective, such restriction must be instituted very early. For this reason, early detection is imperative. This is a complex test, and the nurse will need the aid of a good laboratory technician and a well-equipped laboratory. The procedure can be done on capillary blood; therefore the examiner will need to draw up blood into heparinized capillary tubes. Equipment includes a calibrated pipette, centrifuge, freezer, water bath, and certain chemicals. The blood specimens from the child and one control are mixed separately with some well-chilled chemicals and centrifuged for 5 minutes; additional chemicals are then added and this mixture is centrifuged for 10 more minutes and frozen for several days. Additional test tubes are prepared with specific reagents, and the original test tubes are removed from the freezer, dipped in a water bath for several minutes, solutions added, and the test tubes rebathed. The meniscus is then measured on all tubes, which are then incubated overnight in a water bath. A final reading of the meniscus is taken after removing the tubes from the water bath.

Interpretation is based on changes in the meniscus. A normal (negative) reading is given to the tubes showing a lowered meniscus and an abnormal (positive) reading is given to the tubes showing a meniscus at the same level before and after the final water bath. A positive reading needs further evaluation promptly.

Hematocrit The hematocrit is the comparison of packed red cell volume and the volume of the whole blood. It does not tell the examiner the quality of red blood cells, only the number. Generally this test is used as a screening device for nutritional anemia. A child showing a low hematocrit is given several weeks of medicinal iron and rechecked. If the anemia was nutritional the second hematocrit will be improved. If there is no improvement and the examiner is certain the child has been getting the medicinal iron, further diagnostic tests are needed to determine the cause of the anemia.

This is a very simple test that every nurse should be able to perform. Equipment needed includes two heparinized capillary tubes, puncture apparatus, a centrifuge, and a gauge for reading. Many nurses in outlying well-baby clinics draw up the blood at the clinic and transport the tubes back to the local laboratory for centrifuging and reading. Using the procedure for obtaining capillary blood described earlier, the nurse should draw up two tubes of blood. Depending on the type of reading gauge available, the nurse should fill one half to three quarters of the tube. One end of the tube is sealed with the clay for transporting. The capillary tubes are placed in the centrifuge with the sealed end out. The nurse should remember to balance the wheel with extra empty tubes if necessary and to tighten the screw lid before closing the top so that the tubes are held snugly in place. After centrifuging for 3 to 5 minutes, the tubes are removed and read on the gauge. There are two types of gauges: one is a small plastic card and the other a metal, multiwheeled device (see Fig. 4-25). The card is handy for traveling but difficult to read because the lines are so closely spaced. It also requires three quarters of a tube of blood for reading. The multiwheeled device is much more precise and easier to read and can be used on less than three quarters of a tube of blood. In either case, the capillary tube is lined up with the 100 percent mark at the top of the serum and the top of the red cells at some point below the 100 percent mark.

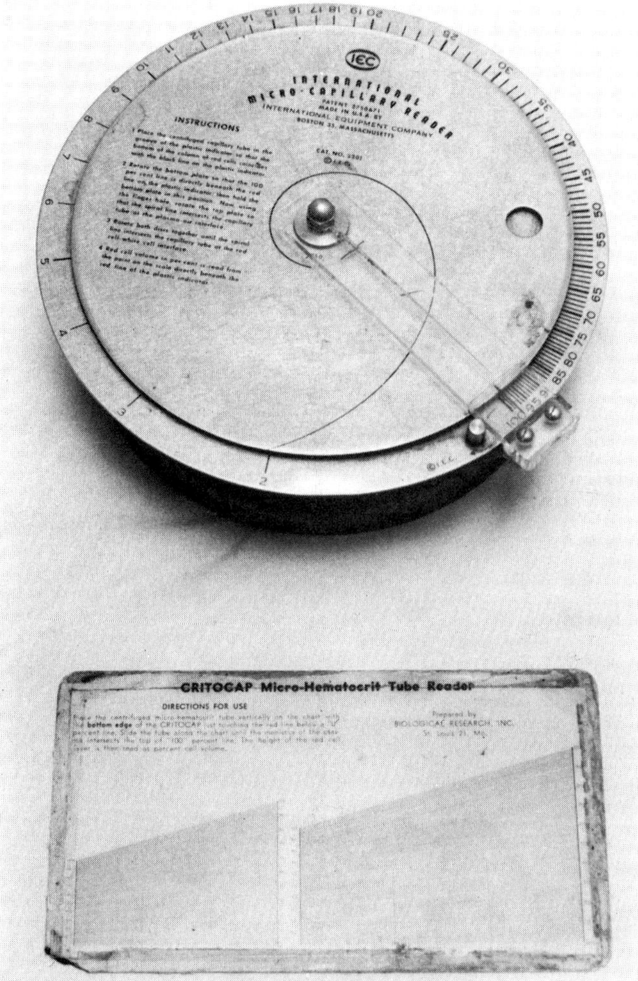

Figure 4-25 Two methods of reading hematocrits.

Remember that whole blood is 100 percent; the normal values are given in percentages since the red blood cells are a fraction of the whole. Depending on age, normal hematocrit values are around 32 to 35 percent and abnormal values are anything below 32 percent or over 50 percent (see Table 4-5).

Accepted norms vary from clinic to clinic and state to state, and so the nurse must be familiar with the prevailing standards.

Hemoglobin A hemoglobin reading refers to the measurement of hemoglobin (a protein) within each red blood cell. There are at least 12 different kinds of normal hemoglobins and as many as 150 abnormal types. The abnormal hemoglobins include anemic hemoglobin and the sickle cell hemoglobin. Some children with anemia have enough red blood cells, but not enough hemoglobin in each cell. Thus it is often important to know both the hemoglobin and the hematocrit of a certain child (see Table 4-6).

This can be a very simple test, and nurses may want to include it in their routine. Many hospitals now perform the test by electrophoresis, which is much simpler and more accurate, but the older methods can be used in the clinical area. Several different tests are used for determining hemoglobin. The colorimetric methods include the direct matching (Tallquist and Dare) and the acid hematin methods (Sahli, Haden-Hausser, and Spencer). Iron concentration can be determined with a chemical method and specific gravity with physical methods (see Fig. 4-26).

Table 4-5 Lower Limits of Hematocrit Values for Definition of Anemia

Age	Lower limit of normal, %
Birth	45
3 days to 1 month	33
1-2 months	30
2-4 months	30
4-8 months	32
8-12 months	32
12-18 months	34
18-36 months	35
3-8 years	36
8-10 years	37
11-18 years	38
Males	
14-15 years	42
16 years	44
Females	
14-15 years	38
16 years	39

Printed by permission of Dr. Burris Duncan at Colorado General Hospital.

Table 4-6 Normal Values for Hemoglobin and Hematocrit

	Hemoglobin, gm/100 ml		Hematocrit, %	
	Full-term	Premature	Full-term	Premature
Cord	15.3-18.9		47-57	
1 day	17.3-21.5		51-65	
2-6 days	17.4-22.2	14.2-18.6	58-74	55-61
14-23 days	14.2-17.2		47-57	
24-31 days	12.2-16.0	9.8-11.4	38-52	27-37
38-50 days	10.9-14.7		36-45	
2-2½ months	10.3-12.5	8.7-10.4	34-42	24-32
3-3½ months	10.4-12.0	9.0-11.0	34-40	28-34
5-7 months	11.8-12.2	10.8-12.3	35-41	33-39
8-10 months	11.1-12.3	10.7-12.3	31-41	33-39
11-13½ months	11.3-12.5	11.0-12.8	37-41	34-40
1½-3 years	11.3-12.3	11.0-12.7	37-41	35-41
5 years	11.7-13.7		34-40	
10 years	12.0-14.4		36-42	
Adult				
Male	14-18		40-54	
Female	12-16		38-47	

Printed by permission of Ross Laboratory, *Children Are Different,* Columbus, Ohio: Ross Laboratories, 1970, p. 110.

Depending on the method being used, either capillary or venous blood is needed. If capillary blood is used, it must be drawn up into a pipette with tubing. The Tallquist method uses a kit with specific absorbent paper and a color scale. After capillary blood is collected, the first one or two drops are discarded and a large drop released onto the absorbent paper and allowed to saturate a large area. A percentage reading is obtained by comparing the blood spot with the scale provided. The other direct matching test is the Dare. This also can be performed on capillary blood drawn into a pipette. The first two drops are discarded and the remainder drawn into a pipette within the Dare hemoglobinometer. Immediately the scale is adjusted to match the specimen and a reading is taken from the standard. The test must be read in artificial light and before the blood clots.

The Sahli, Haden-Hausser, and Spencer tests change the hemoglobin to acid hematin before a reading can be obtained. The Sahli test comes in a small, compact kit containing pipettes; graduated, marked test tubes; a meter; rubber tubing; and three bottles (1% acetic acid, dilution of HCl, and Hayem's solution). Capillary blood is withdrawn into the pipette, two drops discarded, and the remainder blown into the graduated test tube which has been filled to the #10 line with HCl. This mixture is allowed to settle for 10 minutes within the special holder and is then diluted with water until the color matches the standard and can be read. The Haden-Hausser test is similar and comes in a kit containing a hemoglobinometer, white cell dilut-

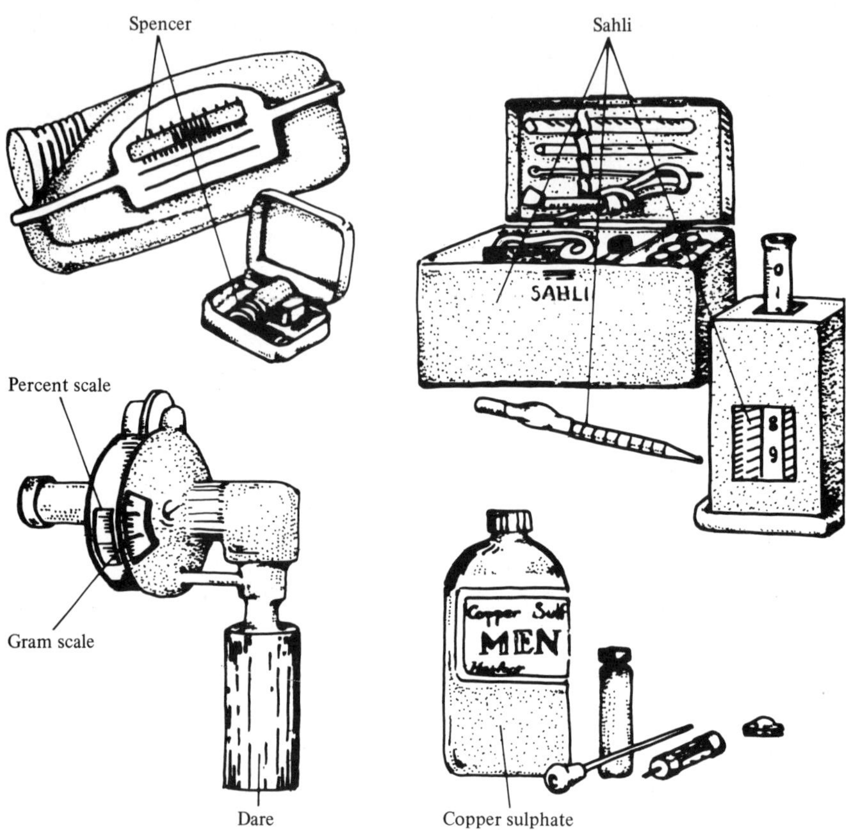

Figure 4-26 Instruments for measuring hemoglobin.

ing pipette, and glass slide and cover. The slide is cleaned and slipped into the hemoglobinometer. Capillary blood is collected in the pipette and diluted with HCl. After a brief wait the acid hematin appears and the specimen can be dropped onto the slide and matched to the provided color standard. A special filter must be used for daytime readings and a different filter for artificial light readings. The Spencer test is a further modification of the same process. The kit includes the Spencer hemoglobinometer, blood chamber, cover glass, and a hemolysing solution. Capillary blood is obtained by puncturing the finger, discarding the first few drops, and then applying the blood chamber directly over the wound. The hemolysing solution is dropped on the chamber, and the cover glass placed over the mixture. The slide is inserted into the hemoglobinometer, the lighting switched on, and the specimen matched with the color standard. Because of the color-matching requirement, all these methods have the disadvantage of being somewhat subjective.

Iron concentration measurements can be obtained by using the Wong method in a laboratory setting. Capillary blood is withdrawn, and 0.5 ml of the heparinized blood is mixed into a 50-ml test tube with digestion solution. It is flamed, several chemicals are added, and the readings are applied to a formula to get the microgram percent of iron in the whole blood.

Specific gravity is easily measured and is used in many blood banks to determine the gross normal hemoglobin content. A stock solution of blue copper sulfate is prepared with a known specific gravity of 1.053 for women and 1.055 for men. Capillary blood is drawn into a pipette and one drop allowed to fall into the solution from 1 cm above the surface. The blood specific gravity will remain stable for 15 to 20 seconds and can be compared with the known copper sulfate specific gravity if read within that time span. Generally, the blood droplet sinks toward the bottom for 5 seconds and then suddenly rises if lighter, continues to fall if heavier, and remains stationary if at the same specific gravity as the copper sulfate. If the blood droplet goes to the bottom in 1.053 solution, that is equivalent to 12.5 gm hemoglobin for women; in 1.055 solution, this signifies 15.5 gm for men.

Hemoglobin values are expressed in grams per 100 ml of blood. Normal values change with age, as seen in Table 4-6, with the general area being around 10 to 12 gm/100 ml of blood throughout most of childhood. As with hematocrits, most clinics establish a cutoff of a certain age when iron supplements should be tried. If possible, both hemoglobin and hematocrits should be done, since the comparison gives the examiner more information than either test singly.

Sickledex Sickle cell anemia is a hematological condition found in 8 to 10 percent of the Black American population. It is a defect in the hemoglobin structure, and stress or lack of oxygen will cause the cells to lose their usual rounded shape and become sickled. Sickled cells do not pass through capillaries like normal cells; instead, they become clogged, causing many clinical signs of vasoocclusion: pain, ulcers, delayed maturation, etc. Sickledex is a simple test for screening children with Hb-S—the defective hemoglobin. This is an easy procedure, and the nurse will not need laboratory help in performing it.

Two test tubes, a special holder, and two bottles of solution are needed. The two test tubes are positioned in the holder. Test tube A is filled with solution A, containing the control Hb-A working solution, and test tube B is filled with solution B. The capillary blood is drawn into a heparinized capillary tube and then blown into test tube B for 2 to 5 minutes of incubation time. A reading is taken by observing the amount of turbidity present in each of the two solutions.

A negative result shows both test tubes remaining clear and a positive result shows test tube A clear and test tube B cloudy. According to one study (Loh, 1968), the Sickledex was performed on 600 patients and compared with the metabisulfite test and electrophoresis with favorable results. However, if the test is positive, the child should be referred to the medical center for a more diagnostic test. The test should be done on every Black child over 6 months. It is not accurate before this time because of the amount of fetal hemoglobin still present.

Serum Hexosaminidase Assay In Tay-Sachs disease ganglioside accumulates within the blood serum, which causes muscle weakness, blindness, mental retardation, and death. It is caused by an autosomal recessive gene found generally (60 to 70 percent) in the children of Ashkenazic Jewish descent. If both parents are carriers, they have a 25 percent chance of having a child with Tay-Sachs disease. It is difficult to detect this disease by symptoms alone before 6 to 12 months of age. However, there is a new test available that can detect both the disease and the carrier state—the serum hexosaminidase assay. Presently there is much controversy over whether this test is a screening test or a diagnostic test since it requires a specially equipped laboratory, specially trained technicians, and a good deal of technical time and it is fairly expensive. However, it is the only method available now, and within specific populations, on an experimental basis, it has been used as a screening tool. The nurse working within such a community should be aware of the test and know how to contact a laboratory for the information needed to do the screening.

Freezers, special ice baths, and complicated chemicals as well as the usual laboratory equipment of test tubes and centrifuges are needed. The test requires 5 ml of venous heparinized blood and takes 24 hours to run.

Interpretation is based on the percentage of hexosaminidase present; one study (O'Brien, 1970) reported the normal range to be 49 to 68 percent, the abnormal range 0 to 4 percent, with carriers showing 26 to 45 percent. These values may change with laboratories or as more studies are completed.

Because there is as yet no known cure for this disease, many authorities feel screening is useless. Some genetic counselors, however, feel that knowledge of the carrier state is important to couples planning families.

Testing for Venereal Disease There are several tests for syphilis, but one of the more common screening tests is the flocculation test developed by the Venereal Disease Research Laboratory (VDRL) of the United States Public Health Service. There are two variations of this method, and they are named after the persons responsible for developing them: Kline and Kahn. Flocculation tests are not specific to one venereal disease. All the tests are based on precipitation caused by antigen-antibody reactions. New to the screening area are two rapid screening tests: the plasma crit (PCT) and the rapid plasma reagin (RPR); these may become more popular in the next few years.

In the older methods (VDRL, Kline, and Kahn), blood can be drawn in clinics but the tests are usually processed in a laboratory by specially trained technicians. Equipment includes a centrifuge, slides and slide holder, chemicals, and buffered solutions. After 5 ml of venous blood is taken, it is centrifuged, heated, and the serum removed. The warm serum is dropped onto a glass slide and emulsified. Antigen is then added, and the slide gently rotated and examined microscopically for clumping of short, straight, rod-shaped substances.

Interpretation is based on the clumping. No clumping is seen in normal (negative or nonreactive) reading, and many large clumpings are seen in an abnormal (positive or reactive) reading. There is also a slightly reactive reading in which several small clumpings are seen.

Diagnostic Tests

The above tests are usually considered screening tests even though some of them are too complicated for the nurse to perform; however, the nurse may be ordering them frequently from the laboratory and should know something about their mechanics and use. The following blood work is usually termed diagnostic and is ordered only where there is some reason to suspect a specific disease or condition. There is no reason nurses could not learn how to do some of these diagnostic tests, but in a general ambulatory clinic they would probably be responsible only for ordering them and participating in the follow-up with the pediatrician. Here again, the normals are given, but there is a wide variation from source to source; therefore nurses are encouraged to check with the laboratory for the clinical averages.

Bleeding Time A child who is suspected of having some bleeding disorder or thrombocytopenia might have a bleeding time taken. Generally the Ivy method is considered the most reliable. The blood pressure cuff is applied and elevated to 40 mm of mercury, and a 2.5-mm-deep incision is made on the forearm. Blood droplets are blotted at 30-second intervals until the bleeding stops. The normal range is 3 to 6 minutes.

Blood Smears Blood smears allow the examiner to differentiate the various types of cells present and their stage of development. Fresh blood is placed on a slide and allowed to air dry. Wright's stain is applied for 3 minutes, and then a buffer is applied. The slide is left to dry for 3 to 6 minutes and then washed with clear water. The slide is slipped under the microscope and the size and shapes of the different cells are noted. Usually the red blood cells stain a light pink, the white blood cells a chrome color, and the platelets a lavender color.

Blood Typing Blood typing is a method of matching antigens and antibodies between two different sets of blood; this becomes important for newborns with hemolytic diseases, children with hemolytic anemias, and anyone with the possibility of requiring a transfusion. The blood is typed (A, B, AB, or O, and Rh positive or negative) and cross-matched (tested for compatibility with the other blood). A blood that is compatible does not clump when mixed with the other blood and can be safely given to that person.

Blood Urea Nitrogen (Bun) This test is done to ascertain the functioning of the kidney in producing urea and maintaining a low blood urea level. It requires 5 ml of heparinized venous blood; according to a standard procedure the blood urea is reduced to ammonia which is then titrated and measured. Many drugs (Garb, 1971) such as bacitracin, chloral hydrate, kanamycin, polymyxin B, salicylates, etc., can affect this test and give false readings. A normal BUN is 9 to 20 mg/100 ml of blood, and any reading over 20 mg/100 ml of blood is a positive or abnormal result.

Bilirubin Hemoglobin is destroyed within the liver, and one of the byproducts of this destruction is bilirubin. If something is wrong with the hemoglobin production or the liver, this balance is destroyed. Thus it is important to check bilirubin levels in children with jaundice, certain anemias, liver damage, and similar problems.

There are several ways of checking the bilirubin: direct, indirect, and total. The direct method tests for free bilirubin and requires 5 ml of venous blood, which is allowed to clot, serum is then extracted and chemicals added to produce a colored reaction that can be measured. The indirect method (van den Bergh test) tests for bilirubin which is bound to a protein. Venous blood (5 ml) is allowed to clot, the serum is extracted, and alcohol and a special reagent are added; the protein then precipitates out and the color is matched to a standard chart. With this test, the patient must be questioned about ingestion of foods and drugs, since many substances can affect the outcome, such as carrots, Vitamin A, and salicylates (Garb, 1971). Total bilirubin measures the concentration of both blood and unbound bilirubin in the serum. This test requires 5 ml of heparinized venous blood which has the serum removed and a special reagent added to produce a color that can be matched to a standardized color chart. Certain drugs and food can also alter these readings.

All three of the tests produce different normal ranges. A normal direct count should be 0.05 to 1.4 mg/100 ml of serum, an indirect count around 0.4 to 0.8 mg/100 ml of serum, and the total count 0.1 to 1.0 mg/100 ml of serum.

Clotting Time Clotting time (or coagulation time) is simply an indication of the blood's ability to clot. Using the Lee-White testing method, 4 ml of venous blood is withdrawn and divided into four test tubes. Test tube A is tilted every 30 seconds until clotting occurs; test tube B is then tilted every 30 seconds until clotting occurs, followed by test tube C and finally test tube D.

Interpretation is made by calculating the average time from collecting the specimen to the clotting of the blood in test tubes B, C, and D. Normal ranges are between 10 and 25 minutes.

Complete Blood Count A complete blood count is a count of all the solid elements in the blood: red blood cells, reticulocytes, white blood cells (including types of white cells), and platelets. Generally the test can be done on capillary blood, but it may be run from venous blood.

For the red blood cell (RBC) count, the blood is diluted with a special solution and the mixture channeled through a counting chamber. By using the microscope the cells are counted within the chamber and calculated for the entire sample. This formerly was done by hand, but many laboratories now utilize an electronic counter which speeds up the process considerably. A normal RBC count is usually 4 million to 6 million cells per cubic millimeter, with a higher count suggesting polycythemia and a lower count indicating anemia.

The young red blood cells, reticulocytes, are also counted, since this gives some indication of the production of red blood cells. A fresh drop of blood is placed on a slide containing dried cresyl blue dye. With the microscope and a counting chamber, the cells are then counted and calculated. This also is now being done electronically. The normal range is 0.1 to 1.5 cells per 100 red blood cells.

Total white blood cells are counted by diluting fresh blood with a special solution, channeling the mixture through the counting chamber and microscope, counting the cells, and calculating the entire number. This can also be done electronically. The normal range is 4,000 to 11,000 cells per cubic millimeter. An increase generally indicates infection; a decrease may signify certain infections or blood dyscrasias.

Sometimes it is important to know the white blood cell differential, that is, the numbers of different types of white cells present. This count requires that a fresh drop of blood be spread evenly over a glass slide and allowed to dry before it is stained with a special solution and placed under the microscope. By means of a special counting chamber, 100 white cells are counted and calculated into percentages. There is a wide variation in normal range as seen from the chart on page 239 and the normal range as listed by Garb (1971).

Neutrophils, 54 to 62 percent
Eosinophils, 1 to 3 percent
Basophils, 0 to 1 percent
Lymphocytes, 25 to 33 percent
Monocytes, 0 to 9 percent

Shifts to the higher or lower percentages can sometimes signify specific disease; for instance, increased monocytes may indicate Hodgkins disease; an increase in the number of eosinophils is usually caused by allergic reactions or parasitic infestations; measles will cause increased basophils.

Generally the platelet count is now done electronically; however, if the older method is utilized, a drop of fresh blood is diluted with a special solution, mixed into a counting chamber, and counted through the microscope. The normal range is 200,000 to 500,000 cells per cubic millimeter. A low count may indicate septicemia, and a high count is seen with broken bones, anemias, and polycythemias.

Coomb's This is a measurement of antigen-antibody levels and can be done directly or indirectly. The direct Coomb's requires 2 ml of fresh, clotted venous or umbilical cord blood. A mixture of red blood cells is dropped onto a Coomb's serum plate and observed for agglutination. Interpretation is read on a 1-to-4 scale, with a negative or normal reading indicating a complete lack of agglutination. Drugs such as penicillin, other antibiotics, and antihypertensive drugs can give false readings (Garb, 1971). An abnormal (positive) direct Coomb's is seen in erythroblastosis fetalis in the newborn. The indirect Coomb's is used to measure Rh and other blood-type factors. Fresh, clotted venous (5 ml) blood is mixed with a special serum and allowed to stand. The red blood cells are removed from the slide and rinsed, and additional serum is added. The slide is then observed for agglutination. Interpretation is again read on a 1-to-4 scale, with a normal (negative) reading showing no agglutination and an abnormal (positive) reading showing agglutination and indicating that the Rh factor is present.

Erythrocyte Fragility The erythrocyte fragility test (osmotic fragility test) measures the destruction rate of the red blood cells. Several milliliters of fresh blood are dropped into numerous test tubes which have differing hypotonic saline solutions. The cells are then observed for rupture. A normal reading is 0.85 to 0.44 percent; an abnormal reading shows a lower rate, indicating acquired hemolytic anemias; a higher rate may suggest congenital anemias.

Fibrinogen Level The protein fibrinogen is needed for the clotting process, and one way of assessing the clotting mechanism is to measure the amount of fibrinogen present. This test requires 5 ml of heparinized venous blood, which is centrifuged to separate the solid from the fluid parts. Only the plasma is tested by adding sodium sulfite and observing the precipitation. The fibrinogen precipitates to the bottom and can be calculated from the biuret procedure. A normal range is 200 to 600 mg/100 ml of plasma.

Glucose The level of glucose is measured to detect certain glucose metabolic disorders such as diabetes, liver disease, and endocrine problems. The patient must fast for 12 hours prior to the test; 5 ml of venous, heparinized blood is then withdrawn. The proteins are precipitated and the glucose oxidized and the result is compared with a color chart for reading. The normal range is 65 to 120 mg/100 ml of serum or 105 mg/100 ml of whole blood. A high level can indicate diabetes, liver disease, or endocrine problems, and a low level may suggest hypoglycemia from coma, convulsions, or endocrine problems.

Glucose Tolerance A measure of the patient's reaction to a certain amount of glucose is particularly useful when diabetes mellitus is suspected. Two tests are used: the standard test and the Exton-Rose test. For the standard test the patient is put on a 150-gm carbohydrate diet for 7 days prior to the testing. For 12 hours prior to the test the patient must have no food, but can drink water. At testing time a single dose of 100 gm of glucose is given at one time. There are two commercial preparations for this: Glucola and Gel-a-dex. Urine and blood samples are collected at regular intervals for the following 4 to 5 hours. For the Exton-Rose test the patient must consume a high carbohydrate diet for 3 days prior to testing, fast for several hours, and have blood and urine samples drawn. Then 50 gm of glucose is given and 30 minutes later blood and urine samples are taken and a second 50 gm of glucose given. Blood and urine samples are again taken after 30 minutes. The values of both these tests are shown in the Table 4-7.

Guthrie Phenylketonuria (PKU) is a metabolic disorder which develops when the enzyme phenylalanine hydroxylase is absent and the amount of phenylalanine in the blood is increased to toxic levels, causing damage to the brain. The usual screening test for PKU is a urine (ferric chloride or Phenistex) test; however, some states use the Guthrie also as a screening test. It is performed on the 3d day of life and after 48 hours of ingesting any protein substance (usually milk formula). The infant's heel is pierced with a lancet and three drops of blood absorbed on a special filter paper. Once the filter paper has been autoclaved, a small sample is punched from the middle of the blood spot and placed on a specially prepared agar plate. The agar has been prepared with Bacillus subtilis. Interpretation is made by observing the Bacillus growth after incubation. A normal (negative) response shows no Bacillus growth near the blood spot, and an abnormal (positive) response shows Bacillus growth up to the blood spot.

Table 4-7 Normal Values for Glucose Tolerance Tests

Standard 100-gm dose

Condition	Fasting	30 min	60 min	120 min	180 min
Normal	80	150	135	100	80
Diabetic	160	250	300	380	290
Mild diabetic	130	200	280	225	180
Hyperinsulinism	80	95	50	60	70

Exton-Rose test

Condition	Specimen	Fasting	30 min	60 min
Normal	Blood	80	150	160
Normal	Urine	Negative	Negative	Negative
Diabetic	Blood	130	225	250
Diabetic	Urine	Negative	Variable	Positive

Printed by permission of Ruth M. French, *The Nurse's Guide to Diagnostic Procedures*, New York: McGraw-Hill, 1971, p. 115.

Hemoglobin Electrophoresis This is a modern, electronically performed test to discover any one of the 150 different types of hemoglobin, some of which are abnormal; it is particularly useful in looking for Hb-S in sickle cell disease. The test requires 5 ml of heparinized, hemolyzed venous blood to which electrophoresis is applied (i.e., the solution is run through by an electric current) and which is then compared with a standard measurement. Normally the adult will show hemoglobin A and the infant will show hemoglobin A and F. Abnormal results show any of the 150 different hemoglobins present.

Heterophile This is an antigen-antibody test generally ordered to aid in the diagnosis of infectious mononucleosis, Hodgkin's disease, or serum sickness. There are three kinds of heterophiles: monospot, presumptive, and diagnostic.

The monospot is really a screening test that is not very sensitive or specific. It requires 0.1 ml (2 gtts) of serum which is mixed with several reagents and spread on a slide with a control smear. The slide is then observed for agglutination in the test and control areas. A positive test shows agglutination and can be a sign of mononucleosis, Hodgkin's disease, hepatitis, or lymphoma. A negative test shows no agglutination.

If the monospot is positive, the examiner must order a presumptive test. This requires 0.2 ml of unheparinized blood from which the serum is extracted, mixed with different dilutions of sheep serum, and observed for clumping. A titer of 1:56 is considered positive for mononucleosis and serum sickness and should be followed by the diagnostic test.

The diagnostic heterophile requires 5 ml of venous blood which is allowed to clot, after which the serum is withdrawn. The serum is mixed with varying dilutions of red blood cells from sheep and is then incubated and observed for agglutination. Interpretation is read as a titer. A normal (negative) result is indicated by a lack of agglutination. An abnormal (positive) is signaled by agglutination of a titer of 1:28 to 1:36 or higher. There is a wide range of what is considered diagnostic for mononucleosis, but serum sickness generally gives a titer of 1:22 to 1:56.

Lead If the screening test for lead is positive, a diagnostic test, usually including both a blood and urine test, is needed. The diagnostic test requires 10 ml of heparinized venous blood to which a series of chemicals are added, and various procedures are performed. The normal reading is 0 to 5 mg/100 ml of whole blood, and anything over 5 mg/100 ml is considered abnormal.

Prothrombin Time This is another indication of the ability of the blood to clot. This test requires 4.5 ml of venous blood which is placed in a specially prepared oxalated solution and a mixture of calcium and thromboplastin added; a stopwatch is used to time the formation of the threads of fibrin. The procedure is then repeated using normal blood. The normal range is 11 to 18 seconds. Abnormally low counts may be caused by liver diseases, vitamin K deficiencies, and certain drug ingestions; abnormally high ranges are seen in barbiturate ingestions.

Salicylate Level This test is used most frequently when children are suspected of ingesting an overdose of aspirin. Occasionally it is also used in ascertaining blood levels in rheumatic fever. It requires 5 ml of venous blood in a heparinized tube. The serum is separated and a ferric ion added before running the specimen through a colorimeter or spectrophotometer. A normal specimen shows no color. An abnormal or positive result shows a purple color. Salicylates of 35 mg/100 ml of blood are considered toxic in children.

Erythrocyte Sedimentation Rate There is some controversy about the reliability and specificity of this test, which simply measures the time it takes for the red blood cells to precipitate to the bottom of the test tube. Usually 4 ml of venous blood is withdrawn, heparinized, and placed in an upright test tube to be monitored for a period of time. The interpretation depends on the method used (Cutler, Wintrobe, or Westergren) and the sex of the patient. A normal range for the Westergren method is 0 to 15 mm/hour for men and 0 to 20 mm/hour for women.

Serological Tests for Syphilis (STS) In general there are two types of testing for syphilis: flocculation and complement-fixation methods. Flocculation includes the VDRL, Kline, and Kahn tests, which were described under screening tests. Complement-fixation methods include the basic tests

(Wassermann, Reiter protein-antigen, and Kolmer), the Treponema Pallidum Immobilization Test (TPA), and the Fluorescent Treponemal Antibody Absorption Test (FTA).

The basic complement-fixation tests require 5 ml of venous blood which is allowed to coagulate with certain additives and is then observed for antigen-antibody reactions. A normal (negative) reading shows no reaction or agglutination. An abnormal (positive) reading shows agglutination and reaction. These tests can give false readings. False negatives are seen in early syphilis. False positives are seen with treated syphilis, yaws, malaria, pellagra, infectious mononucleosis, and leprosy and when equipment used to run the test was not cleaned properly.

The Treponema Pallidum Immobilization Test has a high specificity and sensitivity for syphilis and gives very few false readings. It requires 5 ml of venous blood to which live Treponema pallidum organisms are added and organism immobilization observed. Unfortunately it is a very complicated test to perform and not well suited for general, small laboratories. The normal result shows no organism survival, and the abnormal (positive) finding shows organism immobilization.

The Fluorescent Treponemal Antibody Absorption Test is also highly specific and sensitive to syphilis and gives very few false readings. It is difficult and expensive to perform and best done by large, medical center laboratories. Venous blood (5 ml) is withdrawn and permitted to clot so that the serum can be extracted. The serum is prepared through a heating, diluting, and washing process, mixed with T. pallidum antigen, fluorescein-labeled antihuman globulin, and placed on a slide. The slide is then examined with a fluorescent microscope for fluorescence of the organisms. A normal (or negative) reading has weak or nonfluorescent particles and an abnormal (or positive) reading shows strong to minimal fluorescence.

Sickle Cell Smear If the Sickledex screening is positive, the child must be referred for further evaluation, including a sickle cell smear. There are several methods for performing this test, one of which is McGovern's method. Only 1 to 2 ml of capillary blood is drawn into a pipette with certain chemicals added. After three drops are discarded, one drop is positioned on a glass slide, covered, bordered with petroleum jelly, and heated to seal off oxygen. Generally the slide is examined microscopically after 2 hours for sickled cells; however, some sources feel that sickling will show immediately. A normal reading shows no sickled cells, and an abnormal (positive) result shows the familiar sickled cells.

These are but a few of the thousands of diagnostic and screening tests available using blood. More rapid and more sensitive tests are being developed all the time, and the reader is encouraged to watch the current literature for these developments and to use a good laboratory manual when working with the different tests.

URINE TESTING

One of the most complex and highly structured systems in the human body is the urinary system. As a highly efficient and effective filtering system, it can influence the functioning of the entire body. One of the most painless but effective ways of assessing urinary tract function is to examine the by-product of the urinary tract system—urine. There are many screening tests that can be performed on urine. This chapter will list some of the screening tests and a few of the diagnostic tests most commonly used. As with blood, standards will be given, but these vary from clinic to clinic, and examiners must check the norms in their own settings.

The Renal System

Before discussing examination of the urine, it is important to review the normal anatomy and physiology of the renal system, which includes two kidneys, two ureters, one urinary bladder, and one urethra. Most infants are born with two kidneys, which are rounded, firm, small, lima bean-shaped structures lying deep within the upper pelvis. These are difficult to palpate, but are best felt with deep palpation within the first few hours of life before the GI tract fills with material. Anatomically the right kidney is lower than the left kidney, and by adulthood the kidneys measure 4 to 5 in. by 2 in. The kidney has a *cortex* (covering) and *medulla* (inner surface). The medulla is subdivided into 10 to 16 smaller portions called *pyramids,* which finally unite to become one ureter leading from the kidney.

The basic renal unit is the *nephron,* and there are 1 million nephrons which begin in the cortex and empty into the pyramids of the medulla. As the nephron leaves the cortex it widens into a clump of vessels (called the *glomerulus*) which are covered by Bowman's capsule. From there the nephron twists and turns, becoming the proximal tubule, the loop of Henle, the distal tubule, and finally the collecting tubule. The collecting tubule empties into the kidney pelvis.

From the kidney pelvis, the urine is drained into the ureters, which are long tubes of circular and longitudinal muscle fibers. By adulthood the ureters can be up to 14 to 16 in. long. They display spontaneous contractions which are a form of peristaltic movement which keeps the urine flowing into the bladder.

The two ureters attach on the superior portion of a large hollow balloon called the *urinary bladder.* The bladder lies behind the pubis and low in the pelvic girdle and consists of a series of muscular levels allowing for both contraction and relaxation. The bladder shape and capacity vary with age, sex, health, and certain diseases.

Urine leaves the bladder through the urethra. In the adult female the urethra is a narrow, 1½-in.-long tube opening anteriorly to the vagina and used solely for the passage of urine. The urethra of the adult male is generally about 8 in. long, opens at the tip of the penile shaft, and is used for the discharge of both urine and semen.

The kidneys have many functions, but one of the most important is their filtering action. Within the kidney, substances are either reabsorbed for continued use within the body or discarded as waste. Large amounts of blood plasma (about 1,200 ml/minute in an adult male) are filtered through the glomerulus and into the nephron tubules. As the fluid passes through the tubules, substances are selectively reabsorbed (such as water, urea, phosphates, creatinine, vitamin C) or discretely discarded (such as sodium chloride and dextrose); the discarded substances are passed into the collecting tubules and kidney pelvis. Some substances are always discarded, and some are discarded only when the level circulating in the body reaches a certain level.

Through the peristaltic movement of the ureters the urine is continually passed from the kidney pelvis to the bladder. When 1 to 8 oz. (depending on age) is collected within the bladder, the nerve endings cause the bladder to constrict and force the urine into the urethra. As Table 4-8 shows, bladder capacity changes with age.

Urine is a mixture of organic and inorganic substances; the proportions of these substances may change slightly with each voiding since the kidneys are maintaining a specific chemical level within the body. Macroscopically, urine is a bright, golden, clear liquid with a distinct aromatic odor. Substances normally found in urine are listed in Table 4-9.

Specimen Collection

The method used to obtain the urine specimen depends on the age of the subject and the type of test to be performed. For accurate results, it is important that the examiner collect the specimen in the proper way, at the correct time, and store or preserve it correctly.

Table 4-8 Normal Bladder Capacity and Voiding

Age	Number of voidings in 24 hours	Average quantity at each voiding, oz.
Under 3 months	13.5	1
3-6 months	20.0	1
6-12 months	16.0	1½
1-2 years	12.0	2
2-6 years	8.7	3
6-8 years	7.4	5
8-11 years	7.1	7
11-13 years	7.9	7½
Adults	7.0	6½

Printed by permission of Louis Gershenfeld, *Urine and Urinalysis,* New York: Romaine Pierson, 1948, p. 35.

Table 4-9 Substances Found in Urine

Substance	Amount, gm	Substance	Amount, gm
Water	1,200.0	Chloride (as NaCl)	12.0
Solids	60.0	Sodium	4.0
Urea	30.0	Phosphate (as P)	1.1
Uric acid	0.7	Potassium	2.0
Hippuric acid	0.27	Calcium	0.2
Creatinine	1.2	Magnesium	0.15
Indican	0.01	Sulfur (as S)	1.0
Oxalic acid	0.02	Inorganic sulfur	0.8
Allantoin	0.04	Neutral sulfur	0.12
Amino acid nitrogen	0.2	Conjugated sulfates	0.08
Purine bases	0.01	Ammonia	0.7
Phenols	0.2		

Printed by permission of Ruth M. French, *The Nurse's Guide to Diagnostic Procedures*, New York: McGraw-Hill, 1971, p. 17, and B. L. Oser (ed.), *Hawk's Practical Physiological Chemistry*, 14th ed., New York: McGraw-Hill, 1965.

For a single, clean-catch specimen on an older girl, the nurse need only give the patient a wide-mouthed, clean specimen bottle and instructions on how to hold the labia apart while wiping from front to back over each side of the vestibule, using a fresh cotton ball each time. Finally, with a third cotton ball, the meatus is wiped, also in a front-to-back direction, and urination is begun. The first few drops are discarded and the rest of the urine collected in a clean container. Some institutions insist on a sterile container, but this is probably not essential. Some authorities advocate special soap and sterile water but this is probably not necessary either. Urine from older boys can be collected in a similar manner.

Clean catches on infants are less reliable, but can be attempted. The genital area is cleansed with damp and dry cotton and a small plastic urine bag with adhesive is attached around the penis or between the labia majora. If the bag is applied as the child is weighed in, the infant will generally void sometime during the examination and the bag can be removed. If not, giving the infant a few ounces to drink will usually produce the desired results. Once a child is toilet-trained, a specimen can be obtained in the adult manner, but with direct supervision and help from the nurse.

Specimens may be collected as a single catch or as a total of all urine voided over a period of time. Single specimens are best collected and examined promptly; if that is impossible, refrigeration is necessary. Specimens collected over 24 hours need some type of preservative to prevent bacterial contamination. Some of the more commonly used chemical preservatives are toluene, glacial acetic acid, formaldehyde, and commercial preservative tablets (Urokeep). Some tests require specific preservatives: 17-ketosteroid examinations require a larger amount of glacial acetic acid, and urobilinogen examinations require sodium carbonate. Specimens may also require refrigeration. This is usually done by refrigerating a large container and bringing each new specimen to the container as it is obtained.

Urine Screening Tests

Since urine is so easily obtained, it is used for many screening tests. The majority of the tests described in this section are easily done and read by the nurse. Basically urine is screened macroscopically and chemically.

Macroscopic inspection of urine includes observation of clarity, color, and odor. All urine specimens should be observed before any testing is done. Fresh, normally voided urine should be clear and transparent. It should contain no sediment, clouding, or mucous. Cloudiness can be caused by bacteria; blood; pus; casts; a large, all-vegetable meal; or epithelial cells. Freshly voided normal urine should be some shade of yellowish-amber. Small fluid intake, vomiting, diarrhea, or excessive perspiration may show a darker, more burnt-yellow-orange color, while large fluid intake may produce dilute, pale, or colorless urine. Many drugs and diseased conditions can cause urine to change color dramatically. Povan, used in the treatment of pinworms, for instance, may turn the urine a brilliant red. The mother of the child should be warned of this occurrence before it happens. Table 4-10 shows some of the other conditions that can change urine color.

Odor is another important characteristic of urine. Due to the organic acids, fresh, normal urine has a definite aromatic smell. With time and pathological conditions, the odor can change drastically. As urine is allowed to stand and decompose, there is a strong ammoniacal aroma. Freshly voided urine that has bacteria present may have a foul, putrid odor. Acidosis caused by diabetes, severe vomiting, or prolonged fever may produce urine that smells sweet and fruity. This is due to the increased acetone present in urine. Decomposed, diabetic urine can smell acidy like vinegar or yeasty like dough. Urine smelling like a rotten egg (hydrogen sulfide) may contain cystine. Fecal contamination, from either accidental or pathological causes gives urine a foul, fecal odor. Some foods (e.g., onions and asparagus) give a specific, definite odor, and some strong-smelling drugs (e.g., peppermint, turpentine, and menthol) will carry their odor through the urine. Table 4-11 lists some of the odor changes found in urine.

Chemically there are several simple procedures that can be performed to gather more data about the urine specimen. When screening urine, the examiner can test for pH, specific gravity, and presence of protein, glucose, ketones, bilirubin, blood, phenylalanine, and sulfite. Many of these tests can be done simply with commercial products that require no more than a special filter paper briefly exposed to the specimen. The tests come in many varieties, and the examiner is wise to pick the test that gives the most information for the least amount of money.

Table 4-10 Common Causes of Urine Color Changes

Color	Cause of coloration	Pathologic condition
Nearly colorless	Dilution or diminution of normal pigments	Nervous conditions; hydruria; diabetes insipidus; granular kidney
Dark yellow to amber	Increase of normal, or occurrence of pathologic, pigments; concentrated urine	Acute febrile diseases
Milky	Fat globules; pus cells; amorphous phospate	Chyluria; purulent diseases of the urinary tract
Orange	Excreted drugs, such as santonin, chrysophanic acid, pyridine	
Red or reddish	Hematoporphyrin; hemoglobin; myoglobin; erythrocytes	Hemorrhage; hemoglobinuria; trauma
Brown to brown-black	Hematin; methemoglobin; melanin; hydroquinone; pyrocatechol	Hemorrhage; methemoglobinuria; melanotic sarcoma
Greenish-yellow or brown, approaching black	Bile pigments	Phenol poisoning; jaundice
Dirty green or blue (dark-blue surface scum, blue deposit)	Excess of indigo-forming substances; methylene blue medication	Cholera; typhus (seen especially when urine is putrefying)

Printed by permission of Ruth M. French, *The Nurse's Guide to Diagnostic Procedures,* New York: McGraw-Hill, 1971, p. 19, and B. L. Oser (ed.), *Hawk's Practical Physiological Chemistry,* 14th ed., New York: McGraw-Hill, 1965.

pH This is a test for the amount of acid or alkaline present in the urine. The blood pH is controlled by the kidney, which filters all excessive ions into the urine. Thus pH of the urine varies according to blood levels. The pH is easily tested with the use of special filter paper, sometimes built into such tests as the Bili-Labstix. A filter paper is dipped into freshly collected urine and immediately matched with the color-coded chart for acidity or alkalinity. The standard matching is orange = pH 5, tan = pH 6, light green = pH 7, dark green = pH 8, and dark blue = pH 9. A normal pH is between 4.8 and 8.0 on the scale.

Specific Gravity Specific gravity is a measure of the concentration or dilution of dissolved substances within the urine. The test can be performed by using a hydrometer (or urinometer); the newer method uses the refractometer. The hydrometer is a small, glass-enclosed tube, fat at the bottom

Table 4-11 Odor Changes Found in Urine

Disorder	Compound	Odor
Phenylketonuria	Phenylacetic acid	Musty odor
Maple syrup urine disease	Branched chain *a*-keto acids	Maple syrup or burned sugar
Isovaleric acidemia	Isovaleric acid	Cheesy or sweaty feet
Oasthouse disease*	*a*-Hydroxybutyric acid	Oasthouse or brewery
Methionine malabsorption*	*a*-Hydroxybutyric acid	Oasthouse
Hypermethioninemia	*a*-Keto-γ-methiol butyric acid	Rancid butter or rotten cabbage
Butyric/hexanoic acidemia	Butyric and hexanoic acids	Sweaty feet
Trimethylaminuria	Trimethylamine	Stale fish

*It has been suggested the methionine malabsorption syndrome and the oasthouse disease may be identical disorders.

Source: G. H. Thomas and R. R. Howell, *Selected Screening Tests for Genetic Metabolic Diseases,* Chicago: Year Book Medical Publishers, Inc. Used by permission.

and thin at the top. The top portion contains demarcated spaces and numbers. The hydrometer method requires 20 ml of urine, which is poured into the cylinder holding the hydrometer. The hydrometer floats free until it stabilizes, and a reading is taken at the level of the urine. The new method requires only a drop of urine, which is placed on the slide of the refractometer. This instrument looks like a small flashlight with a flapping door on one side. Once the urine is dropped on the slide, the door is held firmly in place; the examiner looks through one end while pointing the other end toward a light source. A reading is taken by observing the sharp line seen through the lens at the end of the refractometer. A normal specific gravity is 1.003 to 1.030.

Specific Elements There are many commercial products for screening for specific elements present in urine.

Bili-Labstix is probably one of the most complete; one filter paper gives six readings: pH, protein, glucose, ketones, bilirubin, and blood. The papers come in a dark bottle containing 100 reagent strips, and the standardized color chart is on the bottle. The strips must be stored at room temperature in the tightly capped bottle. Freshly voided urine is preferable for testing, but urine preserved with Urokeep or Kingsburg-Clark urine preservative tablets can also be used. Other preservatives give false readings. The reagent strip is removed from the bottle with care to avoid touching the filter areas and the strip dipped completely into the urine sample. Any excess urine is removed by gently shaking or tapping the strip. The filter portion can be matched immediately against the color-coded chart on the bottle. pH may be read immediately and should give a reading around 5 to 8. Protein may be read immediately and should be negative (a light yellow). A trace calls for a repeat test with a second urine specimen. Glucose can be read at 10 seconds and should be negative (a brilliant pink); a reading at "light" (light purple) indicates 0.25 gm/100 ml of glucose present, and the test must be repeated. Ketones can be read at 15 seconds and should be negative (a light tan). Occult blood is read at 30 seconds and should be negative (a soft tan). Bilirubin is read at 20 seconds and should be negative (a light tan).

Clinitest is used to test for glucose in urine. The test comes as 100 reagent tablets in a dark brown bottle. The procedure involves setting one tablet on a dry, clean surface, placing 2 drops of urine on the tablet, adding 10 drops of water, and waiting 15 seconds for the reaction. Interpretation is based on a color chart provided with a scale of 0 to 5 percent. Thus:

Dark blue = 0 (negative)
Dirty green = trace
Olive green = 0.5 percent
Yellow-green = 1 percent
Yellow-brown = 2 percent
Yellow-tan = 3 percent
Orange = 5 percent

Clinistix is a similar product for testing urine for glucose. It consists of reagent strips which are dipped into fresh urine and read after 10 seconds. Results are interpreted according to a color chart on the bottle. Clinistix is not considered as sensitive as other tests since it will give a false negative with sugars other than glucose.

Combistix is similar to Bili-Labstix but tests for only three elements: pH, glucose, and protein. It is a special reagent filter which is dipped in fresh urine. All the tests are read immediately, with pH ranging from 5 to 9, glucose being negative, small, medium, or large, and protein being negative, trace, 1+, 2+, and 3+.

Keto-Diastix is a fairly new screening test for detecting glucose and ketones in the urine. The urine must be at room temperature. The reagent strip is dipped into the urine for 2 seconds and withdrawn. Excess urine is removed and the strip is read at 15 seconds for ketones and 30 seconds for glucose. Interpretation is made according to the color chart on the side of the bottle. The color code is:

Soft-buff = negative ketones
Light pink = positive ketones (small amount)

Darker pink = positive ketones (moderate amount)
Light purple = positive ketones (large amount)
Pale blue = negative glucose
Darker blue = positive glucose (trace)
Deep blue-brown = positive glucose (1+)
Dark blue-brown = positive glucose (2+)
Brown = positive glucose (4+)
Dark brown = positive glucose (4+)

The Keto-Diastix is intended only for use as a screening tool; it can give false readings due to chilled urine, oral hypoglycemic agents, etc.

Uristix is another product which tests for glucose and protein. The reagent strip is immersed in the fresh urine specimen and immediately withdrawn. Protein is determined immediately by comparing the strip with the color chart on the bottle. Lack of color indicates no protein, and traces of color show little, moderate, or large amounts of protein. Glucose is read at 10 seconds, and by color comparison a reading of small, medium or large is made.

All these tests are easy to administer, inexpensive, and can be very useful screening tools when used appropriately.

PKU Testing PKU is a serious disease, and many states now require some form of screening on all infants. Blood testing for PKU has already been discussed; there are also two very simple screening devices for testing urine for PKU: the Phenistix and ferric chloride test.

Phenistix reagent strips must be stored at room temperature in a dark, tightly capped bottle. The strips should be used on fresh urine or urine preserved with the Kingsbury-Clark urine preservative tablets. The procedure calls for the strip to be pressed between two areas of freshly wetted diaper (avoid diaper with fecal soiling) until the strip is well-saturated. Interpretation is made by comparing the strip with the color chart on the bottle after a 30-second interval. A negative reading shows no change in the strip colors, and a positive reading shows shades of blue-gray (meaning 15, 40, 100 mg of phenylpyruvic acid per 100 ml of urine).

The ferric chloride test can be used to screen for PKU, histidinemia, tyrosinemia, alcaptonuria, maple sugar disease, and oasthouse disease and for the presence of some medications (i.e., salicylates, antipyrine, isoniazid, etc.) (Thomas and Howell, 1973). A squirt bottle or eye dropper is filled with a 10 percent solution of ferric chloride (10 gm of $FeCl_3$ in 100 ml of water). One to two drops of the solution is squirted on fresh urine (usually on the diaper) and the color observed after 30 to 60 seconds. No color change (a slight yellowing on the diaper) indicates absence of disease. A positive result shows a different color for each of the specific diseases listed. Phenylketonuria turns the diaper a dark green color and histidinemia will show a dark green, blue, or purple spot. Tyrosinemia may show no color or a transient green or blue. Alcaptonuria shows either no color or a transient blue, and maple sugar disease gives no color or a purple discoloration. A dark green spot can be the result of oasthouse disease. The drugs also give different colors: salicylate, purple; antipyrine, red; and isoniazid, yellow-green to lavender. It must be remembered that this is a screening test and should alert the examiner to more diagnostic, definitive testing.

Sulfite Screening This test is used to detect a urinary sulfite disorder which leads to damaged eye lenses, neurological defects, and mental retardation. A special reagent strip is placed in a freshly voided urine specimen and withdrawn to be read after a 10-second interval. The presence of sulfite results in a brilliant pink; its absence is indicated by a light pink.

Testrip This relatively new screening device is a VMA-sensitive reagent strip to test for neuroblastoma and pheochromocytoma. The test requires freshly voided urine in a clean container or on a clean diaper. Urine that has been preserved can be used, but must have the pH adjusted to between 5 and 7. The reagent strip is thoroughly saturated in the urine and then positioned on a clean, hard surface for 7 to 10 minutes. Interpretation is made by matching the strip to the color chart on the bottle. A negative reading shows a yellow or brown color. A positive reading shows a purple color indicating the presence of at least 20 micrograms of VMA per milliliter. False readings are obtained if the child has ingested vanilla, coffee, bananas, specific fruits, and some medications within the previous 24 hours.

These are a sampling of the many urine screening devices available to the nurse. Most of them are easily run and fairly inexpensive and within certain ranges give reliable results as screening procedures.

Bactiuria Screening By far the most useful of the products available for urinary screening tests are the recently released bacteriological screening agents. These can be used to screen for the most common urinary problem of childhood infections. Almost all the tests currently available from United States manufacturing companies are based on the principle that bacteria will multiply on agar plates under incubated situations. Most of these tests are quite inexpensive compared with a complete urinary culture and for this reason are more practical for screening purposes. They do not, however, give all the information that a complete culture will give; they tell only whether bacteria are present in the specimen and if so, in what amounts they are present; they do not tell what specific bacteria are present, and they do not tell the antibiotic sensitivity of the bacteria that are present. Most of them consist of a small agar plate and a dipstick which is dipped into the urine and then brought in contact with the agar plate before incubation. After incubation, bacterial colonies are visible to the naked eye and are counted.

A specified number is interpreted as minimal and considered to be due to skin contamination; a slightly higher number is considered suspicious, and the test should be redone; colony counts over that number are said to be infections, and a complete culture should be taken. The two most common tests available in the United States are Testuria and Quantikit. Uricult is a similar product manufactured in Finland. All are well below $1.00 in cost. They do, however, have several disadvantages. The first is that although the manufacturers claim they are quite easy to read, this has not always been the authors' experience; the second is that incubation is necessary, and this may be a handicap in certain clinic situations; finally, there is the problem of obtaining clean catch in younger girls. Anyone who has had the experience of performing the meticulous preparatory ritual for a clean catch (i.e., having the little girl spread her legs and hold her urine while the examiner holds her labia apart, washes carefully from front to back three times, and then rinses carefully in the same manner) knows that the most common response is for the child to decide she no longer can urinate. The rate of skin contamination with this procedure in young girls is very high and can invalidate some of these screening tests. There is one test available which circumvents these problems. This product is Uriglox manufactured only in Sweden at the time of this writing. This is a much easier test to use since it is based on a different underlying principle. Schersten (1969) reported that healthy individuals will excrete a minute amount of glucose in their urine (about 2 mg/ml); the only time this is not excreted is when bacteria are present in the bladder long enough to ingest the glucose. He then devised a simple dipstick that could accurately measure the amount of glucose present. If at least 2 mg/ml (the normal) is present in the urine, the stick will turn blue, indicating that no infection is present; if less glucose is present, there will be no color change, indicating that an infection is highly probable and a complete urine culture should be done. For screening purposes, the nurse must be certain to follow the directions carefully. It is essential that subjects eat or drink nothing after 7 P.M. the preceding night and bring the first morning specimen for the screening. If children eat anything after this time, they may excrete excess glucose and a false negative test will result; if they drink anything, they may dilute the amount of glucose in the urine and a false positive will occur. In clinical practice, this problem is usually less severe than the problem of the clean catch, particularly with little girls. These devices are extremely useful tools, since Kunin (1972) has shown that a full 5 percent of young girls will have urinary infections with no symptoms. The only way these infections can be detected is by periodic checks of the urine. A complete urinary culture is far too expensive to be practical for this purpose, but these inexpensive screening devices, particularly Uriglox, are ideal. Routine screening of little boys is probably not worth the effort since so few of them will be found to have urinary tract infections (Kunin, 1972, found only 0.04 percent of little boys to be infected). At any rate, this is by far the most useful of the urinary screening devices currently available, and the nurse should consider using it routinely at periodic intervals for all girls.

Urine Diagnostic Tests

Once a child has been screened and there is a positive reading or some question about the results, more specific laboratory work and a more complete history and physical examination are necessary. While urine is screened macroscopically and chemically, it is diagnostically tested both microscopically and chemically. The following diagnostic urine tests are not all the tests that can be performed on the urine, but only a sampling of some of the more popular procedures.

The microscopic examination is done after the urine has been examined macroscopically for color, clarity, and odor. The specimen should be freshly voided and obtained by the clean-catch method. About 15 ml of urine is poured into a centrifuge tube and spun for 3 to 5 minutes at medium speed. The supernatant fluid is poured off the top by inverting the tube quickly and returning it to its upright position. By quickly tapping the bottom of the tube against the finger or palm, the sediment and remaining urine are mixed. One drop of this mixture is placed on a glass slide and a cover glass dropped over the specimen. The slide may be viewed under the microscope by using a low light, beginning with the 16-mm lens (or low power) for finding casts and proceeding to the 4-mm lens (or high power) for the smaller substances.

Various cells are the first substances to be observed for: epithelial (renal, transitional, squamous), glitter, neoplastic, inclusion bodies, red blood cells, and white blood cells. Epithelial cells are simply the sloughed cells from different parts of the urinary tract. Usually the 16-mm lens is used and all types of cells are lumped together for a count of 1+ to 4+ or more. Renal cells are small with a large nucleus and come from the renal pelvis. These should not normally be seen. Transitional cells have large odd-shaped diameters and come from the pelvis, ureter, or bladder and are seen only in certain pathological conditions. Squamous cells show a tiny nucleus in a large, flat diameter and can be seen in normal specimens. Glitter cells require a special dye for easy observation and are seen only in pyelonephritis. Neoplastic cells and inclusion body cells are seen only in certain pathological conditions and usually require special preparations of the slide for easier viewing. Red blood cells can be seen with both high and low power and appear as roughly rounded cells with no nucleus. Red blood cells should not be present in normal, voided specimens. A catheterized specimen may show a few red blood cells, but generally any presence of such cells means kidney disease or trauma. White blood cells are absent in normal urine; however, with the 4-mm lens adult male urine may show one white blood cell and the urine of adult females and all children may show one to five white blood cells and still be within normal ranges. Both red and white blood cells look the same in urine as they do in a blood smear. They should definitely be absent from multiple voidings, catheterizations, and bladder taps. Pus cells are frequently confused with white blood cells since their appearance is somewhat similar. The presence of pus usually indicates a tumor, trauma, or infection somewhere within the urinary tract.

Casts are abnormal plasma-protein gel produced by the renal tubules after trauma or damage. There are several kinds of casts: hyaline, blood, and epithelial. Degeneration of an epithelial cast forms a granular cast which may be fine or coarse. Other types of casts degenerate to form fatty casts, waxy casts, and amyloid casts. Casts are usually seen with the 16-mm lens, and their presence is reportable and needs further investigation (see Fig. 4-27).

Parasites are rarely seen in urine and are never normal. Trichomonas, schistosoma and filaria are those most likely to be observed.

Sediments are another abnormal substance to be observed for when examining the urine. Colorless, bumpy substances are amorphous phosphate sediment which can be dissolved in acetic acid and is seen in alkaline urine. Bumpy, granulated substances are calcium carbonate sediment which can also be dissolved in acetic acid. Yellow, diffuse granulated sediment is amorphous urates found in acid urine and dissolved with heating and alkali.

Crystals should not be present in freshly voided, warm urine, but they will form in normal urine as it cools. Acid urine shows calcium oxalate crystals and uric acid (or urate) crystals. Alkaline urine shows ammonio-magnesium phosphate, calcium carbonate, and ammonium biurate crystals.

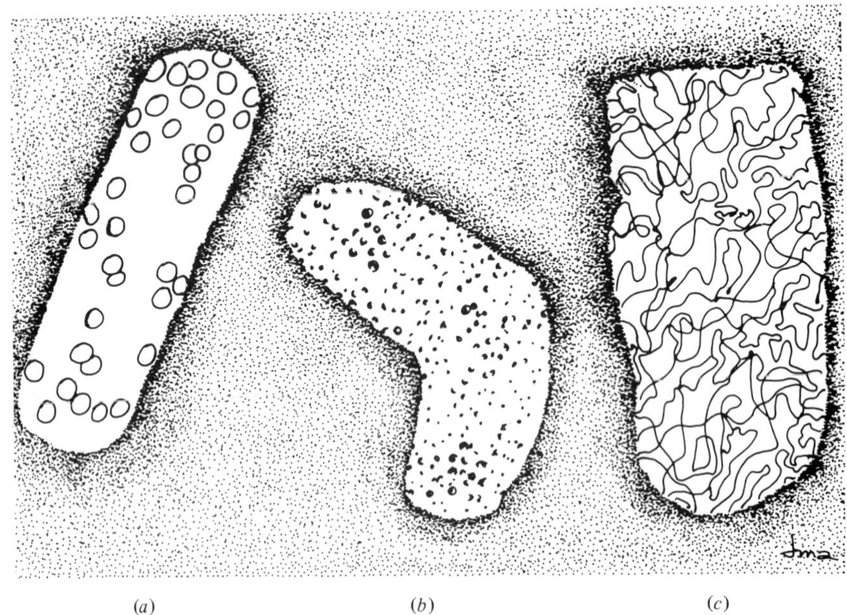

Figure 4-27 Casts seen in urine. (*a*) Blood cast. (*b*) Granular cast. (*c*) Renal cast.

Various other particles can be seen such as thread fibers from panties and cotton left from washing the area. Either external or internal contamination will show bacteria in the specimen (see Fig. 4-28).

Once the urine has been examined for visible particles, it can be tested chemically for the presence of other substances.

Acetone There are three types of ketone bodies found in urine: acetone, acetoacetic acid, and beta-hydroxy-butyric acid. Ketones and incomplete ketones are formed in the metabolism of fat; when low or no carbohydrate intake occurs, fat may be used as an energy source; when this happens, the breakdown products of fat metabolism—ketones—will appear in the urine. A high production of ketones is known as ketosis and leads to acidosis, which is most often associated with uncontrolled diabetes mellitus. Ketosis is also seen after the administration of ether or after severe vomiting or starvation. If a screening test shows ketosis, a diagnostic test for acetone is indicated. Some authorities feel that the presence of acetone indicates the

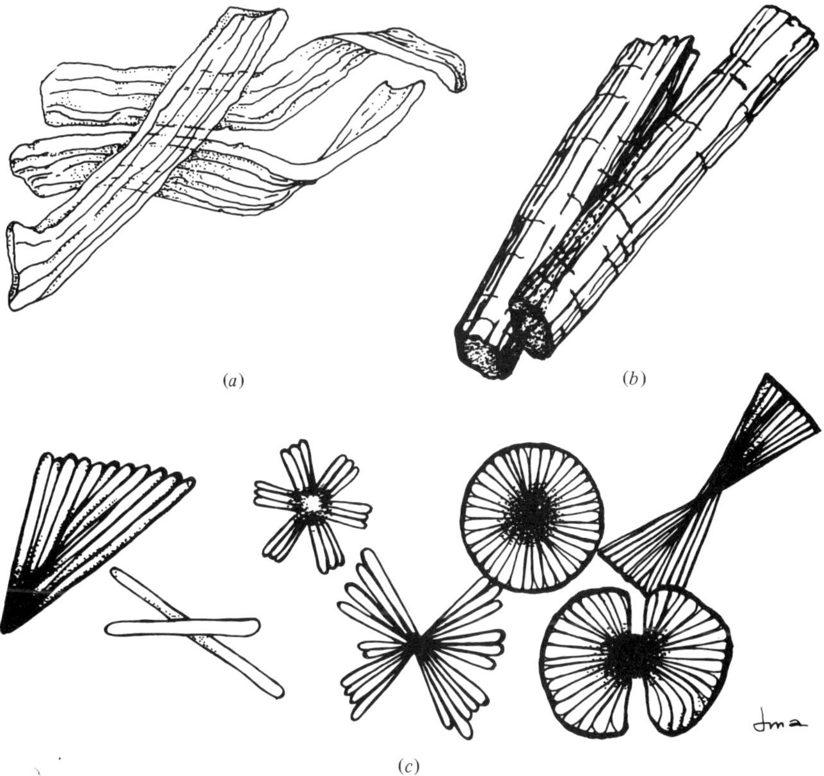

Figure 4-28 Sediment found in urine. (*a*) Cotton fibers. (*b*) Hair. (*c*) Sulphonamide crystals.

presence of the other two types of ketones as well. A fresh sample of urine is mixed with a solution of ammonium sulfate and nitroprusside and additional ammonia is carefully poured on the top surface to give a layered effect. A positive reading (acetone present) shows a reddish-purple ring between the layer of ammonia and the solution. A negative reading indicates absence of acetone. False positive tests can be obtained if the patient has recently taken certain drugs such as L-dopa, Levodopa, or Phenformin, (Garb, 1971) or has been exposed to bromosulfonphtalein or phenolsulfonphthalein testing.

Addis Test The Addis test (Table 4-12) is done to diagnose a specific kidney disease by counting the cells and casts present in the sediment. For reasons of safety, this test is not to be performed on any patient of known renal pathology. For 24 hours the patient may eat but consume no fluids. After 12 hours the patient voids one specimen, which is discarded. For the remaining 12 hours the patient collects all the urine voided (generally around 800 to 1,600 ml). During the collecting period, the urine must be refrigerated. The urine is completely mixed and then centrifuged; the sediment is then examined through the microscope. The diagnosis of nephritis is based on the number of red blood cells, white blood cells, and casts present.

Amylase In some pancreatic pathology, the pancreatic digestive enzymes may ooze into surrounding tissues and serum and finally overflow into the urine. Depending on the laboratory, the test for amylase can be done with a 2-, 12-, or 24-hour collection of urine. The urine is hydrolyzed and observed for the development of a blue color. Interpretation is made by comparing the color of the urine with a standard color chart, with readings of 270 units per hour being in the normal range. Many drugs such as codeine, morphine, demerol, and ethyl alcohol (Garb, 1971) give false positive results. Such conditions as intestinal obstructions, mumps, and salivary gland pathology will also give false readings.

Table 4-12 Addis Test Values

Condition	RBC/mm^3	WBC/mm^3	Casts/mm^3
Normal	0–5,000	0–500,000	1,000,000
Acute nephritis	690,000	405,000,000	48,000,000
Chronic nephritis (active)	1,850,000	34,000,000	14,000,000
Chronic nephritis (latent)	48,000	16,000,000	2,000,000

Source: Opal Helper, *Manual of Clinical Laboratory Methods,* 4th ed., 1954. Courtesy of Charles C. Thomas, Publisher, Springfield, Illinois.

Bilirubin If there is an increase in the destruction of red blood cells or a malfunction within the liver, the bile pigments and bilirubin will increase and overflow into the urine. A single urine specimen can be used to measure this. It is important for the patient to avoid several specific drugs such as acetophenazine, phenazopyridine, and ethoxazene prior to the testing, since these invalidate the test results (Garb, 1971). There are several different tests (Gmelin's, Rosenbach's, Smith's, etc.); they all depend on oxidation of the bilirubin to produce a specific color, which is then compared with a standard. A negative, or normal, result indicates the absence of bilirubin or bile; a positive, or abnormal, result indicates the presence of those substances.

Hormonal Studies There are many complicated, esoteric tests that can be done on urine for the presence of specific hormones; only two are mentioned here: 17-hydroxy-corticosteroid and 17-ketosteroid. The 17-hydroxy-corticosteroid test measures the amount of corticosteroid being produced by the adrenal cortex. The patients must be instructed in the 24-hour collection of urine. The specimen is then processed to extract the corticosteroid with butanol and buffered with a special reagent which produces some color changes which are matched to standard charts. Many drugs will give false readings—cortisone, digitoxin, estrogens, iodides, reserpine, etc. (Garb, 1971)—and the patient must be questioned closely before attempting the test.

The 17-ketosteroid test measures a specific male hormone produced by the adrenals or the testes. Again a 24-hour collection of urine is necessary, as is the avoidance of such drugs as cortisone, meprobamate, penicillin, and oral contraceptives before and during the testing period. In the laboratory, the urine is processed by adding a special chemical and measuring the depth of the red color that results. A result of 8 to 20 mg/day for men and 5 to 15 mg/day for women is considered within the normal range.

Kidney Function The normal kidney has the ability to excrete certain substances, and by measuring these substances some idea of kidney condition can be obtained.

The creatinine clearance test is a measurement of the amount of creatinine (a by-product of metabolism) excreted through the kidney; this directly reflects the adequacy of glomeruli functioning. During the test the patient may eat a normal diet omitting certain beverages (i.e., coffee and tea) and all meat, fish, and poultry. The patient saves all urine for 24 hours and must drink 100 ml of water per hour during the test. Blood is drawn and tested chemically for the amount of creatinine present. A mathematical formula is then used to calculate the amount of creatinine clearance. The normal range is 100 to 140 ml/minute.

The Fishberg (or concentration) test measures the kidney's ability to dilute or concentrate urine. This is a 2-day test and requires hospitalization.

Twelve hours prior to testing, the patient's food intake is restricted and fluid intake limited to 8 oz. The patient is also on limited activity. The first morning specimen is saved, as well as two additional specimens at 1-hour intervals. The patient is then allowed unlimited fluids and food. After a normal supper on the first day of testing, food and fluid is again restricted until the test is complete. The following morning, the first specimen is discarded and the patient instructed to drink 40 oz. of water within a 45-minute period. Urine specimens are collected hourly for 4 hours. As each specimen is taken, the specific gravity is measured and recorded. Normally the concentration period should show a specific gravity of 1.026 or higher and the dilution period should show 1.003.

The phenolsulfonphthalein (PSP) test measures the ability of the kidney's proximal tubules to excrete a certain dye after it has been injected. There are slight variations in the test, but generally the patient must consume 16 oz. of water at the beginning of the test. After 30 minutes 1 to 2 ml of phenolsulfonphthalein dye is injected. Urine specimens are collected at 15, 30, 60, and 120 minutes. The specimens are processed and each compared with a standardized color chart giving the amount of dye normally excreted within each of those time ranges. Bauer (1962) lists the range of normal as:

At 15 minutes, 30 percent dye present
At 30 minutes, 15 percent dye present
At 60 minutes, 10 percent dye present
At 120 minutes, 75 to 85 percent dye present

Such drugs as penicillin, pyridium and some diuretics will give a false reading on this test (Garb, 1971).

Lead If a lead screening test is positive, the patient must be referred for a diagnostic test. After the patient has been on a low calcium diet for 3 days, a 24-hour urine specimen is collected. The lead level may be obtained by chemical or spectrographic procedures. A normal reading is less than 100 micrograms/24 hours; anything over this is considered abnormal.

Morphine This test is used to measure the amount of morphine or heroin ingested within the preceding 24 hours. Several specific chemicals are mixed with a single voided specimen. The resultant color is matched to a color standard to determine the amount of morphine present.

Pregnancy There are many tests for pregnancy, and newer ones are constantly being developed. Most of the procedures are harmless for the mother and the infant; however, some of the more recent tests requiring the mother to ingest specific substances are still being studied for fetal effects.

The newer, more commonly used tests are of two types: the latex-inhibition slide tests (the HCG test, the Gravindex, and the Pregnosticon slide test) and the direct latex agglutination slide test (the DAP test). None of the tests are 100 percent reliable. In fact, Hobson (1969) relates that they have no more reliability than flipping a coin. Kerber's (1970) comparison shows that the Pregnosticon slide test is probably the most useful.

Porphyrins Porphyrins are pigments which are formed by the destruction of red blood cells; they are excreted through the kidney. By measuring the proportion of porphyrins in the urine, the examiner can get some idea of the amount of red blood cell destruction going on in the liver. A 24-hour urine specimen is needed. The porphyrins are precipitated, dissolved, and examined spectroscopically for specific characteristics. A normal urine shows no or very slight amounts of porphyrins; the presence of even small or moderate amounts of porphyrins is abnormal. Drugs like alcohol, sulfonamides, and barbiturates will give false results (Garb, 1971).

Albumin The terms *protein* and *albumin* are frequently used interchangeably; strictly speaking, this is inaccurate, since there are several kinds of protein found in the urine (albumin, globulin, fibrinogen, etc.).

Albumin is the protein most frequently looked for in the urine; both qualitative and quantitative measurements are possible. There are at least four qualitative tests for albumin. The Heller ring test uses filtered urine which is slowly poured into 3 ml of nitric acid, allowed to stand for 3 minutes, and observed for a fine gray line between the two solutions. The amount and density of the gray ring gives a result of trace, +1, +2, or +3. The heat-acetic acid test requires filtered urine to be heated and observed for cloudiness. Several drops of acetic acid are added and cloudiness is again observed. The cloudiness is rated on a scale from 1 to 4. The refined heat-acetic acid test is used to rule out cloudiness caused by any substance other than albumin. The procedure is the same, but sodium chloride and glacial acetic acid are added before the first heating. The sulfosalicylic acid test requires that acetic acid be added to the urine before it is filtered and divided. Half this solution then has sulfosalicylic acid added and is observed for cloudiness; the other half is heated and is also observed for clouding. Cloudiness of either specimen indicates albumin. Such drugs as neomycin, vitamin D, and salicylates will invalidate this test (Garb, 1971).

Quantitatively, there are at least two tests for albumin. The Tsuchiya test requires a 24-hour collection of urine. The urine is diluted to a certain specific gravity, acidified, added to a special reagent, and observed for precipitation. The amount of albumin is measured by the depth of the precipitation. The Kingsbury and Clark test also needs a 24-hour urine specimen. A specific amount of filtered urine is mixed with a certain reagent and allowed to stand for 5 minutes before being compared with a commercial standard.

Both of these tests can be invalidated by many drugs (e.g., bacitracin, aminophyllin, penicillin), and a thorough history of drug ingestion should be obtained before the testing (Garb, 1971).

Sugar Sugar may also be tested for quantitatively and qualitatively. If a screening test has detected the presence of sugar in the urine, a quantitative test is necessary to find out exactly how much sugar is present. One such test is Benedict's test, which requires a 24-hour urine collection. The urine must be preserved by refrigeration and Toluol. When Benedict's solution, sodium carbonate, and a pebble are added together they produce a blue color. The urine is then heated, filtered, and dropped into the Benedict's solution until all the blue color is titrated out. The results can be calculated and interpreted into percentages and gm/24 hours. Steroids, penicillin, and chloral hydrate can give false positives (Garb, 1971).

Sometimes it is important to know what kind of sugar is present; in this situation, qualitative tests must be used. One such test is the fermentation sugar test. The urine from a single specimen is boiled, mixed with yeast, and incubated for 24 hours. Interpretation made is by measuring the amount of carbon dioxide gas present. If only carbon dioxide is present, the test is positive for glucose. If Benedict's test is done and is negative, the test is positive for lactose, glucose, and pentose. Further tests can be performed for additional sugars.

These are a few of the laboratory tests done on urine; there are many more, and the reader is referred to the bibliography for more details and tests. Many of these tests are now being done electronically, with a specimen fed into the computer and any number of tests run automatically, speedily, and inexpensively. Not all laboratories are so equipped, and some continue to use the older, slower, but equally accurate methods.

BIBLIOGRAPHY

Screening in General

American Academy of Pediatrics: *Standards of Child Health Care,* Evanston: American Academy of Pediatrics, 1972.

Browder, J. Albert, Richard B. Hood, and Lloyd B. Lamb: "The Physician and the Child with Hearing Impairment," *Rocky Mountain Medical Journal,* vol. 70, no. 9, September 1973, pp. 42–46.

Burch, George E., and Nicholas P. DePasquale: *Primer of Clinical Measurement of Blood Pressure,* St. Louis: Mosby, 1962.

Christensen, Jacob: "Rapid Haematocrit Determination," *Journal of Medical Laboratory Technology,* vol. 25, March 1968 pp. 383–384.

Downs, Marion P., and Henry K. Silver: "The A.B.C.D.'s to H.E.A.R.," *Clinical Pediatrics,* vol. 11, no. 10, October 1972, pp. 563–565.

Frankenburg, William K., Bonnie W. Kamp, and Pearl A. Van Natta: "Validity of the Denver Developmental Screening Test," *Child Development*, vol. 42, April 1971, pp. 475–485.

Garb, Solomon: *Laboratory Tests in Common Use,* New York: Springer, 1971.

Harper, Paul A.: *Preventive Pediatrics: Child Health and Development,* New York: Appleton-Century-Crofts, 1962.

Joint Study Committee of the American School Health Association and the National Society for the Prevention of Blindness, Inc.: *Teaching about Vision,* New York: National Society for the Prevention of Blindness, 1972.

Loh, Wei-ping: "A New Solubility Test for Rapid Detection of Hemoglobin S," *The Journal of the Indiana State Medical Association,* vol. 61, no. 12, December 1968, pp. 1651-1652.

Moss, Arthur J., and Forrest H. Adams: *Problems of Blood Pressure in Childhood,* Springfield, Ill.: Charles C Thomas, 1962.

O'Brien, Donough, and Frank A. Ibbott: *Laboratory Manual of Pediatric Micro- and Ultramicro-Biochemical Techniques,* New York: Harper & Row, 1962.

O'Brien, John S., Shintaro Okada, Agnes Chen, and Dorothy L. Fillerup: "Tay-Sachs Disease: Detection of Heterozygotes and Homozygotes by Serum Hemosaminidase Assay," *The New England Journal of Medicine,* vol. 283, no. 1, July 2, 1970, pp. 15-20.

Reynolds, Earle, and Lester Sontag: "The Fels Composite Sheet," *Journal of Pediatrics,* vol. 26, no. 4, April 1945, pp. 336-352.

Ross Laboratories: *Children Are Different,* Columbus, Ohio: Ross Laboratories, 1970.

Tanner, J. M.: "Growing Up," *Scientific American,* vol. 229, no. 3, September 1973, pp. 35-42.

Vander Bogert, F., and C. L. Moravec: "Body Temperature Variation in Apparently Healthy Children," *Journal of Pediatrics,* vol. 10, no. 4, April-May 1937, pp. 466-467.

Measurements

American Academy of Pediatrics: *Standards of Child Health Care,* Evanston, Ill.: American Academy of Pediatrics, 1967.

Barnes, Lewis A.: *Manual of Pediatric Physical Diagnosis,* Chicago: Year Book, 1972, pp. 10-18.

Barnett, Henry L.: *Pediatrics,* New York: Appleton-Century-Crofts, 1968.

Burch, George E., and Nicholas P. DePasquale: *Primer of Clinical Measurement of Blood Pressure,* St. Louis: Mosby, 1962.

Chinn, Peggy L., and Cynthia J. Leitch: *Handbook for Nursing Assessment of the Child,* Salt Lake City: University of Utah Press, 1973, pp. 21-22.

Goldring, D., and H. Wohltmann: "Flush Method for Blood Pressure Determinations in Newborn Infants," *Journal of Pediatrics,* vol. 40, February 1952, p. 285.

Gunteroth, W. G., and A. S. Nadas: "Blood Pressure Measurements in Infants and Children," *Pediatric Clinics of North America,* February 1955, pp. 35-42.

Harper, Paul A.: *Preventive Pediatrics,* New York: Appleton-Century-Crofts, 1962, pp. 77-114, 225-233.

Hawke, W. A.: "Elevated Temperatures in Childhood Due to Exercise," *Journal of Pediatrics,* vol. 11, no. 1, July 1937, p. 64.

Heim, Tibor: "Thermogenesis in the Newborn Infant," *Clinical Obstetrics and Gynecology,* vol. 14, no. 3, September 1971, pp. 790-820.

Iliff, A., and V. A. Lee: "Pulse Rate, Respiratory Rate, and Body Temperature of Children between Two Months and Eighteen Years of Age," *Child Development,* vol. 23, March 1952, p. 237.

Kafka, Heinz L., and O. Williams: "Direct and Indirect Blood Pressure Measurements in Newborn Infants," *American Journal of Diseases in Childhood,* vol. 122, November 1971, pp. 426-428.

Kirland, Rebecca T., and John L. Kirland: "Systolic Blood Pressure Measurement in the Newborn Infant with the Transcutaneous Doppler Method," *The Journal of Pediatrics,* vol. 80, no. 1, January 1972, pp. 52-56.

Developmental Screening

Anastasi, Anne: *Psychological Testing,* New York: Macmillan, 1954.

Bayley, Nancy: "Value and Limitations of Infant Testing," *Children,* vol. 5, no. 4, July-August 1958, pp. 129-133

Belmont, Ellian, and Herbert G. Birch: "Lateral Dominance, Lateral Awareness and Reading Disability," *Child Development,* vol. 36-1, no. 1, March 1965, pp. 57-71.

Buros, Oscar K.: *The Sixth Mental Measurements Yearbook,* N.J.: Gryphon Press, 1965.

Cattell, Psyche: *The Measurement of Intelligence of Infants and Young Children,* New York: Psychological Corporation, 1940, p. 274.

Cronbach, Lee J.: *Essentials of Psychological Testing,* New York: Harper & Row, 1970.

Estes, Betsy W., Mary E. Curtin, Robert A. Burger, and Charlotte Denny: "Relationships between 1960 Stanford-Binet, 1937 Stanford-Binet, WISC, Raven and Draw-a-Man," *Journal of Consulting Psychology,* vol. 25, October 1961, pp. 388-391.

Freeman, Frank S.: *Theory and Practice of Psychological Testing,* New York: Holt, 1962.

Fromm, Erika, Lenore Dumas Hartman, and Marian Marschak: "A Contribution to a Dynamic Theory of Intelligence Testing of Children," *Journal of Clinical and Experimental Psychopathology,* vol. 15, no. 2, June 1954, pp. 73-95.

Frostig, Marianne, Welty D. Lefever, and John R. Whittlesey: "A Developmental Test of Visual Perception for Evaluating Normal and Neurologically Handicapped Children," *Perceptional and Motor Skills,* vol. 12, June 1961, pp. 383-394.

Gallagher, James J.: "Clinical Judgment and the Cattell Infant Intelligence Scale," *Journal of Consulting Psychology,* vol. 17, August 1953, pp. 303-305.

Harris, Dale B.: "A Note on Some Ability Correlates of the Raven Progressive Matrices in the Kindergarten," *Journal of Education Psychology,* vol. 50, October 1959, pp. 228-229.

Long, M., J. R. Dunlop, and W. W. Holland: "Blood Pressure Recording in Children," *Archives of Disease in Childhood,* vol. 46, July 1971, pp. 636-640.

Moss, Arthur J., and Forrest H. Adams: *Problems of Blood Pressure in Childhood,* Springfield, Ill.: Charles C. Thomas, 1962.

Nichols, Glennadee A., and Delores H. Kucha: "Oral Measurements," *American Journal of Nursing,* vol. 72, no. 6, June 1972, pp. 1091-1093.

Sievers, Dorothy J. et. al.: *Selected Studies on the ITPA,* Urbana, Ill. University of Illinois Press, 1963, p. 96

Talbot, F. B.: "Skin Temperatures of Children," *American Journal of Diseases,* vol. 42, 1931, p. 965.

van der Bogert, F., and C. L. Moravec: "Body Temperature Variations in Apparently Healthy Children," *Journal of Pediatrics,* vol. 10, no. 4, April 1937, pp. 466-467.

Wold, Robert M.: *Screening Tests to be Used by the Classroom Teacher,* California, Academic Therapy Publications, 1970.

Visual Acuity Screening

Allen, Henry F.: "A New Picture Series for Preschool Vision Testing", *American Journal of Ophthalmology,* vol. 44, July 1957, pp. 38-41.

Bacharach, J., G. Miller, V. Gustafson, et al.: "Vision Testing by Parents of Three-and-One-Half-Year-Old Children," *Public Health Reports,* vol. 85, May 1970, pp. 426-432.

Berens, Conrad: "Kindergarten Visual Acuity Chart," *American Journal of Ophthalmology,* vol. 21, June 1938, pp. 667-668.

Caplan, Bella, and Letha A. Montgomery: "Results of Vision Screening at Seven Years in the Johns Hopkins Collaborative Perinatal Project," *Hopkins Medical Journal,* vol. 128, May 1971, pp. 261-265.

Cunningham, Florence: "Preschool Vision Screening," *American Journal of Public Health,* vol. 49, June 1959, pp. 762-765.

Doster, Mildred E.: "Vision Screening in Schools," *Clinical Pediatrics,* vol. 10, no. 11, November 1971, pp. 662-665.

Ffooks, Oliver: "Vision Test for Children," *British Journal of Ophthalmology,* vol. 49, June 1965, pp. 312-314.

Giles, Conrad L.: "Detection of Amblyopia in the Preschool Child," *Journal of Pediatrics,* vol. 77, August 1970, pp. 309-310.

Green, Morris, and Julius B. Richmond: *Pediatric Diagnosis,* Philadelphia and London: Sannoles 1962.

Hatfield, Elizabeth Macfarlane: "A Year's Record of Preschool Vision Screening," *The Sight-Saving Review,* vol. 36, no. 1, Spring 1966, pp. 18-23.

———: "Progress in Preschool Vision Screening," *The Sight-Saving Review,* vol. 37, no. 4, Winter 1967, pp. 194-201.

Holt, Byerly L.: "Office Preschool Visual Acuity Testing," *The Eye, Ear, Nose and Throat Monthly,* vol. 44, August 1965, pp. 49-51.

Jonkers, G. H.: "The Examination of the Visual Acuity of Children," *Ophthalmologica,* vol. 136, 1958, pp. 110-144.

Krupke, Sidney S., Constance A. Dunbar, and Vivian Zimmerman: "Vision Screening of Preschool Children in Mobile Clinics in Iowa," *Public Health Reports,* vol. 85, no. 1, 1970, pp. 41-45.

Lippman, Otto: "Eye Screening," *Archives of Ophthalmology,* vol. 68, November 1962, pp. 692-705.

———: "Vision of Young Children," *Archives of Ophthalmology,* vol. 81, June 1969, pp. 762-773.

———: "Vision Screening of Young Children," *American Journal of Public Health,* vol. 61, no. 8, August 1971, pp. 1598-1601.

Lo Casciot, George P.: "Preschool-Age Vision Screening," *American Journal of Optometry,* vol. 48, December 1971, pp. 1044-1047.

Nordlow, W., and S. Joachimsson: "A Screening Test for Visual Acuity in Four Year Old Children," *Acta Ophthalmologica,* vol. 40, pp. 453-462, 1962.

Oberman, J. William: "Vision Needs of America's Children," *The Sight-Saving Review,* vol. 36, no. 4, Winter 1966, pp. 217-227.

Osterberg, G.: "A Danish Pictorial Sight-Test Chart," *American Journal of Ophthalmology,* vol. 59, July 1963, pp. 1120-1123.

Press, Edward: "Screening of Preschool Children for Amblyopia", *Journal of the American Medical Association,* vol. 204, no. 9, May 27, 1968, pp. 109-112.

Savitz, Roberta A., Isabelle Valadian, and Robert B. Reed: "Vision Screening of Preschool Children at Home", *American Journal of Public Health,* vol. 55, no. 10, pp. 1555-1562.

Sheridan, Mary D: "Vision Screening of Very Young or Handicapped Children," *British Medical Journal,* August 6, 1960, pp. 453-456.

———, and P. A. Gardiner: "Sheridan-Gardiner Test for Visual Acuity," *British Medical Journal,* vol. 2, Apr. 11, 1970, pp. 108-109.

Snell, Albert C.: "Concerning Observations of the Sharpness of Vision of Abnormal Eyes When Tested at a Distance and at Near Points," *Transactions of the American Academy of Ophthalmology and Otolaryngology,* vol. 32, 1927, pp. 164-182.

Stuart, James A., and Hermann M. Burian: "A Study of Separation Difficulty: Its Relationship to Visual Acuity in Normal and Amblyopic Eyes," *American Journal of Ophthalmology,* vol. 53, March 1962, pp. 471-477.

Taubenhaus, L. J.: "Visual Acuity Testing in Preschool Children," *Journal of the American Medical Association,* vol. 209, no. 13, Sept. 29, 1969, p. 2056.

Trotter, Robert R., Ruth M. Phillips, and Kennetta Schaffer: "Measurement of Visual Acuity of Preschool Children by Their Parents," *The Sight-Saving Review,* vol. 36, no. 2, Summer 1966, pp. 80-89.

Wilhelm, R.: "Evaluating Score Differences on a Visual Acuity Test," *Perceptual and Motor Skills,* vol. 27, October 1968, pp. 419-423.

Withnell A., and Wilson H. E.: "New Method of Screening Young Children for Defects in Visual Acuity," *British Medical Journal,* vol. 4, Oct. 19, 1968, pp. 157-158.

Vision Screening—Heterophoria

Allen, Henry F.: "Incidence of Amblyopia," *Archives of Ophthalmology,* vol. 77, January 1967, p. 1; and *Journal of the American Medical Association,* vol. 199, no. 3, Jan. 16, 1967, p. 211.

Azar, Robert F.: "The Squinting Child," *Journal of the Louisana State Medical Society,* vol. 121, no. 3, March 1969, pp. 81-86.

Burg, Albert: "Horizontal Phoria as Related to Age and Sex," *American Journal of Optometry and Archives of American Academy of Optometry,* vol. 45, no. 6, June 1968, pp. 345-350.

Costenbader, Frank D.: "Symposium: Infantile Esotropia. Clinical Characteristics and Diagnosis," *American Orthoptic Journal,* vol. 18, 1968, pp. 5-10.

Flom, Merton C., and Kenton E. Kerr: "Determination of Retinal Correspondence," *Archives of Ophthalmology,* vol. 77, February 1967, pp. 200-213.

Gundersen, Trygve: "Early Diagnosis and Treatment of Strabismus," *The Sight-Saving Review,* Fall 1970, pp. 129-136.

Henderson, John W.: "The Significance of Vision Problems of Children and Youth," *Journal of Pediatric Ophthalmology,* vol. 6, no. 1, February 1969, pp. 11-14.

Romano, Paul E., and Gunter K. Von Noorden: "Limitations of Cover Test in Detecting Strabismus," *American Journal of Ophthalmology,* vol. 72, no. 1, July 1971, pp. 10-12.

———, and Shinobu Awaya: "Symposium: Sensory Adaptations in Strabismus—A Reevaluation of Diagnostic Methods for Retinal Correspondence," *American Orthoptic Journal,* vol. 20, 1970, pp. 13-21.

Scobee, Richard G., and Earl L. Green: "Tests for Heterophoria," *American Journal of Ophthalmology,* vol. 30, no. 4, 1947, pp. 436-451.

Shaterian, Elizabeth T.: "Significant Aspects of Binocular Visual Acuity in Intermittent Squints," *American Orthoptic Journal,* vol. 18, 1968, pp. 49-51.

Von Noorden, Gunter K.: "Diagnosis and Management of Eye Muscle Problems in Childhood," *Surgical Clinics of North America,* vol. 50, no. 4, August 1970, pp. 885-894.

Hearing Screening

Dale, D. M. C.: *Applied Audiology for Children,* 2d ed., Springfield, Ill.: Charles C. Thomas, 1967.

Glorig, Aram: *Audiometry: Principles and Practices,* Baltimore: Williams & Wilkins, 1965.

———, and H. P. House: "A New Concept in Auditory Screening," *Archives of Otolaryngology,* vol. 66, August 1957, p. 228.

Harper, Paul A.: *Preventive Pediatrics: Child Health and Development,* New York: Appleton-Century-Crofts, 1962.

Jerger, James: *Modern Developments in Audiology,* New York: Academic, 1963.

Katz, Jack: *Handbook of Clinical Audiology,* Baltimore: Williams & Wilkins 1972.

Langenbeck, Bernhard: *Textbook of Practical Audiometry,* Baltimore: Williams & Wilkins 1965.

Miller, Maurice H., and Ira A. Polisar: *Audiological Evaluation of the Pediatric Patient,* Springfield, Ill.: Charles C. Thomas, 1964.

O'Neill, John J., and Herbert J. Oyer: *Applied Audiometry,* New York: Dodd, Mead, 1966.

Portmann, Michael, and Claudine Portmann: *Clinical Audiometry,* Springfield, Ill.: Charles C. Thomas, 1961.

Hearing Screening for Infants

Alberti, P. W.: "Glue Ear," *British Medical Journal,* vol. 1, Feb. 14, 1970, pp. 431-432.

Barnet, A. B.: "Evoked Response Audiometry in 241 Normal and Hearing Impaired Children under Three Years," *Archives for Klinische und Experimentelle Ohren-, Nasen- und Kehlkopfheilkunde,* vol. 198, 1971, pp. 154-157.

Bartoshuk, A.: "Neonatal Cardiac Response to Sound: A Power Function," *Psychonomic Science,* vol. 1, 1964, pp. 151-152.

Bench, J.: "Some Methodological Problems and Techniques in Infant Audiometry," *Bio-Medical Engineering,* vol. 5, January 1970, pp. 12-14.

Bench, R. J., and K. P. Murphy: "The Papousek Cradle: A Device for Measuring Babies' Head Movement Responses to Auditory Stimulation," *Journal of Laryngology and Otology,* vol. 84, May 1970, pp. 521-523.

Bierman, C. W., W. E. Pierson, and J. A. Donaldson: "The Evaluation of Middle Ear Function in Children," *American Journal of Diseases of Children,* vol. 120, September 1970, pp. 233-236.

Clark, J. R.: "Testing the Hearing of Children with Noisemakers—A Myth," *Exceptional Children,* vol. 22, 1956, p. 323.

Economopoulou, H., H. J. Krogh, and L. Fosvig: "EEG-Computer Audiometry (ERA) in a Group of Pre-School and School-Age Children," *Acta Oto-Laryngologica,* Supplement, vol. 263, 1969, pp. 248-250.

Fay, Thomas H., Irving Hochberg, Clarissa R. Smith, Norma S. Rees, and Harvey Halpern: "Audiologic and Otologic Screening of Disadvantaged Children," *Archives of Otolaryngology,* vol. 91, April 1970, pp. 366-370.

Harrelson, O. A., D. G. Ferguson, G. P. Killian, et al.: "Comparison of Hearing Screening Methods," *The Journal of School Health,* vol. 39, March 1969, pp. 161-164.

"Hearing Status and Ear Examination Findings among Adults: National Center for Health Statistics Releases Report," *Industrial Medicine,* vol. 38, no. 2, February 1969, pp. 72-73.

Henriksen, O., Kotby M. Nasser, and A. Kayan: "Auditory Evoked Responses: The Basis for a Promising Objective Audiometric Test," *Electroencephalography and Clinical Neurophysiology,* vol. 29, August 1970, pp. 220-221.

Heron, T., and R. Jacobs: "Respiratory Curve Responses of the Neonate to Auditory Stimulation," *International Audiology,* vol. 8, 1969, pp. 77-84.

Holm, V. A., and G. Thompson: "Selective Hearing Loss: Clues to Early Identification," *Pediatrics,* vol. 47, February 1971, pp. 447-451.

Hooker, Paul, and Richard A. Hoops: "A Portable Diagnostic Speech Audiometry Unit," *Journal of Speech and Hearing Disorders,* vol. 34, no. 3, August 1969, pp. 251-252.

Lentz, William E., and Geary A. McCandless: "Averaged Electroencephalic Audiometry in Infants," *Journal of Speech and Hearing Disorders,* vol. 36, no. 1, February 1971, pp. 19-28.

Mencher, George T., and Barbara F. McCulloch: "Auditory Screening of Kindergarten Children Using the Vasc," *Journal of Speech and Hearing Disorders,* vol. 35, no. 3, August 1970, pp. 241-247.

Moghadam, Hossein K., Geoffrey C. Robinson, and Kenneth G. Cambon: "A Comparison of Two Audiometers in Screening the Hearing of School Children," *Canadian Medical Association Journal,* vol. 99, Sept. 28, 1968, pp. 618-620.

Moncur, J.: "Judge Reliability in Infant Testing," *Journal of Speech and Hearing Research,* vol. 11, 1968, pp. 348-357.

Rapin, I., R. J. Ruben, and M. Lyttle: "Diagnosis of Hearing Loss in Infants Using Auditory Evoked Responses," *Laryngoscope,* vol. 80, May 1970, pp. 712-722.

———, and P. Steinherz: "Reaction Time for Pediatric Audiometry," *Journal of Speech and Hearing Research,* vol. 13, March 1970, pp. 203-217.

Roberts, J.: "Objective Assessment of Auditory Function in Infants," *Proceedings of the Royal Society of Medicine,* vol. 63, July 1970, pp. 701-702.

Roberts, Jean: "Hearing Status and Ear Examination," *Selected Examination Findings Related to Periodontal Disease among Adults,* U.S. Department of Health, Education, and Welfare, ser. 11, no. 33, pp. 1-28.

Rockey, D.: "On the Use of the Drowsy State in Testing the Hearing of Infants and Young Children," *The Medical Journal of Australia,* vol. 2, Sept. 5, 1970, pp. 455-459.

Rosenblith, J. F.: "Are Newborn Auditory Responses Prognostic of Deafness?" *Transactions of the American Academy of Ophthalmology and Otolaryngology,* vol. 74, November-December 1970, pp. 1215-1228.

Rupp, R. R., and W. Wolski: "Hearing Testing in Young Children. Simple Technics Adaptable to Pediatric Office Practice for Screening Neonates, Infants and Young Children." *Clinical Pediatrics,* vol. 8, May 1969, pp. 263-267.

Sandt, W. Van Der: "Clinical Application of Evoked-Response Audiometry," *South African Medical Journal,* vol. 43, Jan. 11, 1969, pp. 33-35.

Schulman, C. A., and G. Wade: "The Use of Heart Rate in Audiological Evaluation of Nonverbal Children. II. Clinical Trials on an Infant Population," *Neuropaediatrie,* vol. 2, December 1970, pp. 197-205.

Sohmer, H., M. Feinmesser, A. Lev, "Routine Use of Cochlear Audiometry in Infants with Uncertain Diagnosis," *Annals of Otology, Rhinology, and Laryngology,* vol. 81, February 1972, pp. 72-75.

Tenney, H. K., and C. Edwards: "Race as a Variable in Hearing Screening," *American Journal of Diseases of Children,* vol. 120, December 1970, pp. 547-550.

Tillman, T. W.: "Special Hearing Tests in Otoneurologic Diagnosis," *Archives of Otolaryngology,* vol. 89, January 1969, pp. 25-30.

Tokay, F. H., and E. J. Hardick: "Validity and Reliability of Bekesy Audiometry with Preschool Age Children," *Journal of Speech and Hearing Research,* vol. 14, March 1971, pp. 205-213.

Tyberghein, J. and G. Forrez: "Objective (E. R. A.) and Subjective (C. O. R.) Audiometry in the Infant," *Acta Oto-laryngologica,* vol. 71, February-March 1971, pp. 249-252.

Van Den Horst, P. Kuyper: "Peek-a-Boo Audiometry," *Practica Oto-Rhino-Laryngologica,* vol. 31, 1969, pp. 288-295.

Walton, J.: "Hearing Disorders in the Pediatric Patient: A Major Medical Problem," *The Journal of the Arkansas Medical Society,* vol. 66, no. 3, August 1969, pp. 100-102.

Weber, B. A.: "Validation of Observer Judgments in Behavioral Observation Audiometry," *Journal of Speech and Hearing Disorders,* vol. 34, November 1969, pp. 350-355.

———: "Comparison of Two Approaches to Behavioral Observation Audiometry," *Journal of Speech and Hearing Disorders,* vol. 13, December 1970, pp. 823-825.

Wilmot, T. J.: "Auditory Analysis in Some Common Hearing Problems," *Journal of Laryngology and Otology,* vol. 83, June 1969, pp. 521-527.

Speech Screening

Berko, J.: "The Child's Learning of the English Morphology," *Word,* vol. 14, 1958, pp. 150-177.

Carrow, Sister Mary Arthur: "The Development of Auditory Comprehension of Language Structure in Children," *Journal of Speech and Hearing Disorders,* vol. 33, no. 2, 1968, pp. 99-111.

Carter, Eunice T., and Buck McKenzie: "Prognostic Testing for Functional Articulation Disorders among Children in the First Grade," *Journal of Speech and Hearing Disorders,* vol. 33, 1958,

Fiedler, M. F., E. H. Lenneberg, U. T. Rolfe, et al.: "A Speech Screening Procedure with Three-Year-Old Children," *Pediatrics,* vol. 48, August 1971, pp. 268-276.

Fletcher, Samuel G., Robert L. Casteel, and Doris P. Bradley: "Tongue-Thrust Swallow, Speech Articulation, and Age," *Journal of Speech and Hearing Disorders,* vol. 26, no. 3, August 1961, pp. 201-209.

Fraser, C., U. Bellugi, and R. Brown: "Control of Grammar in Imitation, Comprehension, and Production," *Journal of Verbal Learning and Verbal Behavior,* vol. 2, 1963, pp. 121-135.

Greene, M. C.: "Early Detection of Speech Difficulty: The Role of the Health Visitor," *Nursing Times,* vol. 65, Sept. 4, 1969, pp. 1138-1139.

———: "Early Detection of Speech Difficulty: Danger Signals," *Nursing Times,* vol. 65, Sept. 11, 1969, pp. 1170-1171.

Hutchinson, B. B.: "Rationale and Standardization for a Combined Speech Articulation and Auditory Discrimination Test," *Perceptual and Motor Skills,* vol. 33, December 1971, pp. 715-721.

Illingworth, R. S.: "The Predictive Value of Developmental Tests in the First Year, with Special Reference to the Diagnosis of Mental Subnormality," *Journal of Child Psychology and Psychiatry and Allied Disciplines,* vol. 2, March 1961, pp. 210-215.

Irwin, R. B.: "Consistency of Judgments of Articulatory Productions," *Journal of Speech and Hearing Research,* vol. 13, September 1970, pp. 548-555.

———, and Barbara Wilson Musselman: "A Compact Picture Articulation Test," *Journal of Speech and Hearing Disorders,* vol. 27, no. 1, February 1962, pp. 36-39.

Kirk, Samuel A., and James J. McCarthy: "The Illinois Test of Psycholinguistic Abilities: An Approach to Differential Diagnosis," *American Journal of Mental Deficiency,* vol. 66, November 1961, pp. 399-412.

Kisatsky, T. J.: "The Prognostic Value of Carter-Buck Tests in Measuring Articulation Skills of Selected Kindergarten Children," *Exceptional Children,* vol. 34, October 1967, pp. 81-85.

Knobloch, Hilda, P. H. Benjamin Pasamanick, and Earl S. Sherard: "A Developmental Screening Inventory for Infants," *Pediatrics,* vol. 38, no. 6, December 1966, pp. 1095-1108.

Koppitz, Elizabeth: "The Bander-Gestalt Test for Children: A Normative Study," *Journal of Clinical Psychology,* vol. 16, October 1960, pp. 432-435.

Lee, Laura L.: "A Screening Test for Syntax Development," *Journal of Speech and Hearing Disorders,* vol. 35, no. 2, pp. 103-112.

Lerea, I.: *The Michigan Picture Language Inventory,* Ann Arbor: University of Michigan Press, 1958.

Lyle, J. G.: "A Comparison of the Verbal Intelligence of Normal and Imbecile Children," *Journal of Genetic Psychology,* vol. 99, April 1961, pp. 227-234.

Mood, George, Bryan Weight, and Patricia James: "Interest Correlations of the Weschler Intelligence Scale for Children and Two Picture Vocabulary Tests," *Educational and Psychological Measurements,* vol. 23, Summer 1963, pp. 359-363.

Popplestone, John A.: "Clinical Status and the Draw-a-Man Test: Congruence and Divergence," *Perceptual and Motor Skills,* vol. 9, June 1959, pp. 131-133.

Rogers, W. B., and Robert A. Rogers: "A New Simplified Preschool Readiness Experimental Screening Scale (The Press)," *Clinical Pediatrics,* vol. 11, October 1972, pp. 558-562.

Silver, Archie A.: "Psychologic Aspects of Pediatrics: Diagnostic Value of Three Drawing Tests for Children," *The Journal of Pediatrics,* vol. 37, July 1950, pp. 127-143.

Smart, M. S., and R. C. Smart: *Children, Development and Relationships,* New York: Macmillan, 1972.

Smith, M. K.: "Measurement of the Size of English Vocabulary Through the Elementary Grades and High School." *Genetic Psychological Monographs,* vol. 24, 1941, pp. 311-345.

Snow, K., and R. Millisen: "Spontaneous Improvement in Articulation as Related to Differential Responses to Oral and Picture Articulation Tests," *Journal of Speech and Hearing Disorders,* Monograph Supplement no. 4, 1954, pp. 45-49.

Steer, M. D., and Hazel G. Drexler: "Predicting Later Articulation Ability from Kindergarten Tests," *Journal of Speech and Hearing Disorders,* vol. 25, 1969, pp. 391-397.

Van Riper, C., and R. Erickson: "A Predictive Screening Test of Articulation," *Journal of Speech and Hearing Disorders,* vol. 34, August 1969, pp. 214-219.

Willis, V. P., and R. Massengill, Jr.: "Language Difficulty: An Analysis of Proficiency and Development," *North Carolina Medical Journal,* vol. 30, January 1969, pp. 18-20.

Screening of Blood

Abbott Laboratories: *The Use of Blood,* Ill.: Abbott Laboratories, Chicago, Ill., 1971.

Bauer, John D., Gelson Toro, and Philip G. Ackermann: *Bray's Clinical Laboratory Methods,* St. Louis: Mosby, 1962.

Canning, D. M., and R. G. Huntsman: "An Assessment of Sickledex as an Alternative to the Sickling Test," *Technical Methods,* vol. 12, January 1970, pp. 736-737.

Doxiadis, S. A., P. H. Fessas, and T. Valaes: "Glucosa-Phosphate Dohydrouenas Deficiency," *Lancet,* vol. 1-1, Feb. 11, 1961, pp. 297-301.

French, Ruth M.: *The Nurse's Guide to Diagnostic Procedures,* New York: McGraw-Hill, 1971.

Garb, Solomon: *Laboratory Tests in Common Use,* New York: Springer, 1971.

Goodman, Stephen I.: *Tay-Sachs Facts,* Denver: F. B. Stolinsky Research Laboratories, Denver, Colo., 1973.

Guyton, Arthur C.: *Basic Human Physiology,* Philadelphia: Saunders,1971.

Hughes, James G.: *Synopsis of Pediatrics,* St. Louis: Mosby, 1971.

Loh, Wei-ping: "A New Solubility Test for Rapid Detection of Hemoglobin S," *The Journal of the Indiana State Medical Association,* vol. 61, no. 12, December 1968, pp. 1651-1652.

Morgan, Samuel K.: "Sicklecrit: Microhematocrit Screen for Sickle Cell Anemia," *American Journal of Diseases of Children,* vol. 122, September 1971, pp. 220–222.

Nalbandian, Robert M., Raymond L. Henry, Joanne M. Lusher, Frank R. Camp, and Nicholas F. Conte: "Sickledex Test for Alemoglobin S," *Journal of the American Medical Association,* vol. 218, no. 11, Dec. 13, 1971, pp. 1679–1680.

———, Bruce M. Nichols, Albert E. Hustis, Winston B. Prothro, and Frederick E. Ludwig: "An Automated Mass Screening Program for Sickle Cell Disease," *Journal of the American Medical Association,* vol. 218, no. 11, Dec. 13, 1971, pp. 1680–1682.

O'Brien, Donough, and Frank A. Ibbott: *Laboratory Manual of Pediatric Micro- and Ultramicro-Biochemical Techniques,* New York: Harper & Row, 1962.

O'Brien, John S., Shintaro Okada, Agnes Chen, and Dorothy L. Fillerup, "Detection of Heterozygotes and Homozygotes by Serum Hemosaminidase Tay-Sachs Disease-Assay," *The New England Journal of Medicine,* vol. 283, no. 1, July 2, 1970, pp. 15–20.

Ross Laboratories: *Children Are Different,* Columbus, Ohio: Ross Laboratories, 1970.

Schwarz, V. J.: "Galactosemia," *Journal of Laboratory and Clinical Medicine,* vol. 56, May 1960, pp. 483–485.

Wolf, Paul L., Patricia Ferguson, Irma T. Mills, Elisabeth Von der Muehll, and Mary Thompson: *Practical Clinical Hematology: Interpretations and Techniques,* New York: Wiley, 1973.

Screening of Urine

Bauer, John D., Toro Gelson, and Philip G. Ackermann, *Bray's Clinical Laboratory Methods,* St. Louis: Mosby 1962.

Chapman, Warren H., Ruth E. Bulger, Ralph E. Cutter, and Gary E. Striker, *The Urinary System,* Philadelphia: Saunders, 1973.

Documenta Geigy Synopsis of Urine, Switzerland: Ciba-Geigy, 1970.

French, Ruth M.: *The Nurse's Guide to Diagnostic Procedures,* New York: McGraw-Hill, 1971.

Garb, Solomon: *Laboratory Tests in Common Use,* New York: Springer, 1971.

Gershenfeld, Louis: *Urine and Urinalysis,* New York: Romaine Pierson, 1948.

Guyton, Arthur C.: *Basic Human Physiology: Normal Function and Mechanisms of Disease,* Philadelphia: Saunders, 1971.

Hobson, B. M.: "Pregnancy Diagnosis," *Lancet,* vol. 2, 1969, p. 56.

Hollman, Louis M., and Jack A. Pritchard: *Williams Obstetrics,* New York: Appleton-Century-Crofts, 1971.

Kark, Robert M.: *A Primer of Urinalysis,* New York: Harper & Row, 1963.

Kerber I. J., A. P. Inclan, E. A. Fowler, K. Davis, and S. A. Fish: "Immunologic Tests for Pregnancy: A Comparison," *Obstetrics and Gynecology,* vol. 36, 1970, p. 37.

Kunin, Calvin M.: *Detection, Prevention and Management of Urinary Tract Infections,* Philadelphia: Lea & Febiger, 1972.

Lippman, Richard W.: *Urine and Urinary Sediment,* Springfield, Ill.: Charles C. Thomas, 1957.

Schersten, Bengt: *Subnormal Fasting Urine Glucose as an Indicator of Urinary Tract Infection,* Lund, 1969.

Thomas, George H., and R. Rodney Howell: *Selected Screening Tests for Genetic Metabolic Diseases,* Chicago: Year Book, 1973.

Winter, Chester C.: *Practical Urology,* St. Louis: Mosby, 1969.

Chapter 5

Growth and Development

The nurse working with children in ambulatory settings should have a knowledge of normal growth and development. It is important for assessing the child in order to pick up early deviations, for reassurance and anticipatory guidance of parents, and for relating to the child himself. Five areas of growth and development will be discussed in this chapter: physical; psychological, social, and cultural; cognitive; perceptual; and linguistic. Growth in all these areas is important to the child, and each should be assessed regularly during the scheduled well-child visits.

PHYSICAL GROWTH AND DEVELOPMENT

Because it has been studied the longest, probably the most is known about physical growth and development. Entire books are available which detail this process on all levels, including the cellular level. In this chapter, the authors will attempt to highlight some of the more important aspects of this field and their application to well-child management. This will include some information on general body and organ system growth as well as some information with which to evaluate the development of both gross and fine motor skills.

General Characteristics

As in all organisms, human growth is orderly and predictable, although certain rates and patterns of growth are specific to certain parts of the body. During embryological development, for instance, the head grows much faster than the remainder of the body. From birth to puberty the extremities grow more rapidly. The general pattern of body growth is cephalocaudal, that is, from the head downward, and proximodistal, that is, from the midline to the periphery of the body. Norms are available to show when growth should begin and stop. Problems may develop when there is too much or too little growth or when growth begins too late, begins too early, stops too early, or goes on too long.

Growth occurs in definite phases. Phase I lasts from conception to the birth of the infant. This stage includes cell multiplication, chemical differentiation, tissue formation, and the actual beginning of cell functioning. Cell multiplication refers to the simple increase in cell numbers. Around the 2d week of life, chemical differentiation occurs and the cells begin to develop three distinct layers (endoderm, ectoderm, and mesoderm). By the 3d week, tissue formation begins and the cells develop into specific organs. Actual cell functioning begins around the 5th month after the cells are well formed. Phase II of growth lasts from birth to adulthood. The entire organism grows larger and more functional. Phase III occurs from adulthood to old age. During this stage, growth is related only to repair and maintenance of body cells and tissues. Phase IV occurs in old age when little growth or repair occur and cell degeneration begins.

Growth is influenced by a multitude of factors. Hereditary factors are the major determinant of growth. Children with tall parents have a good chance of growing tall. One historical study of average heights and weights showed that children are growing larger today than was true a century ago. The average 6½-year-old child in 1954 was the same height as the average 7½-year-old child in the 1880s.

Sex also influences growth. Rate and timing of growth as well as ultimate height differ between males and females. Other variables such as prenatal factors (drugs, infections, diet, trauma), faulty physiological systems (endocrine or metabolic imbalances), malformations, and infections also influence the rate and pattern of growth.

Methods of Assessing Growth

There are several methods of observing children and assessing their rate of growth. The most generally used methods involve measuring and recording height, weight, and head circumference, discussed in Chap. 4. The following are some additional methods of monitoring growth patterns.

The human skeletal system shows definite developmental stages in the growth of connective tissue, cartilage, and bone. These stages may be used in assessing growth. Skeletal age is obtained by the radiological examination of the skeletal system. Since x-raying the entire body is dangerous, only the wrist and hand bones are x-rayed. Interpretation is made by noting the ossification centers present, their size, and the morphological stage of each center. This material has been compiled into the Greulich-Pyle Atlas. According to this atlas, children are classified in six different ways: (1) the average child, (2) the child who matures early but is of average adult height, (3) the child who is tall as a child and as an adult, (4) the child who is short as a child but average as an adult, (5) the child who is short as a child and as an adult, and (6) the child who is average as a child and as an adult.

There are problems with this method of assessing growth. After studying the x-rays, a judgment is made by two observers, and agreement between observers is not always found. Each figure given by the Greulich-Pyle Atlas is an average of several children rather than a longitudinal study of one child, and because of this, the usual increases and decreases seen in most children are lost. Furthermore, this method is not used often because of the danger inherent in x-rays.

Dental age is another method of assessing growth. Most human beings develop two sets of teeth during a lifetime. By knowing the average age of eruption of each set, the examiner may be able to assess the general age of the child. Around 6 months of age an infant's primary (or deciduous) teeth begin to erupt; this set is complete around 3 years of age. The primary teeth begin to fall out around 6 years of age and are replaced by a set of permanent teeth which will be complete between 18 and 25 years of age. This method can also be misleading since genetic and environmental factors can alter the timing of tooth eruption (see Fig. 5-1).

Sexual age is another method of assessing growth. While dental growth gives some indication of development during the early years, sexual age becomes more useful during the pubertal and adolescent years. Sexual age is usually associated with general growth spurts. Girls generally show growth

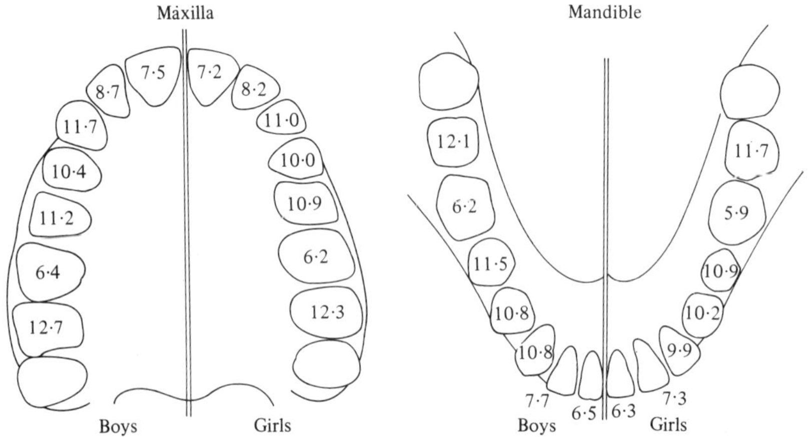

Figure 5-1 Dental age. *(Source: Printed by permission of David Sinclair, Human Growth after Birth, New York: Oxford University Press, 1969, p. 79).*

spurts around 10 to 13 years, with the most intense period lasting about 2 years. Boys generally show their growth spurt around 12 to 16 years, with the most intense period lasting 2½ years. Sexual age is marked by primary and secondary sexual developments. For the female, the primary sexual development involves the uterus, ovaries, hair, and breasts. Around the 9th or 10th year hormonal changes occur which cause the hypophysis to stimulate the adrenal glands to produce androgens and gonadotropins. These two hormones cause the ovary to produce estrogen. Androgens, gonadotropins, and estrogen cause the maturation of the ovaries and uterus. While these internal changes are taking place, there are some external changes that can be assessed. Changes in pubic hair and breast development (Fig. 5-2) are the most noticeable and can be divided into five stages:

Stage I — Pubic area is covered with the same soft, fine hair as the rest of the body, and only the papilla of the breast shows slight elevation.

Stage II — The area around the labia develops several long, pigmented hairs, and the breast papilla becomes slightly erect with some of the surrounding tissue becoming fuller.

Stage III — There is development of additional long, pigmented, coarser hairs from the labia to the mons, and the breast areola and surrounding tissue show continued expansion.

Stage IV — The pubic hair becomes darker, coarser, more curled and covers the labia and mons, while the subareolar and papilla area of the breast becomes distinct from the surrounding breast tissue.

Stage V — The pubic hair becomes more adultlike in appearance and covers the general adult triangular pattern over the pubic area, and the breast shows the projecting papilla with areola and surrounding tissue rounded in contour.

Generally menarche begins during Stage IV of the development of the breast and pubic hair. Knowledge of this sequence is useful in counseling both children and parents about normal sexual development. It can help them anticipate normal body changes.

For girls, the secondary sexual development includes changes in body shape, weight redistribution, and certain hormonal changes. During adolescence the hips become broader, and there is an accumulation of subcutaneous fat in the breasts, upper outer thighs, across the abdomen, and along the inner aspects of the upper arms, and along the thoracic vertebra. The entire body acquires a more curved, rounded, and soft appearance. Once menarche has begun, axillary hair usually appears. The sebaceous glands become more and more active and this, coupled with the increased hormonal levels, often leads to acne.

Sexual development of boys also follows a predictable pattern. They too have primary and secondary characteristics. The primary sexual development for boys involves changes in the penis and testes (see Fig. 5-3). Most of

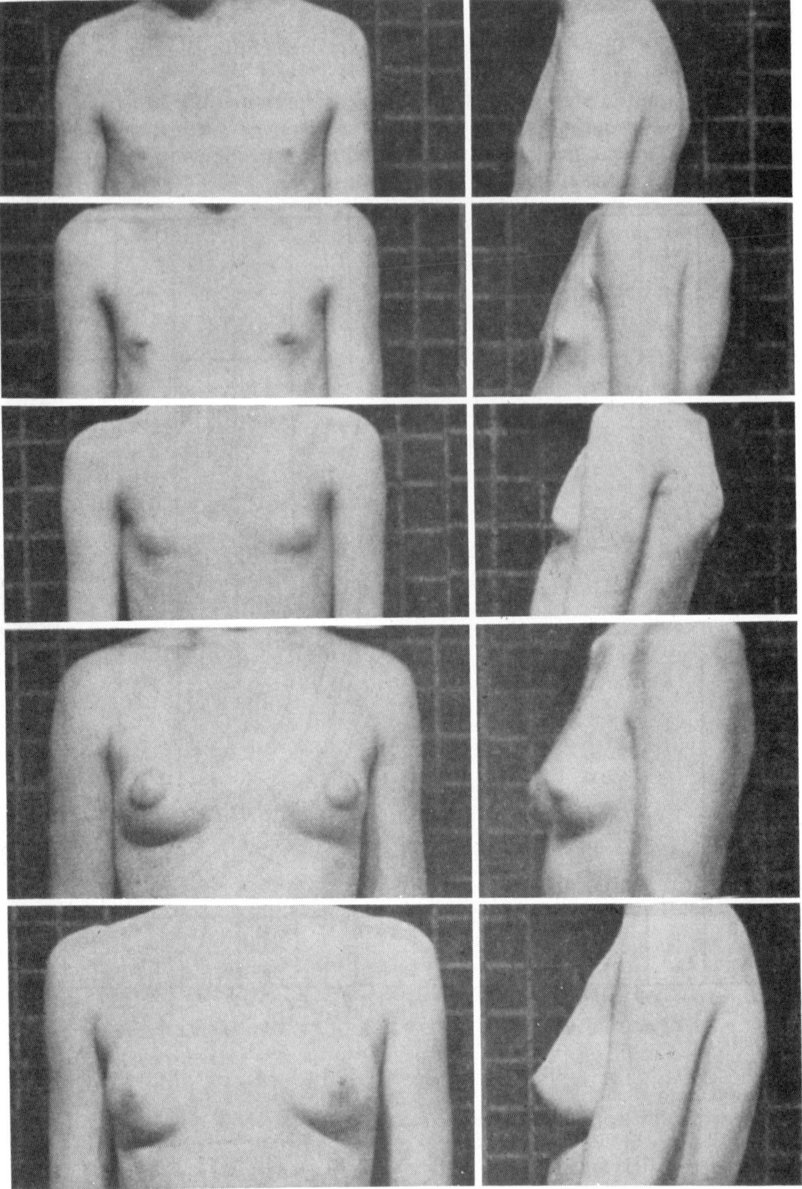

Figure 5-2 Normal breast development. *(Source: E. L. Reynolds et al., American Journal of Diseases, 1948. With permission of the American Medical Association.)*

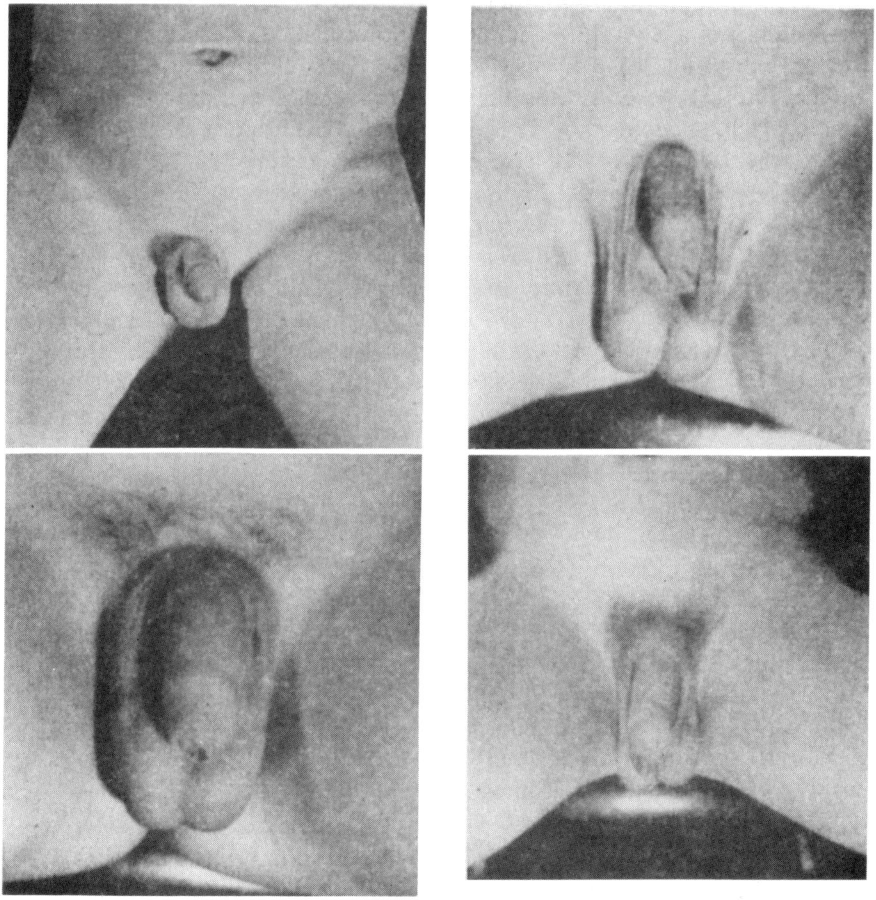

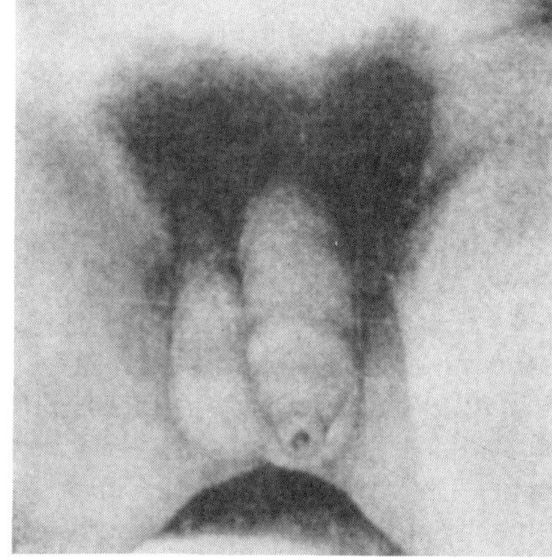

Figure 5-3 Pubic hair development for boys. *(Source: W. W. Greulich, R. I. Dortman, H. K. Catchpole, C. I. Solomon, and C. S. Culotta, "Somatic and Endocrine Studies of Pubertal and Adolescent Boys," Monograph of the Society for Research in Child Development, 1942, 7 (serial no. 33). With permission of The Society for Research in Child Development, Inc.)*

these changes can be seen, as can the development of pubic hair. These changes are also divided into stages:

Stage I	No change is seen in the penis, testes, or scrotal area, and pubic hair is not present.
Stage II	Light-colored, soft pubic hair appears at the penal base, and the penis and testes become enlarged.
Stage III	Dark, coarse pubic hair begins to replace the soft, childish hairs, and the penis lengthens.
Stage IV	Coarse, pigmented pubic hair resembles the adult pubic hair but covers a smaller area, and the testes and penis increase in diameter.
Stage V	Pubic hair, testes, and penis resemble the adult genitalia in size, shape, and texture.

For boys, the secondary sexual development includes changes in body hair, breast shape, and general growth. Axillary hair generally appears after the pubic hair has been present for several months. Facial hair appears at about the same time as the axillary hair. In late adolescence, the hairline recedes bilaterally to form the characteristic bow-shaped male hairline. About 33 percent of all boys go through some breast engorgement during this period. If it is mild and causes no problems, it usually recedes by itself without treatment. The male larynx enlarges during this time to allow the voice to deepen. A generalized increased muscular growth and strength shows broader shoulders, narrower hips, and sudden growth spurts in the length of arms and legs.

A fourth method of assessing physical growth is by measuring various reflections of neural development. This development is reflected in the attainment of skilled motor movements. Basically infants are born with all the potential for the mature central nervous system, but tremendous maturation continues to occur throughout childhood. Generally girls mature much earlier in motor, sensory, and speech skills, while boys, though maturing later, usually develop increased skills in strength and coordination. Growth of the cortex and brain stem as well as myelinization of the entire central nervous system results in the replacement of newborn reflexes with more sophisticated reflexes and coordinated movements. For example, the tonic neck reflex fades as the child begins to roll over, and rolling over becomes less prominent as the child learns to sit upright. Children with reflexes that do not appear and disappear at the appropriate time need further investigation to make sure they do not have central nervous system damage.

The last method of assessing a child's growth to be discussed is the evaluation of the physiological age of the child. As a child matures, many physiological and chemical changes occur within the body. Studies have attempted to take several of these changes and plot them on curves. The Fels Composite Sheet and Wetzel's Grid are examples of such charting. There are entire books describing the changes in organ systems. The following discussion will highlight only a few.

Stages of Growth and Development

For purposes of clarity, the following arbitrary division of growth during the pediatric age range will be used:

Infancy: conception to 1 year old
Toddlerhood: 1 to 2 years old
Preschool years: 2 to 5 years old
School years: 5 to 10 years old
Adolescence: 10 to 20 years old (This may include prepuberty for some children.)

Infancy The period of time between conception and the first birthday is a stage of rapid growth and change. Skeletal development is rapid. By the 8th fetal week most skeletal and muscle tissue has begun to develop. By the 20th fetal week there is enough ossification of the skeletal bones for an x-ray to show fetal position. While the cartilaginous beginning of the hands and feet occur during fetal life, only the phalangeal shafts, metacarpals, and metatarsals have enough ossification at term to show on an x-ray (Fig. 5-4 and Table 5-1).

Although difficult to assess without x-rays, dental development is occurring rapidly during prenatal life. The entire first set of teeth will become calcified before birth. By the 4th and 5th month of fetal life, signs of calcification are seen in the lower central incisors. By birth the first molars are beginning to calcify in the infant's gums, although they will not erupt until the child is 9 or 10 years of age.

Sexual growth is also difficult to assess in this age group since most changes occur before birth. While the sex is determined at conception, the visible signs of femaleness or maleness do not appear until after the 8th fetal week. By birth the infant is fully male or female and capable of response to local stimulation (penile erections are not uncommon in infant boys, for instance).

Neural growth is rapid during this stage. The ectoderm begins to differentiate into the nervous system by the 3d fetal week, and buds for brain and spinal column appear and begin to differentiate by the 7th fetal week. During the 7th to 9th gestational months the outer surfaces of the cortex become more convoluted. At birth the peripheral and autonomic nervous systems are well enough developed to allow the infant to survive outside the protected uterine existence. All cranial nerves except the optic and olfactory nerves are present and myelinated. Brain growth is rapid during the 1st year

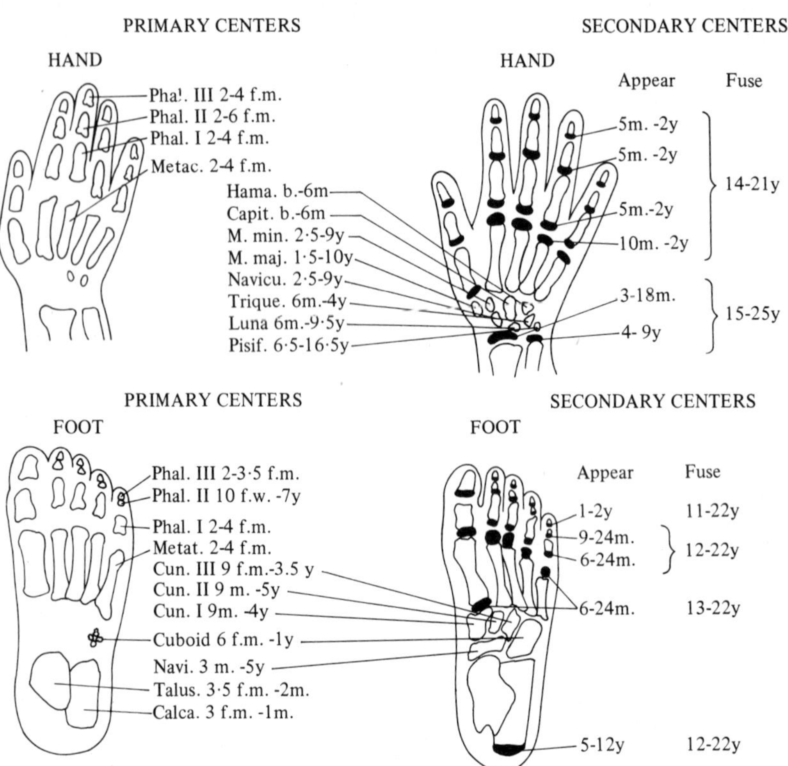

f.m. = fetal months; m. = post natal months; y = year

Figure 5-4 Ossification centers of hands and feet. *(Source: Printed by permission from Ernest H. Watson and George H. Lowrey, Growth and Development of Children, Chicago: Year Book Medical Publishers, Inc., 1967, p. 185.)*

of life, and by the second birthday 90 percent of the total brain growth will have occurred. During this 1st year the cortex develops the deep, distinct folds of sulci characteristic of the area. During this year also, myelinization occurs in a cephalocaudal direction and is reflected in the maturation of certain behaviors corresponding to this head-to-foot progression. An average child can be observed to do the following:

1 month—smiles
2 months—coos
3 months—gains head control
4 months—reaches with the arms
5 months—rolls over
6 months—sits alone
7 months—crawls
8 months—demonstrates a pinch or grasp
9 months—pulls self to standing

10 months—stands alone
11 months—walks holding on to furniture
12 months—walks alone

While the infant is born able to distinguish light from dark, myelination of the visual fibers is not complete until the end of the 3d or 4th month. Within several weeks of birth the infant can fixate both eyes for a short period of time and by 8 months can distinguish details reasonably well. Many cardiovascular changes are occurring at this time. During the last 5 months of gestation the heart grows rapidly, after which it hits a plateau and

Table 5-1 Ossification of Bones of Hands

Order of appearance	Ossification center	Mean average time of appearance in months	
		Girls	Boys
1	Capitate	3.0	4.5
2	Hamate	4.5	6.0
3	Distal epiphysis of the radius	9.8	13.2
4	Epiphysis of the proximal phalanx, digit 3	10.0	15.0
5	Epiphysis of the proximal phalanx, digit 2	10.8	16.1
6	Epiphysis of the proximal phalanx, digit 4	10.8	16.6
7	Epiphysis of the second metacarpal	12.3	18.0
8	Epiphysis of the distal phalanx, digit 1	12.1	18.3
9	Epiphysis of the third metacarpal	13.8	20.5
10	Epiphysis of the fourth metacarpal	15.6	23.3
11	Epiphysis of the proximal phalanx, digit 5	14.3	21.5
12	Epiphysis of the middle phalanx, digit 3	15.4	23.4
13	Epiphysis of the middle phalanx, digit 4	15.6	23.8
14	Epiphysis of the fifth metacarpal	17.1	26.0
15	Epiphysis of the middle phalanx, digit 2	17.2	25.8
16	Triquetral	22.7	29.3
17	Epiphysis of the distal phalanx, digit 3	18.4	27.4
18	Epiphysis of the distal phalanx, digit 4	18.7	27.7
19	Epiphysis of the first metacarpal	19.1	31.8
20	Epiphysis of the phalanx, digit 1	20.9	33.2
21	Epiphysis of the distal phalanx, digit 5	23.7	37.3
22	Epiphysis of the distal phalanx, digit 2	24.1	37.6
23	Epiphysis of the middle phalanx, digit 5	23.6	39.2
24	Lunate	36.0	44.4
25	Trapezium	47.4	68.4
26	Trapezoid	49.4	69.1
27	Scaphoid	50.4	67.8
28	Distal epiphysis of the ulna	68.3	82.4
29	Pisiform	94.6	120.4
30	Sesamoid of adductus pollicis	123.4	152.7

Printed by permission of Dorothy V. Whipple, *Dynamics of Development: Euthenic Pediatrics*, New York: McGraw-Hill, 1966, p. 117.

grows little during the first 4 to 6 weeks following birth. This plateau is followed by rapid growth which allows the heart to double its weight during the 1st year. At birth, the heart lies slightly transverse with a shift to the right side. Fetal circulation is different from infant circulation due to the dependence on the mother's help through the placenta and umbilical cord. At birth, the infant heart contains three additional openings: the ductus venosus, ductus arteriosus, and the foramen ovale. In normal situations the ductus venosus closes immediately at birth due to the changes in atrial pressures. The foramen ovale generally closes within several weeks of birth. There is much controversy over the time of closure for the ductus arteriosus, but studies indicate closure sometime between 1 and 8 days. Since the heart rate is inversely related to the size of the heart, there is a gradual decrease in rate. The fetal heart rate is between 130 and 160 beats per minute; the newborn has a heart rate of 130 to 140 beats per minute; by the end of the 1st year the rate will drop to 90 to 95 beats per minute. Not only does the rate change, but so does the rhythm. During infancy sinus arrhythmia can indicate good heart function, while in later life it can be a sign of heart damage. During infancy, systole and diastole are of short duration, great intensity, and high pitch. One study showed that fifty percent of all children have innocent heart murmurs at some time in their lives. Innocent murmurs are less frequent in the newborn period. Components of the blood show many changes. Fetal hemoglobin, with its great attraction for oxygen, is present until after the first 20 weeks of the newborn period. Adult hemoglobin appears around the 13th fetal week and slowly increases. Hemoglobin levels are high in the newborn period and drop rapidly until around 6 to 8 months of age and then begin a slow rise (see Table 4-6). There are also changes from infant red blood cells to adult red blood cells. Neonatal red blood cells live only 100 days as compared with the 120 days of adult red blood cells. There are many differences in leukocytes, granulocytes, mononucleocytes, eosinophils, basophils, and neutrophils as well.

The gastrointestinal system is a recognizable long tube by the end of the 6th fetal week and fills the abdominal cavity by the 10th fetal week. At birth the newborn has some functioning salivary glands, but the majority mature around 3 months of age, and drooling often occurs at this time. The infantile stomach lies in a slightly horizontal plane and can contain up to 90 ml of fluid at birth. This will increase up to 150 ml by 1 month of age and 360 ml by the first birthday. The liver appears by the 3d week of gestation and grows rapidly during the prenatal period. It shrinks slightly at birth, but is still a large, easily palpated organ filling up to two-fifths of the abdominal cavity. During the first 3 months of life it remains fairly stable and then begins to grow again. During the 1st year it is not particularly efficient and consequently glucogenesis, development of ketone material, amino acid changes, and vitamin storage are limited. At birth the large intestine is filled with sterile meconium, but within hours of birth, bacteria appear in this material. Respiratory movements during infancy are predominantly abdominal with periodic variations in rate and rhythm.

Toddlerhood The 2d year of life is not nearly so dramatic in the number of physiological changes that occur.

Skeletal growth can still be checked. As seen from Table 5-1, the ossification of bone continues during this year, but at a lower rate and in fewer ossification centers. While the epiphysis is being added to the long bones and additional bones are showing in the wrist, the anterior fontanel is closing or almost closed. Many toddlers have no palpable fontanel by 12 months, and all should have none by 18 months.

Dental growth continues but not as dramatically as during the 1st year. By the first birthday the toddler usually has six to eight primary teeth. By the end of the 2d year the child should have a complete set of 20 primary teeth. A few children will be missing their back second molars, which should erupt by their third birthday. During the 2d year calcification is beginning for the first and second bicuspids and second molars.

This is a fairly quiescent time for sexual growth, with little physical or hormonal change occurring.

Neural growth continues but more slowly. By the end of the 2d year myelinization has been completed. While the sulci of the cortex increased rapidly during the 1st year, after the age of 2, additional sulci form very slowly.

Physiological growth is also slower during this year. Little change occurs in the cardiovascular system during this time. The heart rate continues to drop and is usually around 70 to 130 beats per minute. Normal sinus arrhythmia may continue. Components of the blood continue to alter. The toddler's cardiovascular system should contain a total volume of adult hemoglobin, and the hemoglobin should be stabilized at about 12 to 13 gm.

The gastrointestinal system continues to grow, but much more slowly. By 2 years the salivary glands have increased in size 5 times and are as mature as the adult glands. The stomach becomes more bowed and has increased its capacity to 500 cc. Due to diet and maturation, the material in the lower intestine now resembles adult stool material. During the 2d year the liver matures to a more adult level, thus becoming more efficient in vitamin storage, glucogenesis, amino acid changes, and ketone body formation. The lower edge of the liver may still be palpable in some children.

The respiratory tract continues to expand but at a much slower rate, and respiratory movements continue chiefly in the abdominal area. Because the chest wall is thin, they can still be heard clearly and distinctly. The rate is more likely to be steady and slower than in infancy, and the average is around 20 to 30 per minute.

The urinary system is still growing, and the kidneys begin descending deeper into the pelvic area. A normal 2-year-old may secrete as much as 500 to 600 ml of urine a day.

Preschool Years From 2 to 5, children follow their own growth patterns. Some children seem to grow gradually while others have several small growth spurts. Additional ossification centers appear in the wrist and ankle, and additional epiphyses develop in some of the long bones. During this period the legs grow faster than the head, trunk or upper extremities.

During the preschool years visible dental growth is minimal. Most of the growth and calcification are occurring within the gums. Around the 5th, 6th, or 7th year, the child will lose the front primary incisors and replace them with adult permanent teeth. The rest of the primary teeth will continue to be replaced gradually by adult dentition.

The preschool period is a fairly quiescent time for sexual growth, and little physical or hormonal change is occurring.

By this age, neural growth is reflected in fine and gross motor skills by a well-developed central nervous system. Many activities that the preschool child can perform are perfected and made smoother and more coordinated during these years. The child's walking progresses from the stilted, wide-gaited wobble of the toddler to the smooth, coordinated, narrow-based, normal gait of an adult. Visual acuity matures from the 20/70 of a 2-year-old to 20/30 by 5 or 6 years. Fine motor movements become more detailed and sustained. A 2-year-old can easily manipulate fingers to pile two blocks on top of each other, while a 3-year-old can pile at least eight into a tower. Instead of holding the pencil awkardly and scribbling, the older child can grasp the pencil in the normal position and draw certain shapes.

Physiological growth continues at a slower pace. By the end of the 5th year the heart has quadrupled its size since birth and the rate drops to an average of 70 to 110 beats per minute. Innocent murmurs may still be common during this age. Due to the thin chest the point of maximum intensity (PMI) is best heard at the third intercostal space, left of the sternum. The hemoglobin stays stabilized around 12 to 13 gm, and some of the blood solids begin to stabilize while others continue to change. Physiologically the gastrointestinal system is advanced enough for the 4- and 5-year-old child to chew and swallow in the adult fashion. The stomach capacity continues to increase, although at times it is not large enough to carry the child from one meal to the next. Some children may require good snacks between meals to maintain their blood sugar level during their periods of growth. The liver continues to enlarge, and the lower edge can still be felt on a few children during preschool years. The respiratory system continues its methodical growth during these years, and breathing is abdominal until the end of the 5th or 6th year. By this age the bladder is deep within the pelvic area, but the ureters remain short and relatively straight. By the end of this stage, the bladder capacity has increased, and the child will secrete between 600 and 750 ml of urine in a 24-hour period.

School Years In today's society children are frequently in school between the ages of 3 and 25; however, the school-age period is generally defined as the ages between 5 and 10 years.

Skeletally, by this time most of the bones of the hands and feet are present but by no means complete. Ossification of the ends of small and long bones will continue for some years.

During the early years of this period the primary teeth continue to be lost. By the 10th year all primary teeth should be gone from the mouth, and with the exception of the second and third molars, all permanent teeth should be in place.

Sexually these years are the "lull before the storm," and sexual growth is usually quiet and unchanging during these years.

The central nervous system continues to mature slowly, and it is a time in which important cognitive skills such as reading, writing, and manipulating numbers develop.

By 9 years of age the heart has increased six times its newborn size. The rate drops to an average of 65 to 95 beats per minute and is the same for boys and girls. The hemoglobin remains around 12 to 13 gm and the hematocrit around 38 to 41 percent during these years. A few of the other solid elements continue to shift.

Within the gastrointestinal system, the stomach capacity continues to grow. Many of the gastrointestinal changes relate to the psychological factors of eating rather than the physical changes that occur during this period of time. The liver now remains high within the abdominal cavity and should not be easily palpated on examination.

The lungs and respiratory system continue slow, minimal growth and generally assume the adult shape. The respiratory rate is between 17 and 22 per minute.

The urinary system has expanded to allow a child to void up to 1,000 ml of urine per 24 hours.

Adolescence The adolescent period is defined as the years between 10 and 20 and really includes some of the prepubertal years around the ages of 10 and 11. Puberty is sometimes defined as biological growth and adolescence as psychological maturation. This differentiation is useful in certain situations.

The pubertal years (about 9 to 12 years depending on the child and sex) are usually a period of physiological growth and maturation. Girls generally begin their pubertal growth 2 years before boys; thus school classes of 10- and 11-year-olds may have taller girls than boys. The trunk grows more rapidly than the lower extremities, and if puberty begins late, the legs have a longer growth spurt. Up to puberty there is little difference in shape or size of males and females. After this period girls are generally shorter and more curved and rounded, while boys become taller, more solid, and heavier. Skeletal growth appears first, with soft tissue and muscle filling in. Later, this results in the child growing taller before becoming much heavier. All the hand and foot bones are present, but ossification continues until 16 to 18 years for girls and 18 to 20 years for boys. By the end of the 12th to 13th year all four pairs of the cranial sinuses are present and well defined.

During adolescence there is usually little dental growth, although some children have wisdom teeth erupting toward the end of this period.

Sexual growth is rapid during puberty and adolescence. For the girl primary sexual changes begin during puberty when the hypophysis produces ACTH which stimulates androgens and gonadotropin hormones to be produced by the adrenal glands. These stimulate the ovary to mature. In combination with the other two hormones, the ovary produces estrogens which help develop the endometrial lining of the uterus. So, beginning with puberty and throughout the adolescent years the girl moves through the stages of pubic hair and breast development already described. Around Stage IV of breast and pubic hair development she will have her menarche. Once she has menstruated, she may begin periodic cycles every 28 to 32 days; however, these are generally not very regular for the first year or so, and some believe that ovulation takes place only sporadically, if at all, during the first year or two of menstruation.

For the boy, primary sexual changes begin during puberty when the hypophysis produces ACTH which stimulates the androgen and gonadotropin hormones to be produced by the adrenal glands. These hormones cause the testes to produce testosterone. All these hormones produce the primary and secondary sexual changes seen in the male: changes in the penis, testes, pubic hair, body shape, axillary hair, facial hair, and voice. The ability to reproduce appears with the first formation of the sperm. Some authorities feel that the sperm are mature and reproduction can occur when the pubic hair begins to curl.

With the great growth spurt during the pubertal and adolescent years, the central nervous system expands just to keep up with the physical size of the body.

Physiologically the body changes rapidly during this growth period. Along with the other rapid expansions, the heart shows a rapid increase in size during the years from 10 to 20, resulting in the adult-sized, -shaped, and -located heart. Heart rate should stabilize around 60 to 90 beats per minute, with males having a slightly faster rate than females. An adult female rate is expected to be about 60 beats per minute and the adult male rate about 65 beats per minute. Any arrhythmias or murmurs during puberty and adolescence are rare and need to be checked. During puberty there is a rise in hemoglobin and hematocrit levels in boys, generally around 13 to 16 gm and 38 to 47 percent, respectively. Girls show little or no rise, with hemoglobin stabilizing around 13 to 14 gm and the hematocrit around 38 to 42 percent. Other elements in the blood should reach adult proportions during these years.

The gastrointestinal system matures rapidly during the years between 10 and 20. With the rapid growth spurt, the stomach capacity may suddenly increase to more than 900 cc, and it may seem to parents that the child is eating constantly. This sudden increase in appetite to meet the physical growth needs brings many problems (e.g., food fads, diets, skin problems) which will not be discussed here. The liver attains adult size and location and is not normally palpated below the rib cage unless disease is present.

As with the rest of the body, the lungs and respiratory system also show the growth spurt needed to keep up with the oxygen demands of a growing body. The adult-shaped chest is usually attained during these years, and the addition of tissue and thicker chest walls gives the lung sounds a deeper tympanitic sound rather than the resonant sounds heard earlier. The respiratory rate slows to 15 to 20 per minute for both males and females.

During adolescence there is a decrease in extracellular fluid volume; thus the adult proportion of 25 percent of total body weight being extracellular fluid is attained by the end of adolescence. Bladder capacity also increases, and the adolescent can usually void up to 1,500 ml of urine within a 24-hour period.

After this age physical growth moves into Phase III, during which repair and maintenance of bodily cells and tissues is of major importance. This has been only a cursory discussion of some of the physiological changes of growth and development. For further study of this subject the reader is referred to the books listed in the bibliography.

Another important aspect of physical maturation is the growth and development of certain gross and fine motor skills. These are items frequently assessed in developmental screening tests such as those described in Chap. 4 because they are good indicators of neurological and muscular development. A composite of many such skills and their appropriate age of development is seen in Table 5-2.

PSYCHOLOGICAL, SOCIAL AND CULTURAL DEVELOPMENT

Psychological, social, and cultural development is an extremely important aspect of the child's growth process. Not only does the body grow, but the mind and social skills are constantly becoming more refined. Ten years ago, this section would have been labeled "Psychological Development." Today, we realize that not only psychological variables, but also social and cultural ones are highly influential in the child's development. Generally, psycholog-

Table 5-2 Motor Development

Gross motor	Fine motor
Infant: Newborn	
Symmetrical random extremity movements Pronounced head lag Prone—turns head to side and draws knees under abdomen Symmetrical, full Moro reflex Strong, symmetrical tonic neck reflex Full patellar reflexes Walking (or stepping) reflex Crawling reflex Galant reflex (trunk incurvation)	Tight hand grasp Hand predominantly fisted Positive Babinski reflexes Face—Eyes follow to midline Head and eyes move together (by 1 month) Attracted to object with eyes Rooting reflex Sucking reflex
3-month-old	
Symmetrical random extremity movements Little or no head lag Prone—Holds head at 45-90° angle and keeps legs outstretched Symmetrical, full Moro reflex (but fades by 5 months) Weak, asymmetrical tonic neck reflex Full patellar reflexes Walking reflex begins to fade Crawling reflex begins to fade Galant reflex gone	Little or no hand grasp Hands predominantly open, but will grasp rattle Positive Babinski reflexes Face—Eyes follow 180° Smiles responsibly Attracted to and watches own hands Rooting reflex begins to fade Sucking reflex begins to fade
6-month-old	
Reaches with arms Sits—with support comfortably in chair alone briefly Prone—Supports upper chest with arms scoots effectively Rolls over, stomach to back Voluntary crawling appears Parachute reflex appears (7 to 9 months) Moro reflex seen only in Parachute reflex	Crude palmar grasp Can hold small block momentarily Transfers small object hand-to-hand Bangs small object at midline Can release object (drops blocks for noise effect) Positive Babinski reflexes Face—Eyes follow object 180° horizontally Uses small muscles to laugh, squeal Attracted to small object; reaches, grasps, and puts in mouth
9-month-old	
More control over reaching with arms Sits alone for up to 10 minutes Prone—Crawls on hands and knees Rolls over completely when desires	Effective pincer grasp for small objects Positive Babinski reflexes Explores objects with hand and mouth Learns to squeeze, slide, push, pull, rip Can turn small object over

Table 5-2 Motor Development *(Cont'd)*

Gross motor	Fine motor
12-month-old	
Can pull self to sitting position Can twist within sitting position Prone—May walk on hands and feet like a dog Walking—Walking holding onto furniture Standing alone Walking alone Stopping to pick up object at feet Throwing—Deliberately drops or lets go rather than real throw Stepping—climbs on chairs, sofas, beds	Mature grasp—Can reach for, pick up, and give back block (used to initiate social contact) Control over grasp and release Positive Babinski reflex fades
Toddler	
Walking—Alone, with wide, irregular gait even, smoother gait (by 2 years) Sideways and backward (by 2 years) Watches placement of feet (2 years) Stepping—Off one step at a time Can stand on one foot momentarily Climbs up stairs on hands and knees (12–15 months) Climbs up stairs, upright, holding on, one foot at a time (1½–2 years) Throwing—Rigid, underhand toss Begins to throw overhand (1½–2 years) Cannot catch ball Running—Unsteady True, smooth, rhythmical run (2 years) Jumping—Broadjump with two feet (2 years)	Does not distinguish right from left side Holds pencil and scribbles Writing—Scribbles marks in all directions rapidly Slows down and controls scribbles Scribbles in patterns (2 years) Makes crude circle Attempts to close circle Likes to touch, handle, manipulate objects (and name them)

ical development is considered to include intrapersonal variables, primarily mental characteristics (which will be discussed separately under the section on cognitive growth and development) and personality variables such as love, fear, aggression, dependency, and self-image. Social and cultural variables include such things as children's economic situation, their family structure and the cultural and subcultural belief system they are exposed to. A

Table 5-2 Motor Development *(Cont'd)*

Gross motor	Fine motor
Preschooler	
Walking—Tandem walk a line (3 years) Without watching feet (3 years) Stepping—Climbs up stairs alternating feet (3 years) Climbs down stairs alternating feet (4–5 years) Hops down three steps on one foot (3½ years) Hops down four to six steps on one foot (4 years) Crude skip (5 years) Throwing—Throws overhand with ease Begins to shift weight when throwing Catches ball stiffly with extended arms (3½ years) Catches ball with hands (4 years) Running—Adds smooth arm action Adds speed Jumping—Can broadjump a longer distance	Knows there is a right and left side but cannot distinguish (4–5 years) Writing—Recognizes and draws complete circle (2–3 years) Draws crude cross (2½–3½ years) Draws crude three-part man (3–4 years) Recognizes and copies crude square (4 years) Combines two simple geometric forms (4 years) Can combine more than two geometric forms (aggregates) (5 years)
School-age child	
Walking—Can walk a balance board Stepping—Smoother, more regular hop/skip; one foot, then the other (6 years) Can hop on one foot up to 10 seconds Can hop longer distances with more rhythm Throwing—More bodily motion and more accuracy at target Catches ball with hands and body Greater distance throw (8–10 years) Running—Adds speed Jumping—Longer-distance broadjump	Knows and can distinguish right from left side (7–8 years) Writing—Can draw crude three- to six-part man (5–6 years) Draws triangle (6–7 years) Draws diamond (8–9 years) Draws three-dimensional geometrical figures (9 years) Can wind a spool with thread Can drop small objects through a small opening (like pennies in a piggy bank)
Adolescent	
Increases in physical strength and endurance Increases in motor ability Increases in coordination	Same as adult—coordinated, controlled, deliberate, movements

great deal of information is available on many details of psychological, social and cultural development, and the interested reader is referred to some of the listings in the bibliography for an in-depth discussion of them. A summary of some of the more important findings in these areas is included in Table 5-3. The rest of this section will be devoted to some well-known developmental theories which the nurse should be familiar with and which have application to the children she will see clinically.

Psychological, Social, and Cultural Developmental Theories

Many social scientists have observed the normal and abnormal growth and development of children and adults and have created elaborate theories to explain the phenomena they have seen. It should be remembered that these are working theories and not gospel truths. The nurse in ambulatory pediatrics must be aware of these theories, but it is more important that she be attuned to the individual child she is seeing, who may or may not conform to such theories. Although each theory will be helpful in understanding certain phenomena, none of them are totally adequate. These theories range from the lesser known ideas of Adler, Dollard, Jung, and Lewin to the very popular ideas of Freud, Erikson, Maslow, and Piaget. Entire books have been written about each of these theories, and only a brief synopsis of the theories of Sigmund Freud, Erik Erikson, and Abraham Maslow will be presented in this section. Piaget's ideas will be reviewed in the section concerned with cognitive development.

Sigmund Freud is the oldest and most controversial of the theorists. His theories are based on his analysis of troubled people who talked about their life and thoughts. Basically, Freud divided the personality into three parts: the id, the ego, and superego. The id governs the newborn and guides the infant according to the pleasure principle. Because of the id, the child demands immediate gratification of all needs. The superego is imposed by societal restrictions—usually in the form of parental demands that the child conform to certain expectations. Gradually these demands become internalized in the form of the conscience or superego. A compromise between these two extremes (i.e., the permissiveness of the id and the restrictions of the superego) results from dealing with the real world in everyday life, and this compromising capacity is known as the ego.

Freud further divided the mind into the preconscious and unconscious areas. Preconsciousness includes all the thoughts, feelings, or knowledge that we are aware of, either easily or after some reflection. The unconscious includes hidden thoughts, feelings, and desires. These may at one time have been preconscious feelings that have been repressed or they may be thoughts that have never surfaced. These thoughts and feelings may emerge in dreams or after long, meticulous psychoanalysis.

Freud's theory of life development is called the *psychoanalytic theory* and postulates five psychosexual stages of development. The first stage is the

Table 5-3 Social Behavior Development

	Infant: Newborn
Love	Beginning development of a one-to-one relationship with mother. Likes to cuddle, to be held close.
Fears	Dislikes being uncovered, held loosely. May dislike bathing. Dislikes loud noises.
Play	Knows nothing of sharing and giving; infant very taking at this stage. Play consists of someone else doing something to child—stroking, cooing, cuddling.
Dependency	Depends entirely on someone else for meeting basic needs—feeding, clothing, cleaning, shelter, stimulation.
Morality	Has no idea of right or wrong.
Self-image	Knows no difference between self and mother (symbiotic relationship).
Habits	Eating: Frequently (every 2-4 hours) from bottle or breast. May cry when hungry and fall asleep when satisfied. Recognizes bottle and is eager (6 months). Bowels: Frequent movements. Shows no knowledge of activity. Sleeping: Generally most of 24 hours. Most of sleep in spaces of 50 minutes with rapid eye movements. Dressing: Taken care of entirely by mother.
	6-month-old
Love	Has established a one-to-one relationship with mother (or mother substitute). Responsive to looks, gestures, verbalization. Smiles, coos, and babbles.
Fears	Dislikes loss of support, loud noises, strangers (around 6-9 months).
Play	Likes games of "peek-a-boo," "pat-a-cake," "sooo-big." Will play alone or in response to someone else.
Dependency	Still dependent on mother for most activities. Can control some of own movement—rolling over, sitting, reaching.
Morality	Must be totally controlled by external forces (mother and environment).
Self-image	Knows self is different from mother. Knows mother is different from other family members.
Habits	Eating: May eat three meals a day plus bedtime bottle and a variety of solid baby foods. Likes to feed self crackers, but mostly sucks on them. Likes the feel of food oozing between the fingers. Will sit in high chair for a meal. Bowels: Bowel movements and voidings less frequent. Sleeping: May sleep more in night and less during day. Dressing: May struggle against holding still long enough to be dressed. Diapering often awkward because of rolling, crawling.

Table 5-3 Social Behavior Development ***(Cont'd)***

	12-month-old	
Love	Still absorbing a lot of love and returning little. Learning to give love pats, hugs, kisses. Knows mother and can cling to her.	
Fears	Dislikes separation from mother and reacts with crying, upset, irritability.	
Play	Can give and take in game of "give-it-to-me" with block or ball. Likes games with motor action—push, pull, run.	
Dependency	Becoming more independent because of motor control (walking, running, sitting). Tries to do some things for self (feeding, removing clothing).	
Morality	Needs constant external limits and watching.	
Self-image	Can function emotionally as an individual as long as mother is physically present in room.	
Habits	Eating:	Feeds self cracker, getting most of it in mouth. Drinks from a cup. Likes to be with family at mealtime but may need to be fed separately.
	Bowels:	May squirm or complain when diaper soiled.
	Sleeping:	Probably sleeps through night, plus one or two daytime naps. Only 35% of sleep with rapid eye movements.
	Dressing:	Can remove some garments. Helps to dress self by sticking out appropriate extremity.
	Toddler	
Love	Wants and needs love from mother. Can try short separation from mother (across room or in next room with frequent visual and verbal checks on her presence).	
Fears	Dislikes separation from mother and sudden appearance of fears—bath, thunder, dogs, darkness.	
Play	Beginning awareness of ownership "*my* toy," "*my* coat," etc. Solitary play. May have imaginary playmates. Will look at pictures in a book momentarily.	
Dependency	Strives for independence and control (learns one way is to say "no"). If handkerchief is held for him, can blow own nose. Likes to have a choice.	
Morality	Beginning self controls (may say "no" while reaching for forbidden object). Still needs many external controls.	
Self-image	Has little awareness of own body shell (that body has weight, can be an obstacle; knows pain but cannot point to spot). Can name some parts of body—eye, nose, ear.	

Table 5-3 Social Behavior Development ***(Cont'd)***

	Toddler
Habits	Eating: Uses a spoon without spilling. Holds and uses a cup but may drop it or throw it when finished. Can draw through a straw. Eats with family, but cannot sit through entire meal. Bowels: May show an interest in urges, but not reliable. May not fuss at being placed on potty chair, but may have no action. Sleeping: Daytime naps may disappear or become times of quiet play rather than sleep. Bedtime can be a struggle. Dressing: Can put on simple garment. Likes to remove all clothing.
	Preschooler
Love	Parents represent the strength and wisdom in child's life (they can do no wrong). With enlarging world, there are beginning attachments for persons outside immediate family.
Fears	Worries about own body shell (skinned knee, hangnail, bumps, bites; needs bandage and kiss). Worries about outside world (ghosts, bad men, the doctor's office).
Play	Parallel play (3–4 years). Shared play (4–5 years). Everything becomes a game. Tries new roles. Imaginary play ("let's pretend" situations and playmates). Likes games of tag, hide-and-seek, dress-up. Learns to play simple sit-down games (checkers, card games, Parcheesi) but hates to lose and will change rules and cheat to avoid it.
Dependency	Rapid transitions from dependence to independence. Needs security objects for times of stress—thumb, blanket, favorite toy, mother's hand. Strives for independence with "Let me do it."
Morality	Can control some of own urges. May invent imaginary friends to take the rap for own wrong-doing.
Self-image	More aware of others in body and feeling (how they are the same or different). More interested in doing activities within own sex role (girls want to be feminine, boys masculine).

Table 5-3 Social Behavior Development ***(Cont'd)***

	Preschooler
Habits	Eating: Can control and pour from a small pitcher. May be able to sit and eat with family if able to leave when finished. Likes to serve self. Bowels: Completed day and night dryness (3½–4 years). May still announce the event. May still need help in cleansing and clothing. Sleeping: Only at night. May have nightmares. Begins to understand that dreams happen while sleeping. Dressing: Does own buttons. Will dress self if clothing laid out.
	School-age child
Love	Learns parents can be wrong. Sometimes can be disillusioned with own parents and would like to trade them in or is certain he or she is adopted. Learns to share some of own thoughts only with peers. Parents and home a place to return to for some companionship, comfort, and security.
Fears	Is superstitious.
Play	Games show superstitions, teasing, insults. Cooperative play—baseball, jacks, hopscotch. Peers of same sex important. Collections—a type of hoarding.
Dependency	Rejects some ideas of parents and tries own ideas, but usually returns to home base. Reduces need for dependency by using rituals—bedtime, mealtime, bathtime.
Morality	Thinks of own needs first and is out to satisfy them. Can think of relationship between the act and following consequences. Begins to develop an idea of what it means to live by a label (good boy, good girl, bad boy, bad girl). Peer group begins to influence morality with fixed rules and rituals.
Self-image	Begins to see self within a label given by world (boy, girl, mean, nice, bully, cute, etc.).
Habits	Eating: Eats meals with family and can sit through entire meal. Has definite likes and dislikes, but may change suddenly. Has rituals around mealtime—same location at table, same silverware, same food. Bowels: Needs no help from adults. Sleeping: May spend night away from home. Dressing: Can decide on own clothing and dress self. But may ask for help and then ignore it. Can comb own hair.

Table 5-3 Social Behavior Development ***(Cont'd)***

	Adolescent
Love	Vascillating and expanding. Within home: parents wonderful, wise, understanding, and deceitful, dishonest, and stupid. With peers: relationships intense and unstable. With world: idealistic and shallow.
Fears	Worries about loss of identity (bodily, emotionally). Worries about failure (in school, career, friendship). Is uncertain.
Play	Develops skills in individual and group (games, sports, activities). Joins clubs, groups, sports. Cliques important—involve peers of same sex but with activities associated with opposite sex.
Dependency	High ambivalence between wanting limits and freedom. Discovers responsibility that comes with freedom.
Morality	Begins to see that own actions effect a large group of individuals rather than just self. Beginning logical thought about own principles, rights, justice as compared with rest of community.
Self-image	Learned through group contact. Desire to be just like everyone else but more so. Try on many different roles. Hypochondriasis (excessive worry over body and bodily functions).
Habits	Eating: Many food fads. Constant eating. Worry over bodily functions leads to fad diets to correct specific problems. Would rather eat with peers than family. Sleeping: May get so wound up in activities that they sleep very little. May have trouble going to bed and getting up in morning. Dressing: Conformity with peers—clothing, hair, makeup, jewelry.

oral phase, lasting from birth to the first birthday. During this first stage of development the id gratification is sought through oral stimulation. The infant receives pleasure through eating, sucking, and rooting activities. Before the teeth erupt, the child is in the oral-passive stage; after about the 6th month when the teeth erupt, the child enters the oral-aggressive (or sadistic) period. The *anal phase* begins at the first birthday and lasts until the second birthday. During this period of development the id gratification is sought through the anal opening. The infant receives pleasure through manipulation and control of bowel contents. It is a time of great conflicts between parents and children as children learn some control of their own bodies and thereby some control of their environment. The child gets a taste of power. It must be remembered that at the time that Freud wrote, the 2d year was the most common age to toilet train a child.

Between 2 and 5 years the child is in the *phallic phase.* During this stage of development the id gratification is sought around the genital area and includes the complicated development of the Oedipal complex for the boy and penis envy for the girl. Much study has been done concerning the Oedipal complex for the boy, but relatively little has been said about the girl's development during this stage. Freud gave a scanty description of this maturation for the girl. Basically the Oedipal complex directs a 3- to 5-year-old boy to compete with his father for his mother's love. He feels competitive with his father and fears being castrated by him. By the end of the 5th or 6th year the fear of castration becomes overwhelming and the child represses his love for his mother, substituting a strong identification with his father. For the girl the stage involves fears and anxiety over lacking a penis, love for her father, repression of this love, and identification with the mother. The girl believes she has been castrated and becomes attached to her father in hopes of producing a baby and replacing the lost penis. With time this attachment is repressed and the girl begins to identify with her mother and the feminine role.

Freud's fourth psychosexual stage of development is the *latency stage* occurring between the years of 5 and 10. This is a relatively quiet stage following the stormy stage during which children learn to identify with the parent of their own sex (boy to father, girl to mother) and to internalize some of the thoughts, feelings, and styles of their own sexual group. Sexual feelings are kept tightly under control through the development of defense mechanisms such as repression, reaction formation, sublimation, ritualization, projection, and rationalization.

The *genital phase* is the last stage of psychosexual development, and it begins at about age 10. Basically, this is a revival of the phallic stage although on a higher level. During this stage the id gratification is sought around the genital area but is less egocentric and includes tenderness for others. With the phallic stage children are very self-centered and concerned with themselves. By the time the genital phase appears, feelings for the love object are more gentle, tender, and benevolent. The adolescent world encompasses a larger spectrum of people. The adolescent, instead of being restricted to only parents, has a chance to try out many of the earlier feelings on different people in different depths of intensity. Love may be tried out in terms of "I love my best friend" (a peer relationship), "I love that movie star" (an envy of something big, glamorous, and unattainable), or "I love my boy (girl) friend" (heterosexual love relationship).

Freud's psychoanalytic theory gave behavioral psychologists a large amount of material to work with in evaluating behavior. However, as more people worked with the theory, more complaints arose, and many psychologists were motivated to modify the theory. One of the most frequently heard complaints is that it is difficult to explain normal behavior according to a theory based solely on data gathered from pathological behaviors. Nonetheless, Freudian theory has contributed much to our understanding of growth and development, and it is important that nurses working with children be familiar with it.

Erik Erikson is a contemporary psychologist, and while his theory of child development uses Freud's as a foundation, there are some basic differences.

Erikson builds his theory on the process of socialization and acknowledges the evidence of an id, ego, and superego, but emphasizes the ego development in forming stable self-images, concerns, and feelings. He realizes the influences, not only of the child's mother and father but also of siblings, grandparents, aunts, uncles, neighborhood relationships, school, and the society in which the child functions. He is much less deterministic than Freud and believes that environment is very important in personality development. According to Erikson, a personality does not just appear at the age of 5 or 10 or 20; rather a person spends a lifetime building, shaping, and reshaping a personality. Biological, psychological, cultural, and social events all influence the construction and formation of the personality.

Erikson's theory of life development is capsulated in eight stages. The first stage, called *basic trust versus basic mistrust,* lasts from birth to the first or second birthday. The newborn infant is thrust into the world with little more than a body and must rely on others for warmth, love, food, dryness, and shelter. During those early months the mother provides the bodily experiences that bring peace, comfort, and equilibrium to the newborn. If the mother-child relationship is close, warm, and comforting, children develop a sense of trust. If there is no early relationship or it is sporadic, children develop a sense of mistrust and they will suffer from constant anxiety since they are never certain whether their needs will be met.

Stage II, called *a sense of autonomy versus a sense of shame and doubt,* occurs between the ages of 2 and 4, when the toddler begins to discover the difference between dependency and independency. If in Stage I children have developed a sense of trust in one other person (usually the mother) they begin to discover themselves. They find that they and their mothers are separate individuals. They explore not only themselves but their world. They become much more mobile and learn to tolerate short separations from their mothers. Walking, running, climbing, and reaching help them to expand their world and themselves. If basic trust was not accomplished in Stage I, children do not move into Stage II, but remain clinging, dependent persons.

Around the ages of 4 to 8 Erikson feels there is a third stage, which he called *a sense of initiative versus a sense of guilt.* These early school years again reflect the conflict between dependency and independency. Children are pushed to master new skills, tasks, and capacities and to explore the new, bigger world of the school and neighborhood. While they rush headlong into their new exploration, they may also have some guilt feelings of wanting to stay dependent, close to mother, and near home and familiar surroundings.

In a normal, healthy situation, the parents know when to comfort and allow the dependency and when and how to encourage and support the advances toward independency.

Stage IV, called *a sense of industry versus a sense of inferiority,* begins around age 9 and ends around age 12. These are the middle school years, and children work to find their places among their peer group. They want to be good at whatever task they are attempting and thus work diligently to improve their school tasks of reading, writing, and arithmetic as well as the motor activities of running, climbing, and skipping. Peers of the same sex are important for judging one's success or failure. It is nice to have the teacher compliment one's writing skill, but it is even more important to have your best friend admire that skill. Success breeds success, and the child who repeatedly tries but fails soon develops a sense of inferiority rather than industry. Fear of failure is strong during this period, but the need to master skills and be accepted is stronger as long as success generally follows.

Stage V, which Erikson called *a sense of identity versus a sense of diffusion,* occurs between the ages of 13 and 20. This is the time of adolescence when the person must leave childhood behind and become an adult. It is usually a chaotic time, with vast shifts between dependence, independence, idealism, realism, quiet restfulness, tremendous activity, sudden growth spurts, and unpredictability. Both parents and children find this a difficult time. Children who never make the break from home or integrate their inner feelings and thoughts with the outer reality of the world never become full adults. They remain at home, dependent and resentful, in a situation that stifles both their own personality development and that of their parents.

Stage VI, *a sense of intimacy and solidarity versus a sense of isolation,* appears between the ages of 20 and 30 years. This is young adulthood when the person finishes formal schooling, builds a career, chooses a marriage partner, or chooses to live alone. It is a time of contribution and participation in the community and society.

Stage VII, *a sense of generativity versus a sense of self-absorption,* develops between the ages of 30 and 60. This stage shows full adulthood when a person is settled in a career, a family, and a community. Concern for the next generation, the future, the community, and the family are paramount during this period.

Erikson's last stage of development is Stage VIII, *a sense of integrity versus a sense of despair,* and occurs after about age 60. In many cultures this is considered the age of wisdom. During these years, individuals are sought after for leadership and guidance since they have seen most of life's cycles. It should be a time of quiet fulfillment and joy, not a time of despair, isolation, and fear of death.

Erik Erikson is still expanding and reworking his theoretical ideas on development. His writings are presently read with interest and followed by many students of psychology. With time they may show changes and modifications as Freud's work has done.

Abraham Maslow is another contemporary psychologist who has developed a theoretical framework of growth and development. While most of his writings go into great detail about the last stage of development, he does briefly explain some of the stages leading to that final fulfillment.

Maslow's theory is based on a set of basic human needs, and it is often pictured as a rising pyramid with a broad base surmounted by the final goal at the apex (see Fig. 5-5). Maslow does not divide his stages of development by chronological ages since he feels the human organism may be seeking several of these stages at one time.

According to this theory, the basic need of a human being is for physiological well-being and homeostasis. The human body demands certain conditions—food, water, oxygen, elimination, warmth, etc. An adult can probably provide most of the basic needs for himself, while the infant is entirely dependent on outside help. Someone must feed him, clothe him, change him, and protect him. Thus the infant is generally at the first stage of development. Growth into the next stage occurs when the basic needs have been met and the individual is ready to proceed to the next step.

The second stage of development is concerned with the needs for physical safety and includes the necessity for shelter, clothing, stability in the environment, societal rules and laws, and freedom from danger, fears, and anxiety. Infants demonstrate beginning awareness of this stage. When they are warm, dry, and fed, they need a safe place to be held and some continuity of a familiar relationship. The toddlers' world has expanded and they need a safe room, safe backyard, safe car, etc. They also need to know they are safe with their mothers when they are frightened of a big, loud noise or going to the doctor's office. By adulthood, this area of needs includes the laws and rules of society and a country, a job, a community. The world of adults is set up to protect them in many ways, and this need, since it is easily met, is not usually a highly motivating or time-consuming one for the adult.

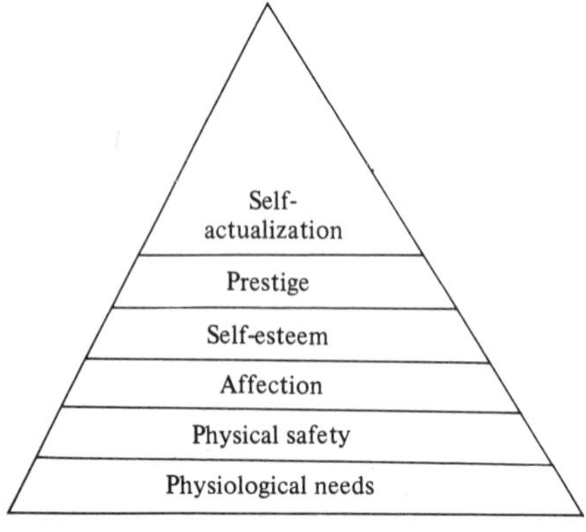

Figure 5-5 Maslow's schematic drawing of human needs. *(Source: Printed by permission of George G. Thompson, Eric F. Gardner, and Francis J. DiVesta, Educational Psychology, New York: Appleton-Century-Crofts, 1959, p. 246.)*

The third stage of development resolves around the need for affection, love, and friendship. Infants begin developing this stage shortly after birth. They must have love and affection to survive. Some of Rene Spitz's early work showed that infants who were provided all the physiological needs but no affection did not survive. No matter how clean and well-fed children were, if they were unloved, they would die. Love begins with a one-to-one relationship between the mother and the child and expands to include other members of the family, friends, and relatives. Love broadens to include relationships of different depths of affection; e.g., an adult woman may love her best friend, but not in the same way she loves her mother or her spouse. This need also includes the feeling of belonging. People need to feel they belong to a certain family, a certain community, and a certain country.

The next stage of development involves the need for self-esteem. All human beings need to feel that they have some control, respect, dignity, and competency. Infants learn very early how to control minor parts of their environment. They know that if they cry, their mothers will pick them up, or if they cry in another manner, their mothers will feed them. There is a sudden desire for power and control around 2 to 3 years of age when children learn that they can control some parts of their bodies and thereby some parts of their environment. They can tell their mothers that they want to go to the bathroom and their mothers make some type of response. Adults need to feel that they are in control of their own lives, that they have the respect of their family, friends and job associates, and that they have some competency in some area of their life.

The need for prestige is the next stage of development. This is tied in closely with the previous need, and sometimes the two levels are combined. Children need to feel that they are important to someone and that they are recognized as something special in some area. Adults frequently have strong needs for being outstanding, important, appreciated, and noticed favorably. Everyone likes a moment of glory, and this can be a very motivating factor in getting certain tasks finished.

Maslow's last stage of development is self-actualization. It really does not apply to children and in many cases not to adults. Self-actualization indicates that people have met all the other needs in the pyramid and have satisfactorily found themselves and developed a certain homeostasis within themselves and their world. They are happy with their jobs, know they can meet problems and crises as they happen, know when and how to seek help if needed, know how to describe their own needs, can be independent or dependent as the occasion demands, and generally find life exciting, stimulating, and full.

Maslow's theories are still being discussed, modified, and applied in different settings. They are different from the other theories since they cannot be divided by chronological age and aspects of each stage appear in all ages. But knowledge of them is important to the nurse working with children as well as to the nurse working with adults.

It may be helpful to look closely at the growth and development patterns of different age groups to see how some of these theories can be applied.

Infancy

During the 1st year of life there are vast changes in the psychological, social, and cultural development of children. Socially, infants spend this year setting the foundation for their acceptance into society. Depending on these early relationships, infants will learn how to love, hate, share, be dependent, and develop morals and will attain some self-esteem and a rudimentary self-image. During this year, infants absorb love, warmth, and caring from a one-to-one relationship, usually with the mother. They take much more than they return during these months. They learn that when they have needs, someone will feed them, clothe them, warm them, comfort them, cuddle them, talk to them, and play with them. If these desires are unmet and no permanent relationship forms, infants learn rejection, fear, and the feeling of being unloved and unwanted, and they fail to grow physically or socially.

Dependency needs are immense during this time since infants really cannot survive without help. They come equipped to do some basic functions (suck, swallow, breath, eliminate), but someone else must prepare the food and get it to them, change their clothing for warmth and cleanliness, change their body positions for varied movements, etc. During this first year they learn some control of their own bodily movements and develop some beginning independency. They can find great joy in being able to turn over by themselves, helping to hold their own bottles and feeding themselves.

Morality, or the sense of what is right and wrong, barely begins during these months. Children are helped into society by having many external reinforcers. Six-month-old children are taught not to bite the mother's nipple by repeatedly removing them from the breast when they bite; gradually they learn this is not allowed. At 10 to 12 months, children are bodily removed from in front of the television set but will return repeatedly. During this time, children have strong urges and they follow these urges to explore and experience their world.

An awareness of self begins to develop during this year. Psychologists believe that during the early months of life infants perceive no difference between self and mother. After the first several months they begin to perceive a separation between their own mouths and the mother's breast. They will fondle the nipple around their mouths and cheeks and against their hands. By 6 to 8 months, children begin to distinguish the mother as a person separate from themselves. They may recognize her face, respond to her, and cuddle more comfortably in her arms. Their concerns are voiced when anyone but their mothers hold them. This is the well-known "stranger anxiety" which seems to be much stronger in some infants than in others. Although unpleasant to experience, "stranger anxiety" is a good sign since it shows that the child is learning to differentiate between familiar and unfamiliar people.

Each of the psychological theories of development considers infancy. Freud felt that infants were in the oral stage of development where all their satisfaction comes through the mouth—sucking, rooting, chewing, drooling, and biting. Erikson felt infants were in Stage I of developing basic trust. Infants learn through their bodily experiences that their mothers bring warmth, food, love, dryness, and shelter. They learn to trust and relate to their mothers, thereby setting the foundation for expanding their trust to other members of the family and society. Maslow would consider infants at the early stages of his first four levels of basic needs: physiological, safety, affection, and self-esteem. By far the most important need during these months is for physiological gratification, and the infants strive to have these needs met promptly and consistently.

The 1st year is a busy year for growing infants, and never again will they show so many vast, visible changes in growth and development.

Toddlerhood

The 2d year is also full of changes and new developments socially. Toddlers no longer spend most of their time in bed sleeping, but are up, running around, verbalizing, and demanding to join in more of the family activities.

Toddlers still need a great deal of love, warmth, and comfort, primarily from their mothers. They also learn to give love and find satisfaction in pleasing their mothers. It is fun to give kisses and hugs and cuddle mommy, especially when she responds with kisses, hugs, and cuddles. Toddlers soon learn they can control some of this. Then they may grant the kiss or withhold it. This increases their sense of powerfulness and control, but may also lead to misunderstandings and hurt feelings if their mothers do not read their moods properly. On the other hand, infants who make their crude attempts at love giving and are rejected or ignored soon stop trying and begin to find pleasure elsewhere. They may find that earlier pleasures of thumb sucking, rhythmical body movements, and body manipulation are more pleasurable than person-to-person contacts. This is a danger sign and may indicate that a child is well on the way to having serious social problems.

Dependency versus independency is very important during this year. The road from depending on mother for everything to doing some things for yourself is rocky and uneven. There are days when children cling to mother's hem and will not let her out of sight, and there are times when they will play for short periods out of sight (next room, back yard) but trot back every so often to see her and be reassured of her presence. Gradually the periods of separation lengthen and the child needs only to hear her voice or check occasionally for security. Separation anxiety is frequent during these years, and it can be very traumatic for both the mother and the child if separation is forced before both are ready for it.

Morality, or the ability to know right from wrong, is still controlled externally during the toddler years. Most control arises from the child's love of the parents and a desire to please them. Much of the morality of this stage has to do with the child's physical safety. Toddlers cannot be expected to make correct choices if left alone in potentially dangerous situations. As toddlers learn some language, they begin to echo the mother's firm "no," but they really do not understand the full meaning of the term. By the end of the 2d year, some toddlers show beginning internalization by saying "no" to themselves and stopping the act or going ahead with the act as they talk to themselves.

Toddlers are often very concerned about body images. As children realize they are separate persons, they begin to take notice of their own bodies. They may become fascinated with the different parts of the body and how they work. Bodily injury becomes a concern, and cuts and bruises elicit much discussion. Toward the end of the 2d year, they may notice the inner feelings of the body, e.g., the urge and tension to move the bowels, the release and relaxation from going to the bathroom, the discomfort of hunger, and the pleasure of eating. They learn the pleasure of control over these situations when they learn to say "Yes, I will go to the bathroom," or "No, I won't go to the bathroom." It is the child's choice and in no way can the mother "make" the child do it. Children are discovering the delights of power and control over others and themselves.

Theoretically the toddler shows many of the characteristics described by the different psychological theories. Freud felt that toddlers progressed through an anal stage, where most of their gratification was sought through the anal opening. Toddlers found pleasure in manipulation of the anal area and controlling their environment by manipulating the control of bowel movements. Erikson felt that toddlers were in Stage II, developing a sense of autonomy and moving away from total dependency into more interdependency. Toddlers discover themselves and explore their own bodies and their expanding world. With their increased mobility, they move away from the mother for short periods of time and look at the world outside their beds, houses, and yards. For Maslow, toddlers were still within the first four stages of development, but with less emphasis on meeting physiological needs and more on physical safety, expanded relationships of affection, and beginning self-esteem.

Toddlerhood is a fascinating period with much psychological, social, and cultural development occurring. It can have many delightful aspects but it may also be a trying time for the mother and the child as they both discover the "terrible twos."

Preschool Years

The years between 2 and 5 also show changes in the child's psychological and social development.

Socially, the preschooler becomes much more like an adult. Parents often find they are more comfortable with children of this age because preschoolers can respond more on their parents' level. Their ability to feed themselves, blow their own noses, go to the bathroom by themselves, etc., means that parents and children can enjoy other activities together.

Love takes on different meanings, and there is a wider range of people "to love" during these years. Children discover that love is not all taking, but comes with certain obligations, responsibilities, and a sense of giving and sharing. Children move away from the very self-centered approach of earlier toddlerhood. Parents are viewed as the epitome of wisdom, power, integrity, and goodness. If earlier stages of the love relationship have not been satisfied, preschoolers may show more fears, inhibitions, explosive behavior, and demands for attention. Children do not actually verbalize their hate of the world, but show many signs that they feel the world hates them.

Preschool children are much less dependent on their parents and frequently can tolerate physical separation for several hours. Peer dependency begins to become much more important. Parents are especially needed during times of stress, frustration, and upset.

Morality becomes more internally controlled during these years. Instead of basing all decisions on the knowledge of what the act will do to them ("If I take the cookie, I will be spanked and that hurts"), children show an elementary understanding of what is right or wrong, fair or unfair in society. They begin to think ahead and become able to plan and avoid punishment by controlling their own urges.

During the preschool years children become increasingly aware of their own self-images and that they are different from their surroundings, their families, and their friends. They begin to realize that their families have feelings, fears, and doubts. As they look at others, they also begin looking at themselves and, in a sense, rediscovering their bodies. Worries over a lost tooth, a removed tonsil, or a skinned knee may concern them. They learn that manipulation of the genital area brings pleasure, and masturbation hits a peak around 3 to 4 years of age. There may also be an interest in looking at the opposite sex and noticing and questioning the difference. All this is related to children's increased knowledge of their own bodies.

The theorists have also studied this age group. Freud felt this is a tremendously active, busy stage of the child's life and termed it the phallic phase. The child's development evolved around the Oedipal complex, with love for the parent of the opposite sex and fear of the parent of the same sex. These relationships were colored by castration anxiety. Erikson thought that preschool children moved from Stage II into the early phases of Stage III.

At this time the children's sense of autonomy was reasonably stable and they began developing a sense of initiative. They learned new skills and began exploring within a larger world than their own homes.

The first four stages of development are still paramount for Maslow, but preschool children have shifted from the lower toward the higher of these levels. Much of their physiological needs had been met and they could control and be responsible for more of their own physical safety. Their needs for affection were still basically met by their immediate families, but they had increased exposure to other relationships and began having opportunities to develop affection outside the home. Self-esteem moved into a higher level as children continued to explore the differences between their own and other bodies. How they were the same or different from mommy, daddy, sister, or brother became important information to gather. The fifth level of development also appeared as children learned the pleasure of being good at something. It was nice to be praised for some special talent, and the first taste for prestige emerges during these years.

The preschool years bring to a close children's protective isolation from the world. Never again will they be so bound within the confines of family members and the boundaries of their own homes. Their world will suddenly expand during the next few years.

School Years

The years between 5 and 10 are often termed the middle childhood or early school years. Socially school-age children move into a much expanded world of neighborhood, church, school, and after-school activities (Scouts, dancing, music). Most of these groups include children of the same sex and age.

Children can now express some feelings of love through verbalization. They learn that they can love their teachers, best friends, grandmothers, and mothers, but not all in the same way. They may discover that their parents are not what they thought they were and look at their friends' parents with interest and envy. Children who lack love during these years learn to seek it in many ways, leading to behavior problems, lying, cheating, stealing, bullying, etc. For them the world is not an easy place, and they learn to grab and take what they can. Some attention, even bad attention, may be better than not being noticed at all.

Children learn to be much more independent of their parents. Within their own peer groups, they learn the rules and limits of their culture. They no longer live totally in the adult world, but have entered the child's world as well. While they may criticize some value or limit placed on them by their parents, they will turn around and defend it if the group takes a different view.

Morality becomes much more than knowing what they can and cannot do. It becomes more abstract, and is involved with conceptualization about the world at large. One researcher has categorized this development into three large stages, two of which happen between the years of 7 and 10. Kohlberg feels that Stage I, which he calls the *preconventional level* occurs around 7 years and includes the first level during which children realize that there is a relationship between punishment and obedience. In other words, children can now consciously think of the external punishment they will receive if they proceed with an act. Stage II, which Kohlberg calls the *instrumental relativist orientation,* means that children are out to satisfy their own needs first and really do not stop to consider or think of others. Stage III, which he calls the *conventional level,* occurs around 10 to 11 years when children develop the idea of what it means to be "a good boy," "a nice girl," "a polite child," etc., and respond to these labels. Children progress into peer groups with fixed rules and rituals which strongly guide them in learning right from wrong.

Self-image continues to grow and change during the school-age years. With increased contact with the outside world, children become aware of how others see them. They know that they are the "neighborhood bully" or the "teacher's pet," rich or poor, black or white, male or female. And they begin to learn what those labels mean and how society expects them to act. Thus their self-images reflect how society (parents, siblings, relatives, peers, etc.) treat them and how they learn the role they must play in the outer world.

Freud called the years between 5 and 10 the *latency phase* because of its quiescence compared with the preceding stormy, turbulent years of the Oedipal conflicts. He felt this was a relatively quiet time when the child learned to identify with the parent of the same sex and became familiar with the role of being feminine or masculine. The child was generally fondest of the parent of the same sex and isolated within a peer group of the same sex.

Erikson felt that school-age children were moving from Stage III into Stage IV. The sense of initiative was still very much present as children learned and expanded their skills within the academic world of school; this merged into the sense of industry when children not only want to try new skills but want to master them, be good at them, and gain prestige and glory from doing them well.

Maslow saw school-age children working well within the pyramid of needs but not yet reaching self-actualization. Physiological needs and physical safety were satisfied more completely at this stage, and children's need for affection encompassed a much larger, more varied group. Children wanted and needed love and support not only from their parents and families, but from their teachers, group leaders, and peers. Their self-esteem broadened to include relationships outside the immediate family, and they began redefining and readjusting their self-images according to different standards. The school-age child learns and remembers the heady feeling of prestige, importance, and glory.

Adolescence

Although this book is considering adolescence to be the years between 10 and 20, many developmentalists would prefer to separate these years into the early preadolescent years (or puberty), adolescence, and young adulthood. Most of the changes during these years are a preparation for adulthood and result from the conflicts of leaving the protected, safe environment of childhood and entering the hectic, ambivalent world of the adult.

During the adolescent years the child's body is growing at such a rapid rate that teenagers frequently state that they feel unhinged and out of joint. Their body is changing so quickly that it seems like a new shell, and children must accommodate themselves to this new structure and inner feelings. This strangeness of one's own body is called *asynchromy*. One researcher documented that during adolescence there is an increase in physical strength, motor ability, and motor coordination. When each of these areas were tested separately, teenagers seemed to do well. The problem arose when they were asked to coordinate several areas. Then they became very clumsy, tripped over their own feet, dropped dishes, and could not quite sit still long enough to accomplish the task (Josselyn, 1972).

By the time children reach middle adolescence, most of their fine motor development is as good as that of adults, and the same tasks expected of adults can be smoothly, easily, and rhythmically performed by teenagers.

Entire books have been written about the changes, conflicts, and adjustments adolescents move through during these years. Only a few topics will be briefly mentioned here, and the reader is referred to a good book on adolescent development for more depth in this area.

During this time the concept of love encompasses many aspects as teenagers prepare for many types of adult love. Conflicts and contrasts prevail during this time as teenagers love their parents, hate their parents, love one girl friend (or boyfriend) this week and another next week. But after all the trials, conflicts, instant joys, depths of despair, and heights of ecstasy, teenagers should emerge capable of handling the many forms of adult love—love for a marriage partner, a close friend, children, etc. During this process teenagers discover that their parents are not pure, lily-white in their values, beliefs, and behavior, and they vascillate between love and admiration and hate and disgust for their parents.

One of the biggest areas of conflict is the need for independence as opposed to the comfort and security of childhood and home. To be fully mature, people must learn to take care of their own needs for physiological maintenance, safety, affection, prestige, and control. But it is a frightening step after one has been cared for and protected for 12 to 14 years of life. One mechanism used in making the break is to find so many faults with the old environment that the new surroundings look more tempting. Needless to say, this solution may be difficult for those from the old environment.

With all the questioning and seeking, adolescents' sense of morality changes naturally. Kohlberg (Holme, 1971) felt that his Stage III of moral development occurred around 16 or 17 years of age. This stage included a level where individuals were guided in terms of the general community, family, and societal rules and regulations. Teenagers begin to see their actions and how they affect a larger group of individuals. By late adolescence they can conceptualize right and wrong logically according to the principles and ethics of their cultural group.

All the struggles and activities of adolescents help them build an image of who they are and who they want to be. They continually measure themselves against the rest of the world and try to find their places in that world. Many hats are tried on during these years, and inconsistency is the only predictable behavior. One time they are idealists, the next, realists; in one situation they want limits, in the next they rebel against any limits; one minute they are in love, the next they cannot tolerate having that person around; one minute they are understanding and compassionate, the next they are totally and intolerably demanding. It is a difficult time for both parents and children, but generally if their struggle is healthy, they will emerge into adulthood secure within themselves and able to handle their world.

Adolescence is looked at differently by different theorists. Freud called the adolescent years and all of adulthood the genital phase. He felt there was a revival of gratification of earlier sexual feelings around the genital area; at this stage, however, gratification was less self-centered and involved more tenderness and concern for others. It also involved a greater number of love objects. While the teenager might be awkward during this stage, by adulthood the needs, and satisfactions settled into a reasonable balance.

Erikson called these years Stage V of development, the stage concerned with developing a sense of identity. He saw the definite struggles of the teenager to let go of childhood and reach for adulthood as an attempt to form one's own identity, separate from that of one's family. He believed that the vast shifts in all realms of the teenager's life (dependency versus independency, idealism versus realism, no growth versus tremendous growth, family versus peers, and so on) were part of this identity crisis.

For Maslow, the teenager was still working primarily within the first five stages of development but probably encountering chaos in each of these areas. While teenagers do not need someone else to take care of their physiological needs, with their changing bodies they are often not aware of their own needs. Sometimes they crave food, and other times they are too busy to eat; sometimes they participate in round-the-clock activity, and other times they crave large amounts of sleep. While teenagers can assume responsibility for their own safety, their occasional feelings of omnipotence and total indestructibility can seriously endanger their safety. Their need for affection expands to include sexual attraction to the opposite sex and a need for approval within their own peer groups. Their self-esteem and self-images change rapidly as they struggle within themselves and their world to find their places. The need for prestige is also strong and is fulfilled predominantly within the peer group rather than in the family or the larger society. With all the turmoil and chaos, self-actualization is not a level achieved during these years. However, from this disorganization should come a knowledge of self and a solid foundation for attaining self-actualization during the adult years.

Adolescence can be an exciting, happy, frustrating, intense, and often intolerable few years because of the immense changes in the psychological, social, and cultural development. But if the storms are weathered, both the parents and the child emerge with a more adult, peaceful relationship.

This brief synopsis of psychological, social, and cultural development should give the examiner some idea of the types of problems that a child may be going through at any one time. Knowing the normal growth and development may help avoid any more traumatic conflicts than are really necessary for both the child and the parents.

COGNITIVE DEVELOPMENT

Certainly one of the areas of child development most studied in this country in recent years has been cognitive development. This is due largely to the work of Piaget, which, although known in Europe for many years, has only recently been translated and become well known in the United States. This research has opened a whole new area in the understanding of children. It is becoming more and more apparent that to communicate adequately with children and help them grow up healthily, it is necessary to understand their thinking—a thinking sometimes postulated on very different premises than adult thinking. This part of the chapter will discuss some of the knowledge available concerning Piaget's theory of cognitive development as well as some other areas of research.

Infancy and Toddlerhood

Because they are so continuous in cognitive development, the periods of infancy and toddlerhood will be discussed as a unit in this section. The younger the child, the more undifferentiated he or she seems to be. It is very difficult indeed to separate cognitive, perceptual, motor, psychological, social, and cultural development in the very young infant. They all seem to blend into one whole. As the child reaches the end of this period, however, differentiation among these types of development is much easier to discern.

Piaget feels that a child from birth to about 18 to 20 months is in a stage he calls *sensorimotor.* This is a very primitive stage during which children lay down the rudimentary beginnings of future cognitive processes. During this stage, they have no way of using mental representations; in other words, they can be aware of an object or sensation that they are experiencing only at the time they are experiencing it. They have no way of forming a mental concept of that object or sensation so that they can deal with it when it is not actually present. Past and future do not exist for them. Their motor activity is more a part of their thinking than it will ever again be. When they kick a pillow, they are not yet aware of the difference between the self, the kicking action, and the pillow. Gradually out of such motor activity will emerge the idea of space—first the space between the self and various objects and much later the space between objects themselves. This first primitive concept of space is called the *action-space concept;* in it only space connected to the self and experienced through the infant's action in it can be conceptualized. Boundaries are blurred; like certain types of regressed schizophrenics, infants are not actually aware of where the boundaries of their own bodies end and those of the world begin.

Their incipient idea of causality is similar. In their egocentricity, they can conceive of no cause except the self. It is their own cry which causes the milk to arrive when they are hungry. It is they who cause sights to be seen simply by opening their eyes; if they close their eyes or look away, the objects will no longer even exist. There are three major cognitive achievements infants will gradually attain during the sensorimotor period. First they will learn to differentiate the self from the environment; objects will be seen as having identity of their own. This will be associated with a less omnipotent view of themselves; i.e. they will begin to realize that there are other wills than their own; they will no longer be able to command the universe. There will be times when they cry for a bottle and cannot make it appear immediately; later they may demand a sharp, pretty knife to play with and be unable to get it. This new realization is related to the second major attainment of this period; the idea of *object constancy,* that is, the realization that objects do not cease to exist merely because they shut their eyes or because the objects are temporarily hidden under a cover. Finally, infants will gradually achieve the very important ability to use symbolization, or as Piaget calls it, *mental representation.* This is a very powerful tool that allows infants to think of objects or situations they are not actually encountering at that moment. It allows them to deal with past and future events and greatly broadens their horizons.

Piaget divides the sensorimotor stage into six phases (or substages). The first lasts from birth to about 1 month, and is composed entirely of innate neurological reflexes like rooting, sucking, and swallowing which gradually become more and more efficient during this phase. From about 1 to 4 months (although Piaget feels the sequence is invariant from child to child, the exact chronological age at which each phase or stage appears may vary considerably) the child enters what Piaget calls the phase of *primary circular reactions.* During this time simple acts are repeated apparently because the child enjoys the action itself regardless of the results of the action. Repetitive fingering of a blanket or opening and closing fists or continual sucking movements may become prevalent during this time. A pacifier or fist may be sucked on with repetitive nonproductive sucking motions apparently just because the child enjoys the sucking activity. During this time also the child's reflexes become more efficient, and certain reflexes begin to show more coordination with each other (for instance, sucking and swallowing reflexes or reaching and grasping reflexes); the eyes follow for further distances, and both strabismus and nystagmus decrease. Infants are more likely now to move toward things outside their own bodies and become interested by various sights and sounds, textures and smells. There appears a very incipient ability to modify a preexisting reflex when it does not quite fit an object; children may be able, for instance, to adjust their sucking to a differently shaped nipple, and indeed begin eating solids (if given during this time) by adjusting their sucking to a spoon rather than a nipple. From 4 to 8 months of age the child is in what Piaget calls the phase of *secondary circular reactions.* This is where intentionality begins. Rather than repeating actions for the sake of the action itself, infants begin to repeat only those actions which produce interesting results. Where they kicked for the sake of kicking during the previous phase, they now kick repeatedly only when they can produce an interesting result, like making the mobile move. Certain previously unrelated activities begin to join; for instance, sucking and prehension, which were previously two distinct abilities, now become coordinated in a hand-to-mouth schema in which everything children put in their hands (or sometimes an empty hand itself) will be placed in the mouth for sucking. Children become more and more interested in the environment and study various phenomena determinedly. An incipient idea of object permanence appears, and rather than believing that when an object is out of sight it ceases to exist, infants will now make rudimentary attempts to follow it; for instance when something interesting is dropped out of view, they will begin to anticipate its movement. This also allows them to attain a very immature idea of causality and further allows them to begin seeing others as distinct from self. They begin to suspect that mother exists even when they do not see her, just as objects do. This is important for a slightly later time period when attachment behavior begins. Toward the end of the 1st year (about 8 to 12 months) the child enters what Piaget calls the phase of *coordination of secondary reactions and application to new situations.* It is during this phase that children begin to solve very simple problems, such as searching actively for a toy when it is out of view and performing certain acts to find it such as knocking down a pillow when they have seen the toy put behind it. This is made possible largely because of their increasing concept of object permanence. They can utilize a response they already know for obtaining specific goals; for instance, they will use the reaching response to obtain many new interesting objects. They continue to see only their own actions as casual, however.

The fifth phase of the sensorimotor stage is called the phase of *tertiary circular reactions* and becomes apparent from about 13 to 18 months. Children are now capable of more complex problem solving and will show actual trial-and-error experiments. They can now modify and vary their movements to suit their purposes and can sometimes be seen to vary an action just to see the variation in outcome. They become more and more differentiated from the environment and can now see outside things as causal. They will search for a hidden object where they saw it last, showing their increasingly thorough understanding of object constancy. They are still not able, however to follow an invisible displacement; in other words, if they see a doll put under a cloth, they will lift the cloth to find it, but if the doll is first put under one cloth and then shifted to an adjacent cloth (without this shift being visible), they will continue to look only under the first cloth.

Finally the child enters the last phase of the sensorimotor stage, the phase called the *invention of new means through mental combinations.* This phase lasts from approximately 18 to 24 months and is intermediary between the sensorimotor stage and the following preoperational stage characteristic of preschool children. Most important, beginning use of mental imagery appears. For the first time, children are able to follow an invisible displacement and can infer a cause when they see only the effect. For instance, at this age a boy may realize that his sister has taken his piece of candy just because he knew it was there before he turned his head away and when he turned his head back, his candy was gone and his sister was happily chewing.

Very little research other than Piaget's has been done on the thinking of infants and very young children. The authors could find only one other useful area of infant cognition that has been investigated and that area is *categorizing.* The ability to sort items into categories is important in later cognitive skills, and Ricciuti (1965) has shown that this skill actually begins in some children by the age of 1 year. In an experiment investigating this skill, he placed four gray balls and four yellow cubes in front of young children of various ages. He found that in the 1-year-old group, over 40 percent of the infants touched either the four gray balls or the four yellow cubes consecutively, indicating some primitive categorizing ability. By 1½ to 2 years, over 70 percent did so. Apparently the bases for categorization cannot be too subtle, however, since none of the children were able to categorize between parallelograms and ellipses.

Anticipatory guidance and counseling of parents concerning the growth of their children's thinking at this age can be helpful. The more the parents understand about how their child is thinking at a particular time, the better able they will be to adjust their expectations and to provide the necessary environmental stimulation. Knowing that a child in the secondary circular reactions phase, for instance, enjoys repeating those actions which bring interesting results will help them understand why such things as a mobile within kicking distance may be useful. Knowing that children in the tertiary circular reactions phase are practicing their new found ability in understanding object permanence may help parents be less exasperated at the constant dropping of toys and food from the high chair. This repetitious and purposeful dropping is not being done from willfulness or to annoy the parents, but to continually retest their new hypotheses that objects which leave the range of vision, still do, in fact, exist.

Preschool Years

In some ways the preschool child's thinking is even more difficult for the parent to understand than that of the infant. This is probably due to the fact that on the surface it has many characteristics which resemble adult thinking. It is easy to assume that it is totally like adult thinking. This is not the case, however; preschool children are in a stage that Piaget calls *preoperational,* and they utilize a very different groundwork for their thinking than do school-age children, adolescents, or adults. A great deal of research has been devoted to this period in cognitive development, and although there are still many unanswered questions, many things are known about it. Piaget feels that the preoperational stage of cognitive development extends from about 2 to 7 years of age. The landmark of this age is language and the ability of mental symbolization which this implies. During this time children are becoming more and more adept at mental representations of the environment and this allows them to deal with past and future ideas—an impossibility during the sensorimotor stage. Children continue to be basically egocentric, however; that is, it is impossible for them to abstract enough to be able to know how things look from another viewpoint. For instance, it is impossible for them to know what an object would look like from any other angle in space than that in which they themselves are. For example, if a girl is seated at one side of a table with her brother on the other side and a doll is standing in the middle of the table, facing her, she will report, if asked, that her brother must see the doll's face also. She is unable to use mental representations well enough yet to place herself in her imagination in her brother's place and realize that only the back of the doll is visible from this viewpoint. This limitation extends to children's concept of time as well. They are totally unable to imagine a viewpoint from any other point in time. They cannot yet grasp historical events, for instance. Another very characteristic attribute of this period of development is that children are almost totally dominated by their perceptions. They do not realize that sometimes perceptions can be misleading. This is why they believe so fully in a magician. Not only are children dominated by their perceptions, but they are unable to consider two aspects of a perception simultaneously, for instance, both the height and width of an object. This is the basis of some of the famous Piagetian conservation experiments that will be discussed later.

The child's reasoning is neither deductive nor inductive at this stage, but is what Piaget calls *transductive;* that is, the child reasons not from the general to the particular nor from the particular to the general but from the particular to the particular. This unique viewpoint of the world is what will enable a 3-year-old boy to announce that he will not eat his applesauce because the beans were burned! In other words, because he did not like one particular vegetable, he will not like another particular fruit. This unadult-like logic is the source of many communication problems between parents and their preschool children.

Time is still somewhat of an elusive concept for children this age. During the sensorimotor stage, children's first experience with time was their own bodily circadian rhythms of hunger and satiation, sleep and wakefulness. During the preoperational stage, some of the culture's methods of reckoning with time become apparent to them although it will not be until later that they can deal really efficiently with all of them. By 4 or 5 years of age, most middle-class children in the United States have learned such time markers as days of the week and seasons of the year and the association of certain holidays with certain seasons. They are not yet able to read clocks, with the exception of one or two important hours of the day, such as eight o'clock if that is their bedtime. Although children of this age may use the words "yesterday," "today," and "tomorrow," they seldom understand the sequence correctly until school age. "Yesterday" often refers to any event from the past, and "tomorrow" to any event in the future. As mentioned before, historical concepts are beyond children of this age group, and it is impossible for them to imagine, for instance, that their own parents were ever children. Many children of this age expect some day to catch up in age to their parents and marry them, a cognitive limitation that encourages the psychological Oedipal stage. By about 5 years, however, children can plan events that will occur in several days, and a special "calendar" made by the children and parents in such a way that each night a day can be crossed off showing how many days are left until the special occasion will help them clarify their concept of time: 1 2 3 4 5 6 7 8 9.

A classic study by Ames shows some of the time concepts children attain at various ages.

18 months: Some sense of timing, but no words for time.

21 months: Uses *now.* Waits in response to *just a minute.* Sense of timing improved. May rock with another child, or sit and wait at the table.

2 years: Uses *going to* and *in a minute, now, today.* Waits in response to several words. Understands *have clay after juice.* Begins to use past tense of verbs.

30 months: Free use of several words implying past, present, and future, such as *morning, afternoon, some day, one day, tomorrow, last night.* More future words than past words.

3 years: Talks nearly as much about past and future as about the present. Duration: *all the time, all day, for two weeks.* Pretends to tell time. Much use

of the word *time: what time? it's time, lunchtime.* Tells how old he is, what he will do tomorrow, what he will do at Christmas.

42 months: Past and future tenses used accurately. Complicated expressions of duration: *for a long time, for years, a whole week, in the meantime, two things at once.* Refinements in the use of time words: *it's almost time, a nice long time, on Fridays.* Some confusion in expressing time of events: "I'm not going to take a nap yesterday."

4 years: Broader concepts expressed by use of *month, next summer, last summer.* Seems to have clear understanding of sequence of daily events.[1]

Space is also a difficult concept for preschool children. During infancy and toddlerhood, children understood only action space, that is, they knew space only from their own activity of moving through it. Although their space concept is gradually becoming more and more refined during this time, they will not reach the next stage of *map space* until the latter part of this period. A classic experiment by Maier (1936) showed that when children this age were taught all the subjects of a maze separately until they knew them well, they were still unable to put the parts together mentally to form the picture of the entire map. As discussed previously, the space concept also remains egocentric in that it is impossible for children to imagine how an object looks to a person standing at an angle in space different from their own.

1 year: Gestures for *up* and *down.*

18 months: Uses *up, down, off, come, go.*

2 years: *Big, all gone, here,* interest in going and coming.

30 months: Many space words are rigid, exact ones: *right, right here, right there, right up there.* Words were combined for emphasis and exactness; *way up, up in, in here, in there, far away.* Space words used most; *in, up in, on, at.*

36 months: Words express increased refinements of space perception: *back, corner, over, from, by, up on top, on top of.* A new interest in detail and direction: tells where his daddy's office is and where his own bed is, uses names of cities.

42 months: *Next to, under, between.* Interest in appropriate places: *go there, find.* Interest in comparative size: *littlest, bigger, largest.* Expanding interest in location: *way down, way off, far away.* Can put the ball *on, in, under,* and *in back of* the chair.

48 months: More expansive words: *on top of, far away, out in, down to, way up, way up there, way far out, way off.* The word *behind.* Can tell his street and city. Can put a ball in front of a chair. Space words used most: *in, on, up in, at, down.*[2]

Categorizing is another important cognitive skill that undergoes some refinement during this time period. In the earlier part of this stage, which

[1] Reprinted by permission from L. B. Ames, "The Development of the Sense of Time in the Young Child," *Journal of Genetic Psychology,* vol. 68, 1946, pp. 97-125.

[2] Reprinted by permission from L. B. Ames and J. Learned, "The Development of Verbalized Space in the Young Child," *Journal of Genetic Psychology,* vol. 72, 1948, pp. 63-84.

Piaget calls the *preconceptual* phase, children have only "preconcepts" and cannot understand the idea of classes. Each snail they see is an individual experience of snail; they cannot group them together into the class of snail. This is one of the reasons children of this age are not disturbed by the experience of seeing a new Santa Claus on every street corner. They are not able to sort well by a common attribute but may sort items on a part-whole basis, often a part-whole basis of family. Thus, if asked to sort a series of blocks which differ in size, shape, and color, they may proceed to put together a small, medium, and large block of any color on the basis that these are the "mama block," "papa block," and "baby block." This is the first level of categorizing skill found at the beginning of this stage and is called *cluster* categorizing. At the next level, children begin to sort by the *chain* method of organizing; that is, they connect each item only to the one preceding it by any attribute present, whether they previously used the same attribute or not. For instance, a child may put a red circle with a red square because both are red; add a blue square to the category because it matches the last item in shape, and then add a yellow triangle because it is the same size as the blue square. The child sees no necessity to remain constant in choice of attribute.

Finally, toward the end of this stage, children become capable of more adultlike methods of categorizing and will be able to pick out one characteristic—usually a rather concrete perceptual one—and use that for the entire categorizing process. It is still impossible for them to use two attributes simultaneously, however, and they will not be able to separate a group of yellow circles from a total category which contains circles of other colors as well as yellow objects of other shapes. This skill will come much later.

Ordering is also very difficult at this age, and only very rudimentary ordering begins toward the end of this period. A child of 3 who is asked to match the order of a yellow block, red ball, and green pyramid, will not be able to do so. This is an important skill for reading, however, since reading requires that the child be aware of the ordering of letters in a word and words in a sentence. More will be said about this under the section on perceptual development.

The development of the concept of causality is not totally understood but it is clear that children of this age are undergoing many modifications in their ability to associate causes with results. Piaget talks about three early stages in the attainment of this concept. The first he calls *realism,* a stage in which infants feel that they personally are the cause of all things. This predominates primarily in the sensorimotor stage. Later comes the stage of *animism* in which the child thinks that actions are caused by an innate personlike quality possessed by all things. For instance, a box might fall off the table because it "wanted" to get to the floor. *Artificialism* is the third phase in which the child feels things are all caused by some controlling humanlike force, a purposeful agent who controls the world. Piaget studied only European children to reach these conclusions, and they have not been replicated well on other cultures. Margaret Meade (1932), for instance, found a very different sequence in the children she studied on a Pacific Island. In summary, then, although this sequence does seem to be exhibited by some children, there appears to be a great deal we still do not know about the concepts of causality in children.

Piaget has studied the idea of conservation extensively in children of this age and the succeeding stage of *concrete operations.* Conservation to Piaget requires the operation of reversibility; that is, a child who has the concept of conservation is able to mentally reverse an operation. For instance, in his studies of conservation of quantity, Piaget shows a child two pitchers that are similar and are filled with water to the same level. He asks the child if the pitchers contain equal amounts of water and the child of course says yes. He then pours the water from one pitcher into a taller, thinner pitcher. Although the child has seen that exactly the same amount of water has been poured into the new pitcher, the child will state that the pitchers no longer contain equal amounts of water; the taller, thinner one contains more. The child is not able to reverse the process mentally to see that the same amount of water remains. Children of this age are so perceptually dominated that the fact that their perceptions tell them that the water level is higher in the second pitcher makes them believe that there is more water in it even though they saw that the same amount was poured into it. They are unable at this stage to consider two separate attributes—height and width—at the same time.

Similar research shows that children of this age are also unable to conserve mass. If children are shown two equal-sized balls of clay and then watch the examiner roll one ball into a flat patty, they will state that the flat patty is no longer equal to the ball, but now contains less clay although they have been watching the procedure and know that no clay has been added or subtracted. Conservation of length follows a similar development. In the early preoperational period, children apparently judge equality of length by matching end points. If two sticks are lined up in such a way that their end points match exactly, children will say that they are of equal length; if they then watch the examiner move one stick to the right several inches, they will state the stick which has been moved is now longer since its end point extends past the other's.

Conservation of number has also been investigated. It is known that children during this period match number by arrangement patterns; thus if one group of eight buttons is clustered closely together and another is spread out, the child will believe that there are more buttons in the group which is spread out.

It is some time before children are able to overcome their strong tendency to be dominated by their perceptions in such a way as to be able to become a conserver. Usually this happens toward the end of the preoperational stage and apparently proceeds in an orderly fashion; at least we know that by 5 years half of the children will be conservers of quantity, by 6 years half of them will be conservers of weight, and by 7 years, half of them will be conservers of volume. This order of achieving conservation—first of quantity, then of weight and finally of volume, seems to be invariant (Uzgiris, 1964).

Because cognitive development achieved during this period is so important for future schoolwork, it is important that the nurse working with children of this age be aware of the processes taking place and able to explain them to parents. Although it is important not to encourage parents to "push" their children educationally, it is also important to help them know what cognitive skills their children should be gaining and some way they may help them to achieve these skills. Several excellent books are available which give suggestions to parents on how to help their children achieve the necessary cognitive skills during the preschool years. *Thinking Is Child's Play* by Evelyn Sharp and *Teaching Montessori in the Home* by Elizabeth Hainstock are two such books.

School Years

Great changes take place in the cognitive skills of children during their early school years. Piaget calls this the stage of *concrete operations;* it begins about 7 years of age and ends at about 12. Certain changes that take place in children's thinking now make it possible for them to understand the basic ideas of mathematics, sciences, humanities, and social sciences. Although they cannot verbalize specific theories, they are able to do problem solving based on these theories. They are much more advanced in being able to see things from a different point of view from their own. This refers to social as well as perceptual and cognitive events. They are now able to tell how a doll in the middle of the table would look from the opposite side of the table. They are also increasing their ability to deal with hypothetical situations. If you ask a boy in the preoperational stage what would happen to him if he were a girl and wanted to play cops and robbers, he would simply reply that he is not a girl. He would be unable to get past the hypothetical part of the problem. This is no longer true during the period of concrete operations.

In this stage, children's notion of causality is also developing. Usually they have largely discarded the concept of artificialism discussed under the section on the preoperational period, and during the school years they first become able to differentiate between the necessary cause and the possible cause; that is, there is a difference in their understanding when they say that A causes B and when they say that A might cause B. A little later during this period the idea of multiple possibilities arises, and toward the very end of the period of concrete operations, children are able to differentiate between the certain, the probable, and the possible (Piaget and Inhelder, 1951). They are not yet able to grasp the idea of relative probabilities, however; this distinction will come during the adolescent stage of formal thinking

The school-age child's idea of time is becoming more specific also. Children are usually able to tell exact time during the first few years of school, and because they are better able to understand relational concepts, their idea of history becomes more realistic, as does their understanding of the human growth and development process. A sharp increase in the ability to judge older persons' ages has been found at the fourth grade level (Lovell, 1968), seeming to indicate an increase in the understanding of the idea of the aging process. Before this time, the child has only one category for older people—adults; and this seems to include anyone from 18 to 92. An understanding of the timing required for rhythms is also increasing, particularly during the early school years, with the child first able to understand the timing of auditory rhythms and only later of visual ones, the latter being a more complex combination of the interrelationships between time and space.

The space concepts of the concrete operational period are still basically those of map space. A child of this age is not yet able to understand the more complex space of geometrics of multiple dimensions; this will become possible for the adolescent who has entered the stage of formal operations. Spatial concepts seem to begin with the perception of the body, and lateralization concepts of the body begin in children during the preschool and early school years, but are only gradually correctly attributed to another individual. Children of 5, for instance, will generally attribute sidedness to another person in mirror-image style. That is, if the mother asks the child to imitate a gesture she performs with her right hand, the child, if facing her, will generally use the hand directly across from the mother's, that is, the left hand. Only slowly does the ability to transpose orientation grow. During this time, the child also begins to be able to use accurate measurements of space, first by comparing them with known spaces on the body (measuring something with the fingers, for instance) and later by using the measuring devices provided by the culture, for instance, rulers and scales in the United States.

Two very important abilities arise during this period: the ability to categorize and the ability to understand relations. Although younger children can also categorize motorically during the sensorimotor stage and perceptually during the preoperational stage, during the period of concrete operations, children take several steps forward in their classifying abilities. For one thing, they are able to classify on more and more abstract criteria: they are no longer dominated by the perceptual qualities existent in the items to be classified. Classifying by perceptual qualities begins to drop off sharply between kindergarten and the first grade; classifying by experience (e.g., grouping some objects together because they all go in a kitchen) begins to drop off around the fourth grade; and classifying on the basis of abstract qualities continues to increase during this entire period. A great deal of energy and interest is invested in this newly emergent ability to classify, as shown by the almost fanatic proclivity for collecting shown during the school years.

The ability to order things according to their relational qualties is another important skill which arises during the school years. Children can now understand relative relations between things—dark, darker, darkest, for instance. This skill appears first as motor skill through which the child is able to serialize things according to their size, hue, weight, or other physical characteristics, but this ability is gradually internalized and becomes more and more abstract. This ability to order is, of course, essential in reading, in which the very essence of the skill depends upon the ordering of letters in words and words in sentences. It is also essential in ordering events in time, such as occurs in history, or ordering places in space, such as occurs in geography.

One of the outgrowths of these two skills (classifying and ordering) is the beginning of a true understanding of the number concept. Although preschool children can usually tell the names of numbers and frequently count to 10 or even 100, this is usually a rote-memory skill with little conceptual understanding present. But when children are able to order, and categorize, they are able to appreciate both the ordinal and nominal aspects of numbers; that is, they can understand both the category of "four" in which there can be "fourness" of many things—four apples, four cows, etc., and the relation of four to three and five. This is the basis for mathematical manipulation.

As was true with the other age groups, knowledge of the cognitive level of the school-age child is necessary both for talking with the child and for counseling the parents. Again, choice of toys and games should be appropriate; for instance, the best possible gift for a young school-age child just beginning to understand measurements might be an inexpensive set of measuring cups and spoons. Likewise, map games in which mother draws a map of the house showing where the cookies are hidden are fun for children who are perfecting their skills in understanding spatial relationships. In giving such suggestions, the nurse can help patients better understand how their children are thinking.

Two other areas of research on cognitive development become important during the school years: the research on intelligence and intelligence testing and the research on creativity.

The concept of intelligence is a confusing one. Some define it as the ability to learn from experience; some, like Guilford, define it as a composite of five cognitive processes: recognition, memory, divergent production, convergent production, and evaluation; some merely state that it is what the intelligence test measures. During the school years, all children will come in contact with intelligence tests, and it is important that the nurse be familiar with them. They were begun by Binet, a French psychologist who was asked to construct a test to administer to mentally retarded children for the purpose of deciding which children would be able to benefit from education. The result was a test including measures of logical reasoning, information from past learning, perceptual-motor coordination, perception, and verbal ability. This is the test which in modified form is today known as the Stanford-Binet Intelligence Quotient Test. This test yields a score called a mental age. The IQ refers to the mental age divided by the chronological age multiplied by 100 (MA/CA × 100 = IQ). Many tests have tried to improve on certain shortcomings of the Stanford-Binet. For instance, the Wechsler Intelligence Scale for Children (WISC) is used more often for older children and is composed of two sections; one section is called the performance scale and is made up of five subtests including copying tasks, comprehension of pictorial representations, complex block designs, recognition of missing parts of pictures, and various puzzles; a second section is called a verbal scale and includes five subtests of various verbal abilities. The ability to separate the two types of skills is an advantage over the Stanford-Binet, which yields only one score. Other tests, such as the Merrill-Palmer, are further attempts at measuring IQs.

The great usefulness of IQ tests is in measuring academic success. High IQ scores correlate well with future scholastic achievement and are good predictors in this sense; they have not been shown, however, to be accurate predictors of anything else, including success in life. It is possible, in fact, that they measure little more than the ability to do well in tests.

Creativity is a subject which is interesting more and more researchers. It is becoming clear that creativity is not the same as intelligence and can exist with it or without it. Creativity in most of experimental research is presumed to show two characteristics: many unique associations and a flexible, permissive approach. The classic work on this was done by Wallach and Kagan (Smart, 1965) and tested creativity in children in several ways. On one test, for instance, a child was asked to tell all the possible ways that certain items could be used; the answers were scored both on number of different answers and number of unusual answers (i.e., answers which few other children had given). Each child then obtained a score for creativity as well as an IQ score derived from a standard IQ test. Some interesting findings resulted from this study. It was shown that children high in both creativity and intelligence manifested self-confidence, peer popularity, and good concentration abilities; they were also easily bored and somewhat disruptive in class. Children high in creativity but low in intelligence had poor self-confidence and difficulty concentrating and were generally withdrawn and unhappy. Children low in creativity and high in IQ had good self-images and good powers of concentration, were not disruptive, but seemed to be socially withdrawn and generally conservative. Children low in both creativity and intelligence scores were fairly self-confident and relatively extroverted. Although there is a great deal we do not yet know about both intelligence and creativity, is is apparent that in some way these are very important in the personality formation of children, particularly during the school years.

Adolescence

According to the Piagetian scheme, most adolescents have reached the final stage of cognitive development—formal thinking. Yudin (1966) finds that adolescents of low intelligence generally reach this level by the age of 14 to 16, while those with above average intelligence reach it by age 12 to 14. Some important changes take place during this stage—some stages which will, according to Piaget, last the individual the rest of his life. One of the most characteristic traits of this stage is the ability to abstract. Adolescents are no longer tied to the perceptual qualities of a situation as are preschool children, nor are they tied to the specifics of a situation as are school-age children. They are able to consider a problem from many different points of view, arrive at several possible solutions, and hold them simultaneously in mind while comparing them and choosing the most appropriate one. They are also able to use abstract rules to solve an entire set of problems, whereas a school-age child was able to apply a rule only to a specific problem. This newly acquired skill further enables their thinking to be purposely deductive and to formulate several hypotheses, test each of them mentally, and choose the most appropriate, much in the way of the scientist. Most characteristically, adolescents are able to abstract enough to be able to think about the thinking process itself, a skill not evident at any earlier level.

The understanding of intelligence and the attempt to measure intelligence through a variety of intelligence testing mechanisms remains essentially the same as was true during the school years. Such measurements at the adolescent level retain all the limitations from the previous levels and maintain their same application; that is, they are useful in predicting future academic success at a statistical level (that is, for a group of individuals, such predictions can be made; for a specific individual, such variables as motivation must be considered). Certain types of measureable intellectual qualities which depend upon what may be called "fluid" mental skills such as perceptual speed, flexibility, and adaptability seem to reach their height during this period and decline thereafter. Other qualities which depend more on experience and judgment, such as tests of vocabulary, comprehension, and information stores, appear to continue to improve into later adult life (Conger, 1973).

Probably the most important thing for the nurse working in this area to be aware of (to help her both in communicating with and understanding the adolescent and in counseling parents concerning the daily stresses of living with an adolescent) is the influence of the adolescent's cognitive level on behavior. Although adolescents' newly acquired ability to look at many alternative solutions to a problem enable them to broaden their intellectual horizons to include such areas as calculus and poetry, it also presents some problems in terms of indecisiveness. It further allows them to realize that their parents' opinions, which they previously regarded as infallible, may be only one of many possible ways to view the world, and, in fact, may be wrong. This sets the stage for the frequent adolescent criticism of parents and can make life with adolescents quite difficult. Furthermore, because, adolescents are now keenly aware that the present way of doing things is not the only way, they may become extremely critical of the political and social situation as well as of any other situation in which they find themselves. They do not yet have enough experience to realize the practical limitations of life, but they do have the cognitive abilities to realize that the situations they find are not ideal. Again, the result is rather severe criticism of those in decision-making capacities.

An adolescent's thinking is characteristically introspective, and this typically results in a new form of egocentric behavior. Because adolescents are able to see things from others' points of view, they are now capable of realizing that others have opinions of them which may differ from their own. Consequently, much of their behavior begins to take on a self-consciousness and they begin to consider their behavior more in relation to how it looks to others. The result is a type of "stage-performance" behavior that can be very trying to adults.

In summary, then, it is important for the nurse working with children, particularly in ambulatory areas, to be well aware of the developmental sequence of cognitive growth and to consider this both in relating to the children and in counseling the parents concerning their relations with their children and their attempts to provide an appropriately stimulating environment for them.

PERCEPTUAL DEVELOPMENT

Less is known about the development of perception than about other aspects of children's development. Most of the research that has been done from a developmental standpoint is on very young children, and even here the findings are somewhat scant. Nevertheless, it is important for the nurse working with children to be aware of what is known in this area and of what implications such knowledge has for guidance and counseling of parents.

The Neonate and Young Infant

Surprisingly enough, the greatest amount of research in the area of developmental perception has probably been done on the neonate. Through a variety of ingenious research approaches, we know a certain amount about what the newborn experiences in terms of perception. Certainly the most thoroughly investigated area has been visual perception. Structurally, the eye is incomplete at birth; the fovea has not yet completely differentiated from the macula. This differentiation will occur at about the same time that most of the myelinization process is finished, that is, at about 4 months. The macula will then continue to mature until about 6 years of age. The ciliary muscles are also immature at birth, and this results in the newborn's limited ability to accommodate; in fact, during the first 2 months, an infant's focusing ability is relatively fixed at a distance of about 8 in. This, of course, has implications for infant stimulation; for instance, the placement of mobiles or toys or even the distance an infant is held from the parent's face while playing should be geared to this limitation of accommodation.

Although strong stimuli are needed to elicit the pupillary reflex at birth, this reflex will stabilize within the first few days, and after that should be readily elicited. Tracking of a bright light source should also be possible for limited distances within the first few days, although actual convergence and binocular vision are thought not to be perfected for the first 7 or 8 weeks (Mussen, Conger, and Kagan, 1974). It is fairly well documented at this time that the most perceptually significant features of visual stimuli for the infant from birth to 2 or 3 months are brightness, movement, and contrast; this is useful information when helping parents choose toys and stimulating experiences for their young infants (Mussen, 1972).

The visual perception and preferences of infants of 4 to 8 months have also been studied rather extensively. Children of this age continue to be attracted by movement, contrast, and brightness, but other characteristics of the stimuli now become more important. It is known, for instance, that meaning is now more important; for instance, an infant of this age will look longer at stimuli resembling the human face than at unfamiliar patterns. (Haaf and Bell, 1967). The question of complexity is still controversial, although it appears that, at least up to a certain point, the infant prefers (i.e., looks longer at) stimuli which are more complex. It is suggested further that infants may prefer curves to straight lines; at least studies utilizing bull's-eye and striped patterns showed that the bull's eye elicited longer gazing (Mussen, 1972). There are also indications that there is an optimal level of discrepancy which the child finds most interesting. For instance, faces that are slightly disorganized will elicit more interest than faces which are completely normal or those which are completely disorganized (McCall and Kagan, 1967). One of the most interesting visual stimuli which combines all the important attributes of movement, contrast, brightness, meaningfulness, and a certain amount of discrepancy is television, and most parents of children this age will report that their infants are intrigued by this stimulus.

The depth perception of young infants has also been studied. It is not certain whether infants are born with depth perception or acquire it later because of experience or because of innate factors. It is known that before 10 weeks a baby is equally attracted to a two- or three-dimensional object; after that, the infant gives preferential attention to a three-dimensional object; this is true, for instance, in regard to a photograph of a human face and a real face (Fantz, 1965). Interestingly enough, this difference is noted whether the baby is using one or both eyes. The classic studies of depth perception have been done with the "visual cliff." This is a construct in which a transparent pattern lies across a certain area. On one side of this platform, a checkerboard pattern is placed directly beneath the transparency; on the other side, the same checkerboard pattern lies several feet below the transparent covering. Since the covering cannot be seen, the impression is given that a drop of several feet exists; this impression would be apparent only to a person with three-dimensional vision, however. Babies of crawling age (about 6 months) are urged to cross this platform. All will refuse to do it when the distance of the drop is quite large. When this distance is less, some of the late crawlers are more easily coaxed across. Those who have been crawling for longer will continue to refuse. This makes some investigators suggest that the role of experience may be important in learning to perceive three dimensions. It is of course possible that this experience is not important in the actual perception of the three dimensions but rather in knowing how to react motorically. An interesting experiment was done by Held and Hein (1963) in which one group of kittens was given a certain type of experience with manipulating three-dimensional situations both visually and kinesthetically; in other words, they were free to move and walk around while they were exposed to visual three-dimensional cues. The second group was exposed visually to the same three-dimensional cues, but were not allowed to move. Later this second group of kittens was found to be defective in the visual-cliff experience. Information from nonhuman animals cannot be directly inferred to humans, but this kind of study does at least raise the question of the importance of both visual and kinesthetic experience for the adequate development of depth perception.

Visual pattern perception and preference has also been studied in young infants. Most of these studies have centered around the pattern of the human face. It is known, for instance, that infants under 1 month will respond to the motion of a bobbing face, but the features of the face are unimportant at this point. By 6 weeks the eyes of the face are important, and an infant of this age will not respond to a representation of a face which lacks eyes but will respond to one which has only eyes and lacks all other features. By 10 weeks both eyes and eyebrows seem to be necessary, and by 20 weeks the mouth is important. At this time, a face without the relevant features (i.e., eyes, eyebrows, and mouth) will not only fail to elicit interest, but will actually elicit withdrawal. By 24 weeks the child reacts to differences in the position of the mouth and will respond better the bigger the smile; pursed lips with wrinkled brows result in withdrawal. By 28 weeks babies respond to female faces more readily than to male faces, and by 30 weeks will respond differentially to familiar and unfamiliar faces (Roe). This corresponds, of course, to "stranger anxiety."

Although less is known concerning the various nonvisual types of perception, some study of this has been done, particularly regarding hearing. It is known that even the fetus in utero will respond to sound stimuli and that by the time the amniotic fluid is drained out of the ears during the neonatal period, the infant's hearing is probably essentially the same as adult hearing. In experimental conditions newborns will react to the difference between 200 and 100 cps (about the difference between a clarinet and a foghorn) (Leventhal, 1964). In one study, the investigators actually elicited different responses to sounds differing only by one musical note (Bridger, 1961). This is a rather fine distinction. Certain things are known about the effect of sound stimuli on the infant. Low frequencies like that of the heartbeat tend to decrease motor activity and crying, while high frequencies elicit an alerting reaction (Mussen, 1972). A study by Salk (1962) shows that newborns exposed to simulated heartbeat, although they ate similar amounts and types of formula, gained weight better and cried less than control infants exposed only to the normal nursery sounds. Other studies have shown, however, that lullabyes and metronomes had similar effects. The length of the sound stimuli also appears to be important. Sounds which are too short (under 1 second) or too long (over a few minutes) fail to attract attention. The optimum length seems to be about 5 to 15 seconds. This information can be useful with certain colicky infants who appear to be quieted by optimum length, tone, and rhythmicity of sounds, such as loud ticking clocks.

Specific sounds other than the heartbeat may also be relevant to the young infant. The sound of the crying of other infants appears to be a distressing stimulus, and a recording of an infant's own crying seems to be even more upsetting (Smart and Smart, 1972). There seems to be an early sensitivity to the human voice (although it is not specific for speech sounds), and infants will turn to the sound of a voice before they will turn to other sounds. Later, usually around about 8 months, probably before the time they can actually understand words, the sound of human speech becomes demonstrably more interesting to children than other human voice sounds such as cooing. Other types of perception have been less studied. We do know that neonates can smell and can localize smells; they will turn their head away from strong smells such as ammonia or acetic acid. One study indicated that the higher the odor saturation, the higher the level of the infant's activity (Disher, 1965).

Infants can also taste, at least by 2 weeks of age, when they will make sucking responses to sugar and will grimace when offered quinine. During the prenatal period, taste buds are found all over the mouth, including the palate and buccal membranes; toward the end of gestation, most taste buds recede and are found primarily on the tongue. During early childhood they appear primarily on the tip of the tongue (perhaps this is why licking activities such as those involved in eating lollipops and ice cream cones are so popular in childhood). Later in life, taste buds seem to recede from the tip of the tongue and are found primarily on the back of the tongue (Nash, 1970).

The neonate also appears to be perceptive of temperature changes and can distinguish 5 to 6° away from a neutral position of 33°C when contacting objects, a phenomenon the nurse will often notice when applying a cold stethescope. Although some investigators (Jensen, 1932) have noted that the infant will squirm and suck irregularly if the milk is colder than 23°C or warmer than 50°C, one study (Holt, 1962) showed that there was no difference in sleep patterns, eating patterns, amount of regurgitation, or weight gain with a group of infants fed cold formulas.

Tactile sensation appears to be present early in fetal development; the fetus is sensitive to tactile sensation in the oral area as early as 3 months. Sensitivity then proceeds in a cephalocaudal direction, and at birth the infant is able to perceive tactile sensation in any part of the body, although the face, hands, and soles of the feet seem to be the most sensitive. It is well known now that early tactile experience (Casler, 1965) is essential to normal growth and development.

Some studies have been done on the newborn's pain perception. It appears that very early in the neonatal period, the infant's pain threshold is relatively high. The number of pin pricks necessary to elicit withdrawal of the leg decreases gradually from birth to about 8 days of age (Sherman, 1925). Girls appear more sensitive to pain than boys. This correlates well with the common observation that newborns cry very little during circumcisions.

Although there is still a great deal that we do not know about the perception of infants, some of the findings discussed above should be useful to the nurse working with families with young infants.

The Preschool and School-Aged Child

Most of the work that has been done in studying the perception of preschool children has been related to the problem of understanding how children normally develop whatever perceptual abilities are necessary to the reading process and what kinds of abnormalities in this development may later result in reading disabilities. Consequently, the bulk of the work done in this area has been concerned with visual development. Some major trends in visual development are evident although we do not know much about the details of such processes. In general, during this period children seem to begin with a global, somewhat vague, gestalt-like way of perceiving visual stimuli; later they become much more precise and differentiated in their perception and will concentrate on details in a more analytic manner; finally, they return to a more holistic perception, but this time include specific articulated details. One of the specific areas of perception in which this trend is particularly evident is in the perception of the whole-part relationship. Elkind (1964) devised a test which illustrated this process quite well. He presented a picture in which a clown was composed of various types of fruits. The younger children saw only the fruit and did not realize that the pieces of fruit seen as a whole constituted a clown. Older children saw only the clown, and the oldest children saw both the clown and the fruit. Children who are at the stage in which they are perceiving only the whole will not be aware of changes of parts within the whole. A similar progression was found in children's responses to a Rorschach inkblot. As Reese and Lipsitt (1970) describe it:

> Up to the age of six years a marked predominance of responses appeared to be based on an undifferentiated perception of the whole blot; these gradually declined in favor of responses based on small details, and subsequently of responses indicating an attempt to encompass the parts of the blot within a single, meaningful whole.

This same process may be at work in learning to read, in regard to both individual letters and whole words. It may be that children first get a global impression of letters and can easily distinguish very different letters such as "H" and "O," but may confuse rather similar letters such as "b," and "d"; only later, when they become more analytical and pay more attention to detail, would they be able easily to distinguish these more similar letters. In the final stage, then, the child would be able to quickly glance at a letter and without specifically studying its component parts be able to articulate the details and the gestalt into the correct recognition of the letter. Errors such as confusing "b" and "d" would drop out at this point. The same process may exist in learning entire words, and this may explain why teaching by the phonetic method, in which each individual letter is analyzed and sounded out, and teaching by the sight method, in which the child is expected to get the gestalt of the entire word without undue attention to the component letters, may each be appropriate methods at different developmental levels.

Gibson (1963) has studied the analytic part of this process in the development of perception of letters. He wanted to find out which characteristic details of letters are perceived at various developmental stages. After extensive study of children of a wide variety of ages, he concluded that by 4 or 5 years of age, most children were capable of what appeared to be the easiest discrimination—open versus closed figures. Children of this age, for instance, were quite accurate in distinguishing an "O" from a "C." The next step was the ability to differentiate straight lines from curves such as would be seen in the letters "U" and "V"; this ability was present in most 5-year-olds. Rotation, that is, inversion from right side up to upside down, such as occurs in the letters "M" and "W" was accomplished next, after which the distinction between right and left directionality occurred. At this stage, the child became able to distinguish between "d" and "b." The most difficult characteristics were the various diagonal slants, and these were difficult even for some 8-year-olds. Many letters require two or more such distinctions simultaneously, such as the letters "A" and "V," which require both diagonals and rotation. It is often helpful to know the developmental sequence of such perception, since most children can discriminate such differences if they are isolated and extra opportunity is provided with the specific problem discriminations. For instance, although most 4- and 5-year-olds will not spontaneously distinguish between mirror images such as "d" and "b," they can do so once their attention is drawn to this difference and it is made relevant to them. Before beginning to read letters, this difference is probably seldom relevant, since most three-dimensional objects are the same whether they face one way or the other. Because of this, prereading children are seldom exposed to the importance of noticing differences in spatial orientation of this kind.

Studies of the movements made by the eye while scanning pictures reveal a similar developmental progression (Reese and Lipsitt, 1970). Young infants show scanning patterns in which only the outline is scanned. There is little organization and much wasted movement in this early scanning. Studies of young children's scanning, however, shows that while they also are inefficient in their scanning movements, they are, as Piaget would say, "centered"; that is, their attention is drawn almost entirely to the center of the picture (see Fig. 5-6). Later they again return to scanning primarily the contour of the form, but this time in a more efficient, systematized fashion. With this increase in efficiency, visual form discrimination increases considerably, and studies of children show that their ability to find embedded figures and recognize small changes in similar patterns increases sharply. In the studies by Zaporozhets (1965) this final stage would take place around the age of 6, the usual time when a child needs this fine discriminatory ability to begin reading. Children older than this change their scanning style, at least temporarily, and will most often be seen to scan in a systematic way from left to right. Presumably this is due to the artificial influence of the process of learning to read which seems to generalize to all visual stimuli.

Although it is known that very young infants perceive three dimensions in the real world, exactly how and when children learn to perceive three-dimensionally in picture form is uncertain. It appears that this is a learned rather than an innate skill, since it never appears in certain cultures, notably in certain African cultures which do not utilize the type of three-dimensional art styles common in the Western world. The implication of this, of course, is that it is quite valuable for children, particularly of the preschool age, to be exposed to pictorial material, especially that which utilizes the Western conventions of depicting three dimensions. Some researchers who have tried to teach African individuals to perceive pictures three-dimensionally later in life have found it impossible to do so and have suggested that there may be a critical period for learning this and that perhaps if it is not learned during the preschool years, it will not be possible to learn it later (Hudson, 1960).

The relation of language to perception has also been studied. The question of this relationship originally arose because of the difference between

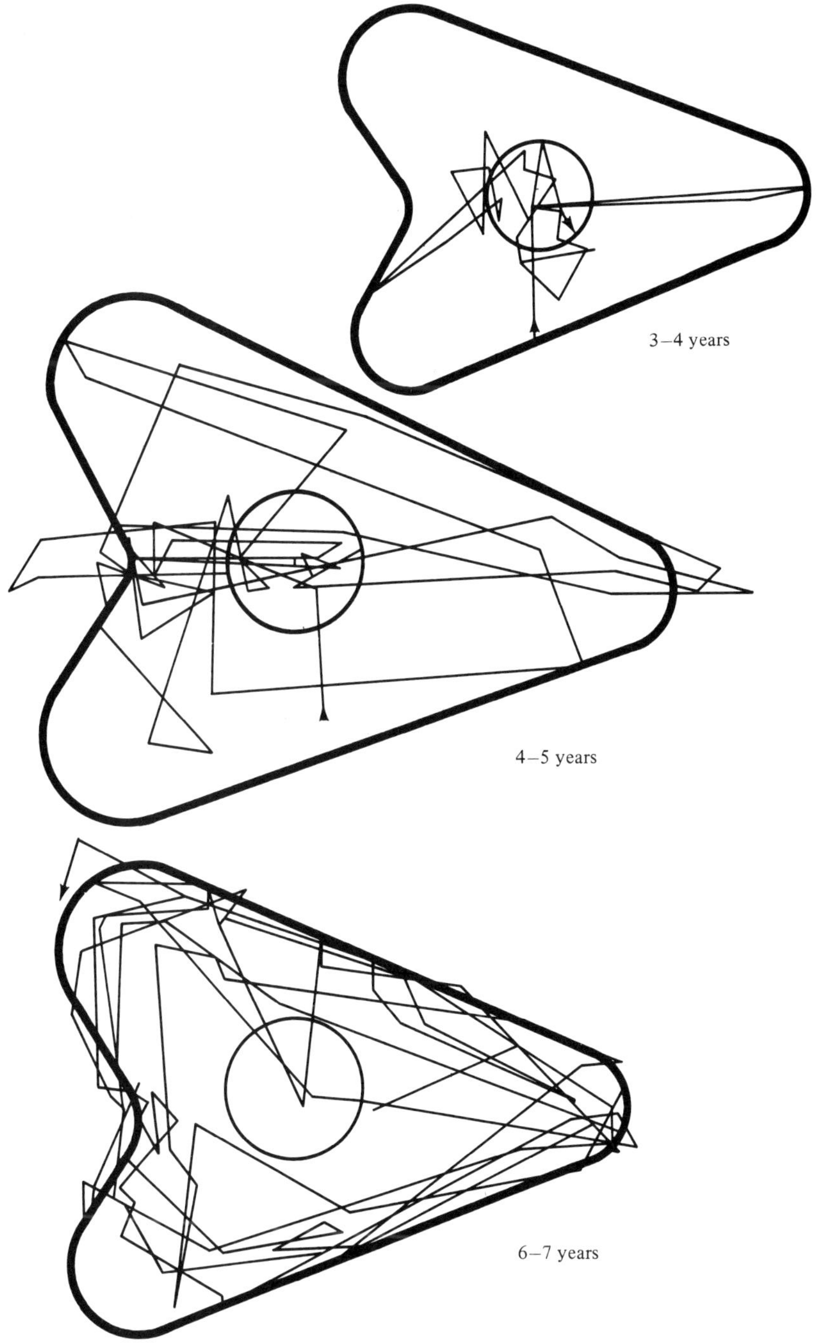

Figure 5-6 Patterns of eye movements. (*Printed by permission of Perceptual Development, p. 396. Source: A. V. Zaporozhets, The Development of Perception in the Preschool Child, in P. H. Musses (ed.), European Research in Cognitive Development, Monographs of the Society for Research in Child Development, vol. 2, whole no. 100, 1965, pp. 86–88.)*

cultures and their color vocabulary. It was known, for instance, that the Navajo language had only one word to describe both green and blue, while it had several to describe that part of the spectrum which we call black. The question was then raised as to whether Navajo individuals were incapable of distinguishing between what we call blue and what we call green. It was found that this is not the case. They are able to perceive the difference in hue even though they do not possess distinct names for the difference. The only time there was a difference in perception between Navajos and Anglo-Americans was when there was a situation of drastic cue reduction (for instance, if the lighting was very poor) or when memory was involved in a color matching test (Brown and Lenneberg, 1954). Apparently, then, language does help in perception but is by no means the determining factor. This is also true for children. In situations in which they have labels for different stimuli, they are more likely to perceptually detect the labeled differences.

The amount of information needed by the child to recognize a stimulus has also been studied. Gollin (1961) constructed a series of cards depicting familiar objects with broken lines. There was a gradation in cards in such a way that the beginning cards had long lines and very short spaces, and the final cards had very short lines and long spaces (see Fig. 5-7). There was a

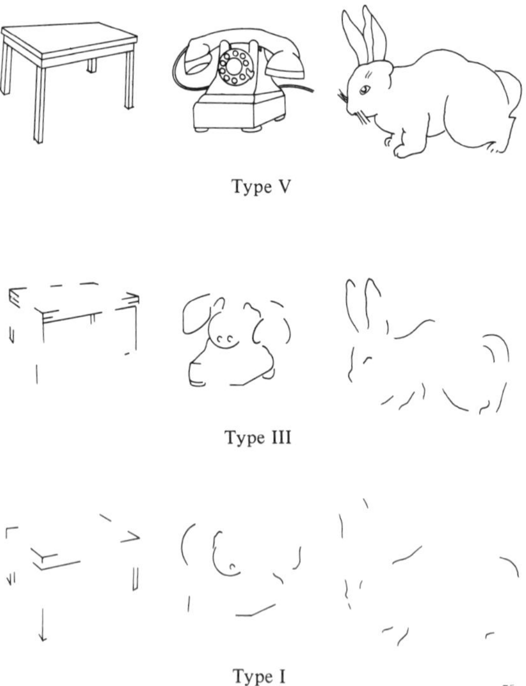

Figure 5-7 Gollin's incomplete figures. *(Source: Printed by permission of S. Gollin, "Further Studies of Visual Recognition of Incomplete Objects," Perceptual and Motor Skills, vol. 13, 1961, p. 307.)*

clear developmental sequence in children's perception of these stimuli. The younger the child, the more concrete information needed to identify the stimulus (i.e., the less able the child was to fill in the blank spaces).

Very little research has been done on other senses, although it is likely that similar developmental sequences exist, for instance, in auditory development. Various Russian investigators (Reese and Lipsitt, 1970) have studied the development of touch and have found its sequence similar to that of vision. The 2- to 3-year-old, when blindfolded and asked to identify an object by touch will palm it with a rigid unpatterned grasp. An older child will use both fingers and palms but still with no pattern; finally, by about 6 years of age, the child will show a systematic patterned exploration of the contour using both fingers and palms. This is highly similar to the studies of eye scanning movements, which also display a gradual increase of patterning. It is interesting to note that visually, while not yet manifesting the patterned eye exploration of the contour, the child will choose to categorize by color rather than by form. For instance, if given a red circle, a red triangle, and a blue circle, and asked which two go together, the child will choose the two red objects rather than the two circular objects. Later, this preference will change, and the child will match by form instead. In a similar fashion, Klein (as quoted in Reese and Lipsitt, 1970) found that at about the same time that tactile exploration developed a systematized pattern, the child changed from tactile matching by texture to tactile matching by form.

Some work has also been done with intermodal sensory abilities, that is, with the ability to coordinate two different senses. One example of testing this is to have children feel various shapes under a covering while looking at other shapes on a table and see if they can match what they feel with what they see. Intermodal sensory abilities seem to increase dramatically between the ages of 3 and 7 years, but continue to become refined until at least 14 (Abravanel, 1968). It also appears that between about 5 and 7 years children switch their primary sensory approach from what Nash (1970) calls the *near-receptor sensations* like tactile, kinesthetic, and proprioceptive senses to the *far-receptor sensations* like hearing and vision. It is interesting to note that this takes place at about the same time that the child is achieving the cognitive stage of concrete operations according to Piaget. The probable importance of intermodal perception is pointed out by Katz and Deutsch (1963) and Beery (1967), who found that retarded readers were likely to have trouble with coordinating their auditory and visual sensations (a skill clearly needed for coordinating the sight of a written word with the sound of that same word).

As can be readily seen, the research in this area is fairly scanty, and it is not entirely clear at this time what application can appropriately be made from this knowledge. Certainly the Montessorian approach which stresses sensory experience would seem to follow well from what is known about the development of perception and the role of experience in this development. If nothing else, it would seem logical at least that a reasonable amount of experience with various sense modalities (visual, auditory, tactile, kinesthetic, and probably olfactory) should be provided for the child.

LINGUISTIC DEVELOPMENT

In this chapter, the child's learning of language will be considered a special developmental process. It actually involves the fine motor development which is necessary for articulation, the auditory perceptual development necessary for understanding words and sentences, the cognitive development needed for understanding and using the syntactical and semantic aspects of language, and the psychological, social, and cultural development which creates the necessity for language. Language itself can be considered the means of communication between people; as such it is a broad term and encompasses spoken language as well as body language, gestures, and other special types of communication such as reading and writing. Speech refers only to spoken language, and this is primarily what the present chapter will deal with. The development of four general areas of speech will be considered: articulation, lexicon, syntax, and semantics.

Articulation

The development of articulation, or the way the structures of the nose and mouth mold the sounds emitted by the larynx, begins at birth. The cry of the newborn is already characteristically human in its articulation, and the nurse should be able to recognize normal from abnormal cries of the newborn. Certain chromosomal and endocrine problems will be signaled by an abnormal cry in the nursery (e.g., cretinism, cri-du-chat syndrome, and others). Mothers will learn to recognize different types of cries early in life—usually these can be seen as different on spectographic analysis by 6 to 8 weeks. Early sounds can be divided roughly into two categories: sounds of comfort and sounds of discomfort. The first discomfort sounds in the delivery room consist primarily of gasps and cries in which the first consonant—an "h"—is clearly audible. The earliest consonants after that are those formed primarily in the back of the mouth like "k" and "g," later followed by labials and dentals such as "b" and "p" (a development enhanced by sucking and swallowing movements which are becoming more coordinated). Discomfort cries originally consist primarily of front narrow vowels nasalized by tension, with the "w," "l," and "h" sounds later giving these discomfort sounds more acoustic variety. The almost universal "mama" is probably produced by a discomfort cry combined with an anticipatory sucking movement of the mouth.

Babbling is an important step in the development of articulatory ability. Responsive babbling should begin by about 3 months. Originally, babies babble in the sounds of all languages; this is apparently an innate development since even deaf babies babble. This is usually followed by a brief period of silence after which more specific babbling occurs. During this second stage of babbling, infants become more particular and selectively babble only in the sounds of the language they hear around them. Between about 4 and 8 months, babies use most of the vowels and about half of the consonants of the adults in their environment. They are also articulating about half of the phonemes they hear (i.e., single sound units which may be vowels or consonants or blends such as "ch" and "bl") and a few morphemes (i.e., one-syllable units of speech which may be simple words such as "me" or other single syllables that add meaning to words like "ing" or "ed"). Vowels predominate through the 1st year in a ratio of about 5:1; this will gradually change until adult life, when the ratio is about 1.4:1 in favor of consonants. Children learning various languages will develop sounds in the same sequence.

Articulatory skill continues to become more refined, and infants between about 8 months and 2 years are usually about 25 percent intelligible to a stranger. The intelligibility rate jumps to about 66 percent during the 2d year, a time when there is much voice play, including playful changes in pitch and loudness. There also occurs a normal hesitance in speech which should be ignored as it will soon be outgrown. By the age of 3, the child's speech should be about 90 percent intelligible to the examining nurse although some medial sounds which are difficult for the child to understand in adults' speech may not be reproduced clearly. This is the time of normal stuttering, and it is important for the nurse to assure the parents that this is a normal developmental phase and is best ignored. The etiology of adult stuttering is unclear, but many speech pathologists feel that it is caused by too much attention being paid to this normal developmental stuttering. Children should not be made to stop and start again or asked to speak more slowly, and should not in any way have their attention drawn to their stuttering. By 4 years of age, speech should be completely intelligible with the exception of particularly difficult consonants like "r," "l," "s," "th," "z," "sh," and "ch."

In general, the developmental sound sequence proceeds in this way:

3 to 4 years of age: lip sounds ("m," "p," "b," "w," and "h") should be intelligible.

4 to 5 years of age: tongue contact sounds "n," "t," "d," "k," "g," "y," and "ng" should also now be intelligible.

5 to 6 years of age: the "f" sound is added.

6 to 6½ years of age: "v," "ch," "l," "sh," and a voiced "th" (as in "then") are added.

6½ to 7 years of age: the "z," "s," "r," and voiceless "th" (as in "thin") are added.

7½ years of age: the child should now have all articulation sounds.

When children are learning new articulation sounds, they usually progress through a regular sequence of mispronunciation. When first learning, they will simply omit the new sound. After they are a little more familiar with it, they will try to substitute another more familiar sound for the new sound (the "w" for "r" substitution as in "wabbit" for "rabbit" is most common; less common are substitutions of "l" for "j," "f" for unvoiced "th," and "v" for voiced "th"). The next most advanced step in learning the new sound is an error called *distortion,* which is simply a lack of clarity (for instance, the classic "hasgetti" for "spaghetti"). Finally, the most advanced type of error, which is a sign that the child will soon be learning the sound correctly, is an error called an *addition,* in which the child adds an extra sound to the word (for instance "gulad" for "glad"). It is useful for the nurse to know this developmental sequence of errors since she can then explain to the parents at exactly which level the child is and reassure them that the child can be expected to progress through various levels before finally arriving at the correct pronunciation. Screening tests as discussed in Chap. 4 are helpful in this type of assessment.

Lexicon

The term *lexicon* refers to what we commonly think of as the vocabulary. Although the least complex of the types of language learning, this is the one most often singled out in assessment of the child. This is particularly true in various developmental and intelligence tests; particularly the latter rely heavily on vocabulary. Although there are norms available for how many words children of various ages are expected to have, many variables can influence this. Environment, stimulation, intelligence, bilingualism, and personality can all affect this measure potentiality in the older age groups. Nevertheless, it is sometimes useful for the nurse to know some rough estimates of norms for various ages. Generally, a boy is expected to say his first word around 14 months of age while a girl generally begins 3 to 6 months earlier. Even at this early age, there is a wide range of normal due to individual variation. Between 8 months and 2 years, the child's vocabulary generally can be expected to expand to include around 200 to 300 words, and by 3 years, 900 is given as the average number; this grows to about 1,500 by 4 years old (3- to 5-year-olds are expected to add approximately 50 words a month to their vocabulary). Their spoken vocabulary will continue to grow, although less rapidly during the school years, and between first and sixth grade, children usually about double the number of words they know, although their reading vocabulary lags behind in the early school years, it is about equal to the listening vocabulary by eighth grade (Smart, 1973).

Syntax

Syntax, or grammar, is a complex skill given a great deal of attention in recent years by psycholinguists. It refers to the complicated ways that languages have of ordering their words into sentences to express various meanings. In some languages the word order in the sentence is important to meaning (e.g., in English, the sentence "John likes Mary" means something very different from the sentence "Mary likes John," and this difference in meaning is indicated by the word order). In some other languages word order is unimportant. In some languages parts added to a word (like our "ing" or "ed" endings on verbs) are important indicators of meaning. There are a great many complicated grammatical rules children must learn in order to master the syntax of their language. It is truly amazing to realize that the child almost totally completes this task in about 2 years (from about 18 months to 3½ years). Again, very definite developmental stages can be isolated. The first is the stage of *receptive language* (sometimes called *competence*) which begins at about 8 months when children can understand but not produce language. Generally even later when learning new parts of language such as new words or sentence structures, children will understand others who use the new word or structure before they will be able to use it themselves.

The next stage usually begins sometime between 12 and 18 months when the child begins to use *holophrases,* or single words to express whole ideas. When a 2-year-old says, for instance, "milk!" this one word actually stands for the whole sentence, "Give me a glass of milk, right now!" In other words, a complex idea which will later be expressed in a series of words structured into a particular sentence is, at this stage, expressed in one succinct word. Most commonly, these holophrasic sentences are of two types; denomination (or labeling) and commanding (or imperative).

Later, usually at about 18 months, begins the stage called *telegraphic speech.* This is probably the most complex and most intensely studied stage of childhood syntactical development. This is the stage of the two-word sentence, but children do not, as was once believed, put any two words together randomly. There appears to be an innate simplistic grammar which emerges at this time and which has only recently been appreciated. In this grammar, the child, rather than possessing many classes of words (nouns, pronouns, adjectives, etc.), possesses only two classes: a pivot class and an open class. The pivot class consists of only a few words each used quite often. Different children may use different words as pivot words, but an individual child is very slow to add new words to the pivot class. The open class consists of more words, and newly learned words are generally readily accepted into this class. During this phase, a child uses only these two classes to structure sentences, which might be diagrammed as P–O, that is, a word from the pivot class followed by a word from the open class. Because the pivot class contains fewer words than the open class, a sample of an individual child's repertoire of sentences might include: "doggy comes," "doggy pretty," "doggy eat," "doggy all gone." In these examples, the child has classified "doggy" as a pivot word, and it will never be used by this child in the open-class position. Other sentences might use a second pivot word with the same open-class words: "daddy come," "daddy pretty," "daddy eat," and "daddy all gone." About 2 to 3 months after the stage in which children use only pivot and open-class words, they begin to further subdivide the pivot class. The original subdivision is into articles, demonstrative pronouns, (i.e., this, that) and a second pivot class. Two or three months after this, the second pivot class will be further subdivided into adjectives, possessives, and a third pivot class. To date, linguists have not yet followed the further development of this grammar. Much is still to be learned about how this apparently innate method of categorizing language develops, but it is at least useful to realize that a child's syntax does indeed seem to progress through predetermined developmental stages. When more is known about this development, it is hoped that screening and diagnostic tests will be developed which can be used by the nurse working in the ambulatory pediatric setting.

Something is known also about the development of sentence types. In general, the older the child, the more likely he or she is to use compound and complex rather than simple sentence structure. In regard to particular types of sentences, it is known that the child understands active sentences first, then questions, then passive, and finally negative constructions. The order is slightly different, however, in regard to production of the various sentence types. Again active sentences are the first to make their appearance. Next come both the negative and question structures. These two have been fairly extensively studied. It is known, for instance, that the first negative sentence structure a child is able to make is made by prefixing the sentence with a "no" or "not." The child then proceeds through three more stages before arriving at the fourth stage of the adult negative structure (see Table 5-4). Studies have also been made of the child's development of the syntax of questions (see Table 5-5). Again, it is hoped that in the future these results will be refined well enough that a clinician will be able to utilize this information to quickly assess a child's developmental level in regard to specific types of sentence structure.

Some information is also available on specific items of syntax, such as pluralization and the use of past tenses. In both situations, children appear originally to learn each word as an individual unit. At this stage, they will use the irregular forms correctly. For instance, they will say "brought" as the past tense of "bring," and "geese" as the plural of "goose." It is only later when children grasp the concept that all plurals and all past tenses have something in common and are governed by similar rules that they begin to grasp the most common rule and overgeneralize it. For a while after children first realize this, they will apply this rule to all verbs, and will now say, "bringed" for the past tense of "bring" even though they have previously used the correct "brought." They will likewise begin to say "gooses" instead of the correct "geese," in an attempt to make it conform to the newly discovered rule of pluralization by addition of an "s." At a later stage they will realize that there are exceptions to the most common syntactic rules and, in fact, that there are lesser rules that apply to smaller numbers of instances. It

Table 5-4 Syntax of Negative Constructions

Rule	Examples
Stage 1 (1.4–1.9 morphemes)	
a. {*no* / *not*}-S	No wash. No mitten. No more. No play that. Not fit.
b. S-{*no* / *not*}	Wear mitten no. Why not?
Stage 2 (3.3–3.4 morphemes)	
a. NP-{*can't* / *don't*}-VP	I can't see you. I don't want it.
b. Demonstrative-{*no* / *not*}-NP	That no fish school. That not milk.
c. *Don't*-VP	Don't leave me. Don't push it.
d. *Why not*-NP-(*can't*)-VP-Q	Why not me sleeping? Why not me go?
Stage 3 (4.8 morphemes)	
a. NP-Aux + *n't*-VP	I don't want cover on it. I won't eat it.
b. NP-(*be*)-*not*-{NP / adj}	That not a clown. He is not a girl.
NP-*not*-VP (with *-ing*)	He not going. I not crying.
c. *Don't*-VP	Same as Stage 2 Don't hit me.
d. *Why*-NP-Aux + *n't*-VP-Q	Why the kitty can't stand up? Why it won't start?
e. NP-Aux + *n't*-VP (with *some* as form of indefinite determiner or pronoun in object position)	I didn't see something. He won't have some.

Table 5-4 Syntax of Negative Constructions

Rule	Examples
Stage 4 (5.7 morphemes)	
a. NP–Aux + *n't*–VP	Same as adult and Stage 3 I doesn't know how.
b. NP–*be* + {*n't* / *not*}–{NP / adj}	He isn't happy. Those are not your tires.
NP–(*be*)[b] + {*n't* / *not*} – {VP (with *-ing*) / adj}	He isn't looking. I not peeking.
c. *Don't*–VP	Same as Stage 2 Don't do it on me.
d. *Why*–NP–Aux + *n't*–VP–Q	Same as Stage 3 Why you couldn't find it?
e. NP–Aux + *n't*–VP (with indefinite determiners and pronouns containing negative element)	He can't have nothing. Nobody won't recognize us.

Source: Hayne W. Reese and Lewis P. Lipsitt, *Experimental Child Psychology,* New York: Academic, 1970.

is at this stage that they will return to correct syntactical usage. This is important to realize when working with parents since they frequently become concerned when they feel that their child is developing worse rather than better grammar. This is an instance where developmental guidance by the nurse can be very helpful.

Semantics

Semantics, or the study of meaning, has been less researched from a developmental standpoint than have the other areas of language already discussed. In general, it appears that a similar progression to that found in other developmental sequences occurs; the child develops from a more global to a more differentiated understanding of the meaning of language. Words used in any language have both a denotative and a connotative meaning. The denotative meaning refers to the specific, concrete referent of the word, while the connotative meaning includes a broader range of feelings aroused by the word. Adults can usually separate these two aspects of meaning, but children seldom can. In fact, it appears that very often, although they are quite adept at using words correctly, they may have only a very vague, diffuse connotative understanding of the word. For instance, it has been found that many children understand the words "happy," "pretty," and "good" as synonyms during the early school years. In one study, 62

Table 5-5 Syntax of Questions

Rule	Examples
Stage 1 (1.8–2.0 morphemes)	
a. S–Q	No ear? See Hole? Mommy eggnog?
b. *What* NP (*doing*) *Where* NP (*going*)	What's that? Where Daddy going?
Stage 2 (2.3–2.9 morphemes)	
a. S–Q	You can't fix it? See my doggie? Mom pinch finger?
b. *Wh*–S	Who is it? What book name? Why not he eat?
Stage 3 (3.4–3.6 morphemes)	
a. Aux–NP–VP–Q	Can't you get it? Am I silly? Does turtles crawl?
b. *Wh*–NP–VP	Why you caught it? What we saw?
Wh–S (object questions; *do* optional, object NP optional and Aux is not moved)	Where my spoon goed?
Wh–VP (subject questions)	Who took this off? What lives in that house?

Source: Hayne W. Reese and Lewis P. Lipsitt, *Experimental Child Psychology*, New York: Academic, 1970.

percent of the first graders believed they were synonymous (Ervin and Foster, 1960). Similarly, young children often use the word "heavy" to refer to anything difficult, weighty, or strong. They may state that the mountain is heavy to climb or ask if the ice is heavy enough to walk on. It is only gradually that the specific denotative meanings become understood.

As more is learned about the young child's understanding of semantics, the nurse should be able to communicate more effectively with children. What is known at least makes it clear that *what* the parent or nurse says to the child is not as important as *how* she says it, since the child relies less on the specific denotation of the words spoken than on the general connotation and feeling or tone of the words, gestures, and manner of the nurse.

BIBLIOGRAPHY

Physical Growth and Development

Boyd, Julian D.: "Clinical Appraisal of Growth in Children," *Journal of Pediatrics,* vol. 18, no. 3, March 1941, pp. 289-299.

Clements, E. M.: "The Age of Children When Growth in Stature Ceases," *Archives of Disease in Childhood,* vol. 29, no. 144, April 1954, pp. 147-151.

Epstein, Nathan: "The Heart in Normal Infants and Children: Incidence of Precordial Systolic Murmurs and Fluoroscopic and Electrocardiographic Studies," *Journal of Pediatrics,* vol. 32, January-June 1948, pp. 39-45.

Fogel, David H.: "The Innocent (Functional) Cardiac Murmur in Children," *Pediatrics,* vol. 19, no. 5, May 1957, pp. 793-800.

Garn, Stanley, S., Arthur B. Lewis, and Rose S. Kerewsky: "Sex Difference in Tooth Size," *Journal of Dental Research,* vol. 43, no. 2, March-April 1964, pp. 306-307.

Greulich, William W.: "Somatic and Endocrine Studies of Pubertal and Adolescent Boys," *Monographs of the Society for Research in Child Development,* vol. 7, ser. 33, no. 3, 1942, pp. 1-85.

———, and S. I. Pyle: *Radiographic Atlas of Skeletal Development of the Hand and Wrist,* Stanford, Calif.: Stanford, 1950.

Harper, Paul A.: *Preventive Pediatrics: Child Health and Development,* New York: Appleton-Century-Crofts, 1962, pp. 77-152, 176-233.

Lee, Marjorie M. C., K. S. F. Chang, and Mary M. C. Chan: "Sexual Maturation of Chinese Girls in Hong Kong," *Pediatrics,* vol. 32, no. 2, September 1963, pp. 389-397.

Maternity Center Association: *A Baby Is Born,* New York: Maternity Center Association, 1964.

McCammon, Robert W.: *Human Growth and Development,* Springfield, Ill.: Charles C. Thomas, 1970.

McIntosh, Rustin: "On Growth and Development," *Archives of Disease in Childhood,* vol. 32, no. 164, August 1957, pp. 261-270.

Meredith, H. V.: "Stature and Weight of Children in the United States with Reference to Influence of Racial, Regional, Socio-Economic and Secular Trends," *American Journal of Diseases of Children,* vol. 62, 1941, p. 909.

Mills, Clarance A.: "Temperature Influence over Human Growth and Development," *Human Biology,* vol. 22, no. 1, 1950, pp. 71-74.

Reynolds, Earle, and Lester Sontag: "The Fels Composite Sheet," *Journal of Pediatrics,* vol. 26, no. 4, April 1945, pp. 336-352.

———, and Janet V. Wines: "Individual Differences in Physical Changes Associated with Adolescence in Girls," *American Journal of Diseases in Children,* vol. 75, no. 3, March 1948, pp. 329-350.

Richards, Mary R., Katherine K. Merritt, Mary H. Samuels, and A. G. Langmann: "Frequency and Significance of Cardiac Murmurs in the First Year of Life," *Pediatrics,* vol. 15, no. 2, February 1955, pp. 169-179.

Root, Allan W.: "Endocrinology of Puberty: Part I Normal Sexual Maturation," *Journal of Pediatrics,* vol. 83, no. 1, July 1973, pp. 1-19.

Ross Laboratories: *Children Are Different,* Springfield, Ill.: Charles C. Thomas, 1962.

Sehan, Max, and Arthur J. Moss, "Electrocardiography in Pediatrics," *Archives of Pediatrics,* vol. 59, no. 7, July 1943, pp. 419-445.

Silver, Henry, Henry Kempe, and Henry B. Bruyn: *Handbook of Pediatrics,* Los Altos, Calif.: Lange, 1969.

Sinclair, David: *Human Growth after Birth,* New York: Oxford, 1969.

Sontag, Lester W., and Earle Reynolds: "The Fels Composite Sheet," *Journal of Pediatrics,* vol. 26, no. 4, April 1945, pp. 327-335.

Tanner, J. M.: *Growth at Adolescence,* Springfield, Ill.: Charles C. Thomas, 1962.

———, and Berbal Inhelder: *Discussions on Child Development,* New York: International Universities, 1971.

———: "Growing Up," *Scientific American,* vol. 229, no. 3, September 1973, pp. 35-43.

Todd, T. Wingate: *Atlas of Skeletal Maturation,* St. Louis: Mosby, 1937.

Washburn, Alfred H.: "The Child as a Person Developing," *American Journal of Diseases of Children,* vol. 94, no. 1, July 1957, pp. 46-53.

Watson, Ernest H., and George H. Lowrey: *Growth and Development of Children,* Chicago: Year Book, 1967.

Weinter, Irving B., and David Elkind: *Child Development: A Core Approach,* New York: Wiley, 1972.

Wetzel, Norma: "Assessing the Physical Condition of Children," *Journal of Pediatrics,* vol. 22, January-June 1943, pp. 329-340.

Whipple, Dorothy V.: *Dynamics of Development: Euthenic Pediatrics,* New York: McGraw-Hill, 1966.

Psychological, Social, and Cultural Development

Asarinsky, Eugene, and Nathanial Kleitman: "Regularly Occurring Periods of Eye Motility, and Concomitant Phenomena, during Sleep," *Science,* vol. 118, Sept. 4, 1953, pp. 273-274.

Baldwin, Alfred L.: *Theories of Child Development,* New York: Wiley, 1968.

Conger, John J.: *Adolescence and Youth,* New York: Harper & Row, 1973.

Cratty, Bryant: *Perceptual and Motor Development in Infants and Children,* New York: Macmillan, 1970.

Erikson, Erik H.: *Childhood and Society,* New York: Norton, 1963.

Espanschade, Anna: "Motor Performance in Adolescence," *Monographs of the Society for Research in Child Development,* vol. 5, no. 1, 1940, pp. 1-125.

Fiorentino, Mary R.: *Normal and Abnormal Development: The Influence of Primitive Reflexes on Motor Development,* Springfield, Ill.: Charles C Thomas, 1972.

Fraiberg, Selma H.: *The Magic Years,* New York: Scribner, 1959.

Frankenberg, William, and Josiah B. Dodds: *Denver Developmental Screening Test,* Colo.: University of Colorado Medical Center, 1969.

Frankl, Viktor: *Man's Search for Meaning,* New York: Washington Square Press, 1965.

Gesell, Arnold and Frances L. Ilg: *The Child from Five to Ten,* New York: Harper & Row, 1946.

———, and Catherine S. Amatruda, *Developmental Diagnosis,* New York: Hoeber-Harper, 1969.

Hellmuth, Jerome: *Exceptional Infant,* vol. 1, *The Normal Infant,* New York: Brunner/Mazel, 1967.
Holme, Richard, et al.: *Developmental Psychology Today,* Del Mar, Calif.: CRM Books, 1971.
Hurlock, Elizabeth B.: *Adolescent Development,* New York: McGraw-Hill, 1967.
Illingworth, R. W.: *An Introduction to Developmental Assessment in the First Year,* London: Heinemann, 1962.
Jones, H. E.: *Motor Performance and Growth: A Developmental Study of Static Dynamometric Strength,* Berkeley: University of California Press, 1949.
Josselyn, Irene M.: *The Adolescent and His World,* New York: Family Service Association of America, 1972.
Lewis, Melvin: *Clinical Aspects of Child Development,* Philadelphia: Lea & Febiger, 1971.
Lindszey, Gardner, Calvin S. Hall, and Martin Manosevitz: *Theories of Personality,* New York: Wiley, 1973.
Maier, Henry W.: *Three Theories of Child Development,* New York: Harper & Row, 1965.
Maslow, Abraham H.: *Toward a Psychology of Being,* New York: Van Nostrand, 1968.
———: *Motivation and Personality,* New York: Harper & Row, 1970.
Mussen, Paul H., John Conger, and Jerome Kagan: *Child Development and Personality,* New York: Harper & Row, 1969.
Oettingen, Katherine B.: *Normal Adolescence,* New York: Scribner, 1968.
Prechtl, Heinz, and David Beintema: *The Neurological Examination of the Full Term Newborn Infant,* London: Spactics Society Medical Education and Information Unit in association with Heinemann, 1964.
Spitz, Rene: "Hospitalism," *Psychoanalytic Study of the Child,* vol. 1, New York: International Universities Press, 1945.
———, and K. M. Wolf: "Anaclitic Depression," *Psychoanalytic Study of the Child,* vol. 2, New York: International Universities Press, 1946.
Stone, L. Joseph, and Joseph Church: *Childhood and Adolescence,* New York: Random House, 1968.
Thompson, George G., Eric F. Gardner, and Francis J. DiVesta: *Educational Psychology,* New York: Appleton-Century-Crofts, 1959.
Watson, Ernest, and George Lowrey: *Growth and Development of Children,* Chicago: Year Book, 1967.
Weiner, Irving B., and David Elkind: *Child Development: A Core Approach,* New York: Wiley, 1972.

Cognitive, Perceptual, and Linguistic Development

Abravanel, E.: "Developmental Changes in the Intersensory Patterning of Space," *Proceedings of the 75th Annual Convention of the American Psychological Association,* vol. 2, 1967, pp. 161-162.
———: "The Development of Intersensory Patterning with Regard to Selected Spatial Dimensions," *Monographs of the Society for Research in Child Development,* vol. 33, ser. 48, no. 2, 1968.

Ames, L. B.: "The Development of the Sense of Time in the Young Child," *Journal of Genetic Psychology,* vol. 68, 1946, pp. 97-125.

———, and J. Learned: "The Development of Verbalized Space in the Young Child," *Journal of Genetic Psychology,* vol. 72, 1948, pp. 63-84.

Beery, Judith, W.: "Matching of Auditory and Visual Stimuli by Average and Retarded Readers," *Child Development,* vol. 38, 1967, pp. 827-833.

Bridger, W. H.: "Sensory Habituation and Discrimination in the Human Neonate," *American Journal of Psychiatry,* vol. 117, 1961, pp. 991-996.

Brown, R. W., and Lenneberg, E. H.: "A Study in Language and Cognition," *Journal of Abnormal and Social Psychology,* vol. 49, 1954, pp. 454-462.

Casler, L.: "The Effects of Extra Tactile Stimulation on a Group of Institutionalized Infants," *Genetic Psychological Monographs,* vol. 71, 1965, pp. 137-175.

Disher, D. R.: "The Reactions of Newborn Infants to Chemical Stimuli Administered Nasally," *Ohio State University Studies of Controlled Psychology,* vol. 59, 1965, pp. 312-316.

Elkind, D.: "Discrimination, Seriation and Numeration of Size Differences in Young Children," *Journal of Genetic Psychology,* vol.104, 1964, pp. 275-296.

Ervin, S. M., and G. Foster: "The Development of Meaning in Children's Descriptive Terms," *Journal of Abnormal and Social Psychology,* vol. 61, 1960, pp. 271-275.

Fantz, R. L.: "Visual Perception from Birth as Shown by Pattern Selectivity," *Annals of the New York Academy of Science,* vol. 118, 1965, pp. 793-814.

Gibson, E.: "Perceptual Development," in H. W. Stevenson (ed.), *Child Psychology,* 62nd Yearbook of National Social Studies in Education Chicago: University of Chicago Press, 1963, pp. 144-195.

Gollin, E. S.: "Developmental Studies of Visual Recognition of Incomplete objects," *Perceptual and Motor Skills,* vol. 11, 1960, pp. 289-298.

———: "Developmental Studies of Visual Recognition of Incomplete Objects," *Perceptual and Motor Skills,* vol. 13, 1961, pp. 307-314.

Guilford, J. P.: "Intelligence Has Three Facets," *Science,* vol. 160, 1968, pp. 615-620.

Haaf, R. A., and R. Q. Bell: "A Facial Dimension in Visual Discrimination by Human Infants," *Child Development,* vol. 38, 1967, pp. 893-899.

Held, R., and A. Hein: "Movement-produced Stimulation in the Development of Visually Guided Behavior," *Journal of Comparative and Physiological Psychology,* vol. 56, 1963, pp. 872-876.

Holt, L. E., Jr., E. A. Davies, E. G. Hasselmeyer, and A. O. Adams: "A Study of Premature Infants Fed Cold Formulas," *Journal of Pediatrics,* vol. 61, 1962, pp. 556-561.

Hudson, W.: "Pictorial Depth Perception in Sub-culture Groups in Africa," *Journal of Social Psychology,* vol. 52, 1960, pp. 183-208.

Jensen, E.: "Differential Reactions to Taste and Temperature Stimuli in Newborn Infants," *Genetic Psychology Monographs,* vol. 12, 1932, pp. 363-479.

Katz, Phyllis, and M. Deutsch: "Relation of Auditory-Visual Shifting to Reading Achievement," *Perceptual and Motor Skills,* vol. 17, 1963, pp. 327-332.

Levanthal, A. S., and L. P. Lipsitt: "Adaptation, Pitch Discrimination and Sound Localization in the Neonate," *Child Development,* vol. 35, 1964, pp. 759-767.

Lovell, L.: "Some Recent Studies in Cognitive and Language Development," *Merrill-Palmer Quarterly,* vol. 14, 1968, pp. 123–138.

Maier, N. R. F.: "Reasoning in Children," *Journal of Comparative Psychology,* vol. 21, 1936, pp. 357–366.

McCall, R. B., and J. Kagan: "Attention in the Infant: Effects of Complexity, Contour, Perimeter and Familiarity," *Child Development,* vol. 38, 1967, pp. 939–952.

Meade, Margaret: "An Investigation of the Thought of Primitive Children with Special Reference to Animism," *Journal of the Royal Anthropological Institute,* vol. 62, 1932, pp. 173–190.

Mussen, Paul H., John J. Conger, and Jerome Kagan: *Child Development and Personality,* New York: Harper and Row, 1974.

Nash, John: *Developmental Psychology: A Psychobiological Approach,* Englewood Cliffs, N.J.: Prentice-Hall, 1970.

Piaget, J., and B. Inhelder: *La genese do l'idee de hasard chez l'enfant,* Paris: Presses University de France, 1951.

Reese, Hayne W., and Lewis P. Lipsitt: *Experimental Child Psychology,* New York and London: Academic, 1970.

Roe, L.: *Developmental Psychology Today,* Del Mar, Calif.: CRM Books, 1971.

Salk, L.: "Mother's Heartbeat as an Imprinting Stimulus," *Transactions of the New York Academy of Science,* ser. 2, vol. 24, 1962, pp. 753–763.

Sherman, M., I. C. Sherman, and C. D. Flory: "Infant Behavior," *Comparative Psychology Monographs,* vol. 12, no. 4, 1936.

Smart, Mollie S., and Russel C. Smart: "Children," *Development and Relationships,* New York: Macmillan, 1972.

Uzgiris, I. C.: "Situational Generality of Conservation," *Child Development,* vol. 35, 1964, pp. 831–841.

Wallach, M. A., and N. Kogan: *Modes of Thinking in Young Children: A Study of the Creativity-Intelligence Distinction,* New York: Holt, 1965.

Yudin, L. W.: "Formal Thought in Adolescence as a Function of Intelligence," *Child Development,* vol. 37, 1966, pp. 697–708.

Zaporozhets, A. V.: "The Development of Perception in the Preschool Child," in P. H. Mussen (ed.), "European Research in Cognitive Development," *Monographs of the Society for Research in Child Development,* vol. 30, no. 100, 1965, pp. 82–101.

Chapter 6

Common Childhood Problems

INTRODUCTION

In growing up, every child passes through different stages of physical and emotional maturity which may cause difficulties within the family setting. Many of these are normal, and most mothers learn to cope with them as they arise. While this chapter is titled "Common Childhood Problems," the items discussed are not really problems in the sense of being abnormal. Most children will develop some of these behaviors. In some families the activity will come and go, hardly noticed; in others the mother may feel she must "do something" to correct or change the situation. The nurse must have some knowledge of these common behaviors in order to evaluate them and counsel the mother concerning them.

The best pediatricians and nurses will listen well and watch the child carefully, before reaching any decision or giving any advice. Some clinicians have a tendency to memorize a list of "recipes" or solutions and apply them to all situations. The truly sensitive practitioner fits each solution to each child. To the careful, highly sensitive observer, the child will give clear clues about the problem.

This chapter will discuss some of the more common situations that come up in working with mothers and children. The creative, sensitive nurse and mother should be able to manage many of these areas. There is a vast library of books written about many of these topics, and the nurse is advised to read widely in the area.

COMMON PROBLEMS

Infancy

During the 1st year of life, the infant goes through vast changes in physical growth and emotional and social maturity. Patterns of eating, sleeping, playing, moving, and making noises will change drastically during this year. Not all babies are the same, as Brazelton has so dramatically pointed out in *Infants and Mothers, Differences in Development.* The quiet baby will prefer a different schedule than the active baby, and mothers may find it difficult to adjust to these differences.

Appetite is a problem for many mothers. They may feel that their infants eat too much, too little, too frequently, or too fussily. Physiological changes and many emotional overtones affect how, when, what, and how much the child will eat. Many infants seem to have a sudden increase in stomach capacity around 5 to 7 weeks of age. This may cause little concern to the bottle-fed baby, but to the mother who is breast feeding and suddenly has a fussy infant whom she is unable to satisfy, this can be a distressing time. A mother can easily think her milk is drying up and decide it is time to stop breast feeding. On the other hand, if she can be encouraged to breast feed more frequently for 2 or 3 days and is helped to understand the basis for this change in behavior, her milk will usually increase to satisfy the infant and the breast feeding will return to its usual 3- to 5-hour intervals. Some children will demonstrate a sudden decrease in appetite around 11 to 13 months of age, and a mother may complain that her child eats nothing all day long and worry about the child's health. The child's growth curve is extremely important at this point, since the child who is really falling off the curve does need a careful work-up to discover why. But if the child is following the usual curve and the examiner takes a careful history, it is usually discovered that the child is eating one large meal every day or every other day and eating on the run at other times. This may be the time the mother needs to discuss finger foods, tiny portions on tiny plates (rather than on a regular-sized plate, which emphasizes the smallness of the portion), pleasant mealtimes, etc.

Biting can become a problem after the child begins to have teeth during the last half of the 1st year. This is particularly a problem for the breast-feeding mother. Most mothers will solve this problem themselves by their reaction to the sudden pain. Some pull the child off and say "no," and after several times the infant gets the idea of sucking without biting. If the infant likes to bite, this may be the time to introduce something else to bite on—teething ring, zwieback, metal spoon, hard rubber toys, etc.

Crying worries a good many mothers. Some mothers can tolerate several hours of crying and some mothers cannot tolerate a few minutes. Babies rarely cry for no reason. They are usually trying to tell the adult world something, although they may outgrow their reason for crying before the mother or nurse can discover it. The nurse must be sensitive in her inquiry into the mother and the child's needs. It is far too easy to label all crying colic and give some pat answer like rocking the baby. True, that will help some babies and mothers, but it will not help all. The examiner needs to look at when the crying starts, what seems to make it start, how the baby cries, how long the baby cries, where the baby is when he or she cries, whether anything seems to comfort the baby, what makes the baby stop, what the mother does when the baby cries, and when the baby stops. A careful inquiry usually gives some clues about where to start in correcting the situation. Some infants need less stimulation (i.e., quietness, darkness, no movement, etc.), others need some particular stimulation (i.e., rhythmical sound or movement, warmth), and some may need more stimulation. A few infants seem to be very distressed with themselves because of their lack of muscle control. They may become quiet each time they are moved, but cry a few minutes later because they cannot roll over, sit up, lie down, etc. For such infants a frequent change in position may help until they learn to perform some of these activities on their own. Other infants cannot tolerate much stimulation (too much noise, light, movement, bodily contact); their world needs more control. Infants also cry because they are hungry or wet, cold or warm, or ill. A good history and physical examination is essential in helping a mother and child communicate their needs.

Relatives sometimes become a problem in child care when the mother finds herself in conflict with a well-meaning but overbearing relative who does not want this child ruined by an unwise new mother. If the nurse finds this situation developing, she can usually discover what the mother wants to do and then give support and encouragement for this decision. Sometimes telling the mother to say, "The nurse said . . ." may give the mother a chance to try her own ways.

Spoiling is usually a topic sometime during the 1st year. No mother wants a spoiled baby, but it is difficult to define what is spoiled. Some feel that no baby can be spoiled and that lavish warmth, security, and love during the 1st months and years are a must for later emotional stability. Others feel that spoiling occurs when the mother is forced to meet some demands of the baby that she does not like meeting, for instance, picking the baby up every time the baby cries. Some feel that there is definite threat of spoiling and that specific rules and regulations should be followed to avoid it. There is no one right answer; the topic should be fully explored with the mother to help her develop a workable arrangement and philosophy.

Some babies spit during the 1st year. There is probably some reason for spitting, but it often goes away before anything can be done. Babies can spit because they are physically ill, allergic to the formula, reacting to specific feeding problems (too large a nipple hole, wrong position during feeding, too much air in the stomach, etc.), or reacting to a general emotional overtone within the home. The reason is often difficult to discover and may take a sensitive, patient examiner some thought, time, and careful listening. Usually if the cause is found and corrected, the spitting will disappear.

Teething also happens during the 1st year. An average baby will begin having teeth erupt around 6 or 7 months of age. Many mothers think that the beginning of excessive drooling around 3 months is the beginning of teething, but this is not true. Drooling has nothing to do with the actual teething, but the child will probably continue to drool while the teeth are coming in. Teething should be accompanied by little more than slight irritability and the desire to bite on hard objects. Infants who are teething and having diarrhea, vomiting, abdominal pain, fever, etc., are sick infants who are teething. An illness can easily be missed if the mother or examiner attributes the additional symptoms to the teething. Certainly an infant who is showing a desire to bite should be given some appropriate objects to bite: zwieback, teething rings, hard rubber toys, cool spoon, etc. Some mothers like to rub teething lotions on the gums, but these should be advocated cautiously since they are not to be swallowed and some contain high percentages of alcohol.

These are a few of the normal problems arising during the 1st year of life and most can be effectively handled by the sensitive examiner and the wise mother.

Toddlerhood

Physical growth is not as dramatic during the months between the first and second birthday as it was earlier. Toddlers tend to walk more smoothly and with more balance, learn to climb, work at controlling their small muscles so they can hold cups, stack several blocks, use spoons, and manipulate many small objects. They work diligently to perfect their motor skills—trying many times and failing many times. Often they are clumsy and awkward, but this does not usually bother them as they start over and try again. Socially they learn about independence and take great pride in doing as many things as possible for themselves. They like having a choice in matters and learn to say "no" with authority even though they may not always know what it means. Their world enlarges, and they explore everything, looking, touching, tasting, and manipulating. They babble a lot to themselves but do say a few words and understand a good many more. Their drive toward independence is not smooth and easy, and frequently they vacillate between being a "big boy (or girl)" and "mommy's baby"; this can be a difficult time for both the child and the mother.

Eating can present many frustrating situations. The bottle sometimes becomes a problem if the child is still attached to it. Many children seem to naturally lose interest in the bottle sometime after the 8th month, but some children do not, and this can be a cause of concern to the mother. The purpose of the bottle is to get nourishment into an infant who has no teeth and cannot chew. Once teeth appear and the swallowing mechanism matures, children can physically take solid food. However, the bottle is more than mere nourishment. It becomes a source of warmth, security, comfort. Thus the child who is adequately nourished in other ways may still hang onto the bottle; removing it removes more than a physical object. The best way to remove the bottle is to have children do it themselves. The mother and nurse must carefully look at the situation and find out when, how, and why the child is still using the bottle. The mother can then begin to substitute other ways of meeting those needs until the child finds as much comfort in these alternatives as in the bottle. Obviously this takes a sensitive nurse, an interested and motivated mother, and some time. One point to keep in mind is that infants who get teeth at 6 months and continue to take a night bottle of milk tend to have a higher frequency of severe dental caries in their deciduous teeth (Shalka, 1974). So if the infant will not give up the bottle, the mother should be encouraged to substitute water. Some infants who are allowed to take the bottle lying down have a tendency to show more ear infections. Their eustachian tubes are so short and the mouth, nose, and ear canals so small and close together that milk taken in the lying position runs up the eustachian tube and gives a fine media for bacterial growth. Therefore, it is wise to encourage mothers from the beginning to hold their babies during feeding. Every mother props the bottle once in a while, but the less often this happens, the better.

Eating patterns during toddlerhood show some other changes. Children learn to use utensils and like to join the family at mealtime. In their drive to perfect their fine motor skills, children learn to grasp spoons properly and get them into their mouths smoothly. They may like trying a fork, but a knife is usually out. If possible, they should have smaller utensils that fit their hands and mouths and give them the satisfaction of mastering their own eating. There should still be plenty of finger foods around, since when they get tired or are really hungry, they may revert to more familiar methods of getting the food into their mouths. If they have a sturdy, comfortable chair that places them at the level of the table and the family eats meals together, toddlers usually enjoy joining these gatherings. They can be fed at the same time, or they may be fed earlier and just allowed to eat nibbles and enjoy the company. By the end of the 2d year they will probably have outgrown their high chairs and want regular or junior chairs at the table. Frequently around this age children like having their own places at the table, having their own utensils, coming to the table with everyone, trying dabs of the food, and leaving after about 8 or 10 minutes. This should be acceptable as long as the child is not snacking on cookies elsewhere and the mother understands the child's short span of attention. Gradually the appetite increases, the attention span lengthens, and the child may eat more and stay longer at the table. But no matter what the pattern, mealtime should be pleasant for the child and the family.

Discipline and limit setting become a problem during this time. All children need limits set for their own safety, well-being, and socialization. The problem arises in knowing how much, when, and how to change as the child matures and can handle more alone. Entire books are written on the subject. Much is said about being consistent, being fair, loving the child and punishing the act, verbal versus physical punishment, etc. Fortunately there is no set of definite rules to be followed which will guarantee a perfect child. A great many methods can be tried and will work. The nurse needs to find out what the parents are comfortable with, how they were reared, and what they hope to produce in their child. If parents were spanked as children, they will probably spank their children; if parents yell at each other, they will probably yell at their children. It sounds good to tell parents to be consistent, but the world is not a consistent place; children learn this early when they are told yes, it is okay to play with the knobs on the kitchen sink doors but no, it is forbidden to play with the knobs on the electric range. Some children even learn to respond positively to the consistency of inconsistency. Thus the toddler does need some limits set, and these should be worked out with the mother, the family, and their setting. Since the toddler is showing such swings between dependence and independence, a sensitive mother can easily become frustrated in her inability to predict her child's responses. Frequently the discipline problem surfaces around a specific area: toilet training, eating, dressing, etc., and the discussion can center on certain ways of helping that specific situation. The nurse should be careful to help parents fit their life style and expectations with the child's particular stage of development and personality rather than handing out dictums.

Negativism is another term frequently used during toddler years. In striving for independence, children learn the word "no" and some of its power for controlling others. So they try to use it as frequently as possible—even in inappropriate situations. For example, asked if she wants a cookie, a little girl may hold out her hand and shake her head while saying "no." Asked if he has to go to the bathroom, a little boy may say "no" and stand there and wet his pants. These situations can be frustrating for the mother and the child. Developmentally, children are learning to control themsleves and others. There is a feeling of power in having a choice and being able to make it. In learning any new activity, one is clumsy, awkward, and frequently wrong, but practice helps. Thus children practice this technique all day long, every day for a period of time—from several weeks to all year.

With time they make better choices, have more success, and feel more powerful; they no longer have to practice as hard or strive as hard to show others their power; the "negative" stage passes. Sometimes giving the child as many choices as possible will help. If the child can have a choice of wearing a blue or a red cap, let the child make the choice. If the child can choose between playing inside or going outside, let the child choose. Do not offer a choice if there is no choice. If the mother has already made up her mind that the child is to go to bed, then the child must be told, not asked. Furthermore, the mother should be prepared that sometimes children will make their choices and then change their mind, and she needs to think about her reaction and what she will do. Most mothers are happy when this stage is passed.

Play is an important part of every toddler's life, and they really do not differentiate play from work. Mothers are frequently concerned about what children should play with or at, and this leads to discussions of toys, play activities, books, records, etc. Within each of those areas there are wide variations of easy, simple, inexpensive activities and items and more formalized, researched, and expensive activities and items. Toddlers are active, exploring individuals whose interests change rapidly as they discover their world and themselves. They can increase their small motor movements by playing in water—tub, sink, dish pan, hose—as long as they are continually and carefully supervised. They like the feel of clay, mud, cookie dough, and finger paints. They can enjoy soft, cuddly toys such as dolls, teddy bears, and stuffed animals. And frequently they have special blankets or toys that accompany them everywhere. As mother works around the house they may want to help or imitate—dusting, wiping, drying dishes, picking up, or sweeping. They may even do some of those things on command, but this behavior is still quite inconsistent. Big muscles can be exercised with push-pull toys like a wagon, duck on a string, or tricycle which they may not ride but just pull around. Balls of varying sizes can also be fun and teach a cooperative type of game. They may like books and magazines, but these have to be of sturdy material since toddlers may have a tendency to shred them. Some children like to be read to, but their span of attention is short (several minutes), and mothers should keep that in mind when picking stories to read. Children's records can also be fun as the child learns to sing or dance with the tunes. Some children will also watch television and some of the children's programs, but frequently they enjoy the commercials better than the program. The nurse would do well to visit local stores (department, discount, record, grocery, baby), library, and day-care centers to see what is available before discussing play with the mothers.

Frequently parents wait until the child is 13 to 24 months before having the next child; the first child then has to be helped to understand that it's possible to share the parents' love without losing it. Jealousy and rivalry are common feelings throughout life; with a new arrival, jealousy is almost always present, but some children show it more openly than others. If the nurse can talk with the mother during her pregnancy and do some planning at that time, the rivalry can be handled much more smoothly and the mother will not be so shocked by her child's abrupt behavior. There is a good deal written on this subject, and the reader is referred to the bibliography at the end of this chapter for more detail. But generally, a 2-year-old needs a good deal of attention to be helped through a difficult time. If any large changes are to be made in furniture, or if there is to be a new bed, new room, or new babysitter, these changes should be made before the infant arrives so that the toddler has a chance to adjust to the changes without blaming them all on the newborn. Some toddlers like to help in the preparations (getting the clothing ready, the new bed made up, etc.), but others show no interest and should not be forced into interest. They should not be asked whether they are wishing for a sister or brother, since they really have no choice in the matter. And they should not be told they are getting a playmate, since they really will not be able to play games with the baby. It is difficult for toddlers to be left by their mothers for several days (which is a *long* time in the life of a toddler), and many children are quite angry with their mothers when they return from the hospital. Sometimes small surprises left at home to be distributed during the absence, or telephone calls, or visits (some hospitals now allow this) will help during this period. Mothers should be prepared for possible anger or rejection on their return and for sudden demands for attention, usually at times when they cannot give it. As they sit to feed the new infants, toddlers demand milk, wet their pants, climb on forbidden furniture, etc. Toddlers may also regress to more infantile behavior and ask for the bottle or breast, wet their pants, or cry more; depending on the situation and the mother, this can usually be handled by ignoring these behaviors while reinforcing the more "grown-up" behaviors. The combination of the newborn's presence, the mother's tiredness, and a demanding and regressive toddler can lead to an explosive few weeks, and the sensitive nurse will make herself readily available as an outlet for the mother. Usually just knowing someone is as close as the telephone and willing to listen and help her work out some small solutions will make the difficult weeks pass more quickly. Some families seem to sail through this period with the toddler showing only occasional firm "love pats" or remarking that infants should be put down garbage disposals; other families have a difficult time, and the nurse should be ready to help.

Sleeping is a problem for some toddlers. They are so active and into everything that they cannot "turn off" and go to bed. Some children need 12 hours of sleep and others need 5, but when a toddler is sleepy and does not know it, there can be friction at bedtime. Again, there are no pat answers, but the nurse and mother must assess the situation, the infant, and the mother's feelings and comfort in order to work out a reasonable solution.

Temper tantrums can make their ugly appearance during this time. They usually consist of mounting frustration, crying, kicking, screaming, turning red and blue in the face, and a lot of commotion. Some children will go as far as holding their breath and passing out. Temper tantrums stem from the child's striving for power and control and sudden loss of both. There is no one good way to deal with the problem, and it may depend on the mother's comfort in the situation. The goal is to restore children to some control and calm, but not necessarily by giving them what they wanted in the first place. Some feel it is best to go to children, hold them, comfort them, and offer some substitute (if not another cookie, perhaps a toy, etc.). Others feel that children should be removed from the stimulation of the situation and placed alone in their rooms or in corners until they can gain their own control. Others feel the child who has a tantrum needs a good spanking. In any case it is hoped that the background of the situation is taken into account so that the mother can deal with the tantrum and show the child better ways to handle frustration.

Thumb sucking or pacifiers can become a problem at birth or in toddlerhood. Some parents do not want their children to suck their thumbs or use pacifiers ever; others think it is fine for a while, but not after a certain age. Before suggesting anything, the nurse must find out the parents' attitude on the subject. One theory has it that all infants need a certain amount of sucking; some are satisfied with the bottle or breast and others need additional sucking. This theory states that if the infant is allowed to suck enough during the early years, the need will pass by the time the child outgrows infancy. Another theory is that we live in an oral society and that people simply change their modes of oral stimulation as they grow, using a thumb or pacifier in infancy. During infancy, a problem arises only if the parents do not want the child sucking a thumb and substitutes have to be found—smaller nipple holes so the child has to suck longer and harder at the bottle, additional breast feeding, etc. Usually by toddlerhood the child sucks the pacifier or thumb only at times of stress or when tired, and if left alone, this habit will slowly recede and usually disappear by 3 or 4 years of age. However, if this upsets the mother, special attempts can be made to "lose" the pacifier, substitute a special blanket or activities at bed time, give the child something else to do with the hand when the thumb goes into the mouth, etc. Attempts to punish the child, applying foul-tasting substances to the thumb, bandaging the thumb, or restraining the arm should be avoided. If the thumb sucking persists to 4, 5, 6, and 7 years, it is best not to work at stopping the thumb sucking, but to find out why the child is having such stress and needs that kind of comfort. If the cause can be found and corrected, the thumb sucking will probably disappear. If only the thumb sucking is looked at, it can probably be stopped with various techniques, but the stress and discomfort will cause other symptoms like nail biting, bed wetting, nightmares, etc. Many dentists feel that persistent, late thumb sucking causes tooth malalignment and must be stopped at all cost. Thus they have devised harsh metal appliances that will injure the thumb when it is inserted into the mouth. This is financially costly and ignores the cause of the problem.

Toilet training is the big activity during this stage for many mothers. Often being a "good" versus a "bad" mother is determined by how early the mother can train her child. Toilet training can be the easiest or most difficult thing to accomplish. Fortunately, few mothers demand that their infants use the toilet by 8 months, but many mothers start working at it by 12 months, and very few are able to wait patiently until 2½ to 3, when the child is ready. If the principles of growth and development are applied, the child is generally ready sometime between 32 and 44 months. Physically, children must have the muscles to sit well and stand well before they can have any control over anal sphincters. Usually bowel control comes first, then bladder control. Children must be able to understand the urge to go, hold it, tell their mothers verbally of their desires, get themselves to the bathroom, have their clothing removed, and then release. Neurologically, this is a very complicated set of maneuvers that most children cannot master until after 2½ years. Psychologically, another complicated process must be accomplished. Children need to know that they have some control and power over their bodies. They will say when they will eat, when they will move their bowels, when they will go to sleep. And while mothers may sit them at the table, there is no way mothers can make them eat; mothers may sit them on the potty, but there is no way mothers can make children move their bowels at that moment. Along with the negativism, learning how to control, and being somewhat independent, the child must have developed a sense of trust and love with someone (usually the mother). The child has learned what pleases her and what displeases her. The child likes to please her but does not always. Once the child has matured psychologically and physically to this stage, toilet training happens almost overnight. However, many mothers cannot wait for the child's readiness. In that case, the wise nurse needs to help make the situation as comfortable as possible for both mother and child during the interim. Since children frequently have little control over this area, accidents are going to be frequent. Harsh methods, such as tying children into potty chairs, forcing them to sit there until they go, and spanking for accidents, should be avoided. Child-rearing books are filled with a variety of helpful hints that may make the situation more pleasant and make the mother feel she is doing something. The use of potty chair or toilet seat, silk panties for girls or training pants, watching others in the bathroom, regular times for pottying, toys versus no toys with the potty chair, etc., all are techniques that may help in one situation or another.

Preschool Years

During the years between 2 and 5 when children are past infancy but not yet going to school, they make refinements in their gross and fine motor movements. They learn to do the tandem walk; run fast; do a crude skip; draw crude circles, crosses, and simple geometric forms; and hold a knife and fork properly. Much of their development is social and psychological. They become much more independent and able to take care of many of their own personal needs, such as dressing themselves, feeding themselves, blowing their own noses, and going to the bathroom by themselves. They move away from their previous self-centeredness and learn about obligations, responsibilities, sharing, and right and wrong; they can now be happily separated from their mothers for short periods of time. This is often a stage where there is less conflict and worry over problems, and the family life surrounding the preschool child is relatively calm.

Some preschoolers have periods of specific food likes and dislikes, and this can sometimes be unnerving for the mother. It may involve the dislike of one food and the refusal to eat that substance. That is easy enough to work around, and with time, if the rest of the family eats the food, the child may return to liking it. Sometimes children take on a food fad and will eat only one food. They ask for peanut butter and jelly sandwiches three times a day. Mothers may find that harder to live with since they expect children to eat a variety of foods. However, if children can be allowed their requests as frequently as possible, maybe for every lunch, or for Saturday breakfasts, the craving usually wears itself out after a while. Children do not starve during this time, but their intake may be peculiar for some days.

Masturbation may be a disturbing activity for the mother. Children have to learn about their bodies in the same way they learn about other things—looking, touching, feeling. Usually around 8 months of age infants will discover their genitals during diapering or bathing, and the fondling gives pleasurable stimulation and may be continued with each diapering; this interest usually subsides as other areas become more important. Then again, some time before children enter school they go through several stages of discovering themselves—who they are, where they live, who their mothers are, what a boy is, what a girl is, what the name of each part of the body is. Most children discover that touching the genital area will bring pleasure, but they soon learn that that kind of manipulation is only done in private or not at all and move on to other forms of stimulation or comfort. The child who is under a lot of pressure or stress, finds little comfort in life, and is having some difficulties in daily life may find masturbation a source of comfort and never move on to other forms of satisfaction. In that case, the nurse must try to find the reasons for the discomfort and attempt to lessen the stress rather than stop the masturbation.

Santa Claus, the Easter Bunny, and other myths sometimes appear as a problem toward the end of the 4th or 5th year. Many families enjoy this form of make-believe and giving, sharing, and loving, but the sensitive mother may suddenly wonder how to tell her 4-year-old that there is no such thing as Santa Claus. The older child may also have the Tooth Fairy to contend with. Children usually let their mothers know they are ready for some more explanation when they begin questioning all the discrepancies in the different stories; some children never ask for an explanation because they are afraid that will end all of Christmas or Easter. It is also cruel to let a child go to school and then be laughed at as the dummy in class because everyone else knows there is no Santa Claus. The nurse does not have to give the mother a one-sentence answer about how to tell the child, but may have to lead the discussion as the mother formulates her own ideas on the topics so that she can convey to the child that Santa Claus is not a man, but rather the spirit of giving. Many children during this time are learning the art of giving—making a birthday present for Daddy or going with Mommy to buy a Christmas present for grandmother—and this can become the exciting thing rather than the idea of one red-suited man. Many families have some form of religious belief. It is important in such a family that the child not equate Santa Claus with God and begin to wonder if God is also a myth. That could be a little disconcerting to a highly religious family. With most of these problems, it is not the exact words that are said, but the attitude that goes with them, and the child very quickly picks that up.

Separation is a process that goes on from the moment children are born until they move away and start their own families. It includes such situations as death, divorce, and hospitalization. Some children take each stage of separation as it comes and move easily into the next; other children fight each new stage; and some mothers never learn to let their children go. The separation process is very much involved with the child's self-image and self-concept, and some theorists are very Freudian in their interpretations. But basically children must learn that they are total, independent persons who are capable of caring for themselves. As children learn about themselves, they are able to separate themselves from others for longer and longer periods of time. Signs of this development are frequently seen around the 7th or 8th month when children display stranger anxiety and suddenly cry if anyone but their mothers hold them. Some children show very strong stranger anxiety, others very little. But they now know they are different from their mothers and their mothers are different from everyone else. Later, around 12 to 24 months, children will go through separation anxiety and will be unable to tolerate more than a little distance between themselves and their mothers. First the distance may be only across the room; then they may be able to let their mothers be out of the room for a minute or two as long as they can hear them; gradually their tolerance for separation increases. Toddlers may frequently play quietly in rooms away from their mothers as long as they can trot in to see or touch their mothers at regular intervals. By the time children are of preschool age they may be able to handle and tolerate from 1 to several hours with the babysitter or in a day-care center. This does not mean that children are never left until preschool age, because mothers do work outside the home and parents do go out for an evening or away for a week-end. However, if the nurse is aware of the different stages of development of the child, she is better able to help the mother cope with the different reactions she may get with separation. In other words, an evening out when the child is 6 weeks old will probably cause very little upset in the child, but 3 days away from the 2-year-old will cause a lot of trauma if it has not been prepared for. For the working mother, separation may come early in the child's life and really be more difficult for the mother than the child. For the mother who is staying home, the question usually arises later in the child's life, when mother is having some time out and the babysitter is left with the child or when the mother is beginning to think about sending the child to preschool or a day-care center for periods of time. Again, there are no set answers, and the nurse and mother must look carefully at the child's stage of development and past experiences, and what is available and possible at the time. A child may be able to tolerate 1 hour at the babysitter or day-care center or 8 hours. A close look will usually tell what the child can tolerate and some ways to help the child tolerate what must be tolerated.

Sharing is a difficult concept to teach a child and probably is best done by example rather than verbal lessons. A family that shares in work, pleasures, and material things probably has little difficulty in getting the youngest child to follow along. Before 4 or 5 years of age, children really have little idea of what sharing means. They may share their cookies before then, but that really means just giving away half the cookies. Children usually do not share in playing until 4 or 5 years. Up until that time they may play in the same room with another child or do the same activity as another child, but playing together, sharing the toys or the equipment, does not come until late in the preschool years.

School Years

During the school years the child's world expands dramatically to include school, school friends, outside activities, and experiences outside the immediate family. Physically, children may have short growth spurts but these do not last the entire time between 5 and 10. Meanwhile they are developing speed, smoothness, and coordination in fine and gross motor activities. Language increases dramatically as the child learns new words, new ways of putting words together, and much better ways of expressing thoughts and feelings. Instead of depending totally on parents the child learns to have relationships with teachers, other adults, and peers. The child begins to see the relationship between right and wrong and to comprehend the cause and effect in disobedience and punishment. Children begin to see others as others see them and to know that they have specific labels according to behavior, cultural background, religious affiliations, and economic and racial situations. They learn more deeply what it is to be masculine or feminine and generally restrict their interactions to their own sexual group—the boys playing with the boys, and the girls playing with the girls. This can be a nice time for both parents and child.

Activities can become a big part of a child's life during this period. In our society it is sometimes possible for school-age children to become enrolled in such a large variety of activities after school that they really never have time to do nothing. While it may be true that children who have too much free time on their hands get into trouble more quickly, it is also true that children who never leave the pressures of striving, trying, and learning are more prone to physical exhaustion and many physical complaints. Children need some opportunity to structure their own time. This is usually not a complaint that is verbalized by mothers or children, but children who show up at the clinic repeatedly with minor complaints and conditions need to have a good history taken and a good listener to help slow their lives down to a reasonable pace.

Cheating can become a problem during these years. Certainly all children are exposed to cheating, and most try it at some time. Attaining adult standards of morality takes time and progresses through universal developmental stages. School-age children become increasingly aware of how their parents may cheat in different ways. By this age children have learned to respect their parents' authority and generally follow their set of rules, but temptations from peers or high pressure from parents may tempt children to break the rules for the desired goal. If children cheat and are never caught, they may continue in their cheating or may set themselves up for other forms of punishment, thus clearing their consciences while continuing to cheat. In other words, they may cheat on their schoolwork and then come home and irritate their mothers with their behavior until finally they are punished. They then feel better, calm their behavior at home, and continue to cheat at school. Some children have developed such strong consciences and receive such great emotional rewards for being "good" that having once tried cheating they feel so guilty they never try it again. Cheating that continues and begins to cause problems in school needs further investigation and a close look at the child's life and needs.

Scatology or the use of dirty words often becomes a problem during the school years. The 2- or 3-year-old learns language by imitating sounds and sometimes hears a dirty word and tries it for sound. This age child has no idea what the word means and will repeat it only if it sounds good or gets a good reaction from the mother. By school age the child can hear dirty words or phrases from a variety of places and may try using them around the house. The child may still have no idea what a word means, but quickly learns how to get a reaction from parents. Normal children usually need only a reminder that those words are not to be used at home and if they must use them, do so with their own friends or in the privacy of their own rooms. However, if the parents use the words all the time, the child will probably follow their example.

Fear is not a feeling peculiar to childhood. Everyone has some fears, and fear of some activities is healthy and life saving. Fears in childhood change as children become more able to handle some of their own activities but must face new challenges. Fears are generally learned from adults, from some experience, or from some inner feeling of diffuse anxiety. Many children have the same fears as their parents, and there is little that can be done without correcting the fear in the parents. A traumatic experience may also cause a child to become fearful in the situation again. For instance, a large, noisy dog may scare a child once and make him fearful of all dogs. Some fears come from learning right from wrong and knowing and fearing the punishment that follows. Some fears protect the child and are necessary; other fears are minor and do not really bother the child or the parents; other fears cause problems in the daily life and need to be resolved. Each fear has to be dealt with separately; the nurse must look closely at what might have caused the fear and what it is doing to the child; she then must help the parent and child to formulate a plan for handling future fear-producing situations.

Fighting usually occurs during childhood. Most siblings fight among themselves. Generally girls do not fight outside the home, but most boys will engage in at least one fight during their school years. Within the family if the parents enjoy and participate in verbal or physical fighting, the children learn this as a way of life. Living in any group of human beings means that everyone is going to have bad days and that hot words will be exchanged sometimes. When siblings tangle, many parents let them work out their own differences or separate everyone for a period of time until the atmosphere cools down and each person regains composure. An occasional fight at school is usually no problem, but children who are continually picking fights or being involved in fights need a closer evaluation to discover why they choose physical assault as a method of resolving their problems. If their other problems can be solved, the fighting should diminish.

Lying is difficult to correct because it is tied in with the large moral issue of truthfulness. Every mother wants her child to tell the truth, but in the real world absolute truthfulness is rarely found or approved of. It is difficult to explain to children of 4 years that they must answer mother truthfully about removing the nickel from her purse, but must not truthfully tell grandmother that they disliked the birthday gift she sent. Children cannot easily grasp why it is okay to make up a story about the big fish they and daddy caught on an outing, but not okay to make up a story about cleaning their room when they did not do it. At this age the real world and the make-believe world frequently get confused, and children should not be punished for this confusion but gently reminded of the facts and helped to realize that everyone knows they are making up the story. Sometimes it is easy to place the child in a position of having to lie. If the parent knows the child did some wrong act and asks the child about it, the child may decide to lie to avoid punishment. Then the parent has the original act plus the lying to contend with. Some psychologists feel that parents can easily explain to the child that they approve of the child and of the child's truthfulness, but that they will have to punish the child for the original wrong act. However, that is difficult to do and can easily get confused in the child's and parent's minds as they perform this I-love-you-but-I-am-going-to-hurt-you routine. Generally by school age children have learned something about the broad concept of telling the truth, and their respect and love of their parents will usually keep lying at a minimum. For children who continually lie, the nurse and mother must find out whether they know right from wrong, what they are gaining by lying, and what it is going to cost them to tell the truth before these children can be helped over their way of dealing with life by lying.

Stealing at a preschool age may mean the child has no concept of ownership. By the time children are in school they know which things do not belong to them, and stealing at this age must be carefully evaluated. Most children will try some form of stealing at some time. For some it may mean a nickel from mother's purse or some candy from the local store or something from another child. For most children, a sense of right and wrong is so strong by school age that their guilt forces them to reveal themselves one way or another. In this situation the parent needs only to show disapproval and help the child return the object, and it probably will not happen again. For the child who continually steals, the reason has to be found. Does the child really need the objects stolen? Is the child trying to show the world that he or she is clever? Is the child attempting to gain attention? Is the child attempting to gain approval or love by buying friends with stolen materials? The act of stealing shows that the child has some unmet needs; if these underlying problems can be found and corrected, the stealing should disappear. Attempting to stop the stealing by harsh physical punishment or scare techniques will not usually work if the child still has a need for stealing. Some teenagers try stealing for the same reasons or for the thrill and excitement of doing something they know is wrong. Stealing can be more dangerous at this stage, since if they are caught, they will be prosecuted much as an adult and end up with a police record for their thrill.

These are a few of the common problems mothers may mention during the child's school years. Usually they occur only for brief periods of time, and most parents have some effective method of dealing with them. Occasionally one area becomes a more serious problem; a close, objective look at the situation will usually show the reasons for the problem and will help the mother think of ways of dealing with the child to correct the problem.

Adolescence

During adolescence there is a lot of activity physically, emotionally, psychologically, and culturally. Physically the child changes rapidly in size, shape, and outward appearance. Emotionally and psychologically the teen years are filled with turmoil and change as the teenager swings between love and hate for parents, close friends, current girl friend or boy friend, and finally marriage partner. There is a lot of questioning and trying of different values, beliefs, behavior, feelings, and activities. The changes and swings can come so swiftly and so drastically that both the teenager and the parents frequently feel frustrated. Teenagers must also move from dependency on their parents to independency and a self-sufficiency. The child's morality is sharpened and redefined. By the 20th year individuals should have come to some definite ideas about their own selves, feelings, and goals and how they will fit into the world at large. Some will meet these objectives by 20, others by 30, and some people will never achieve them.

By the time children reach the teen years, they should be relating directly to the examiner. The nurse should be able to converse with both the child and the parent. The sensitive, objective nurse can easily find herself listening and guiding the teenager through some problem areas.

Dating and social life can be a large part of the worries of junior and senior high school students. They want to know how to get dates, how to avoid certain dates, what to do on dates, what not to do on dates, etc. The child who does not date may worry about it or have a mother who worries and pushes the activity. Very popular children may worry that they cannot continue or that their popularity will fade. The child who wants to date but cannot because of parental limits also has problems. There are no definite answers, but children and parents should be helped to communicate with each other to work out mutually agreeable solutions.

Drinking sometimes becomes a problem during the high school years. If teenagers want to drink, they usually have little trouble finding someone who will help them get the liquor. Peer pressure is tremendous during these years, and no child likes to be taunted or ridiculed for not following the crowd. Some teenagers admit that they would not ordinarily drink but if everyone else is doing it, so will they. Parents and teenagers who worry over the flow of alcohol need to find ways for adolescents to handle themselves, feel confident about their behavior, and still be part of their peer group. In homes where alcohol has always been present and enjoyed without being overindulged in and the parents and child have a good relationship, the drinking situation can probably be weathered by both the parents and child. In other homes, a more serious situation may be created.

Driving the car can also become a problem during these years. Legally a child can begin driving a car at 16 years of age in most states. A car can add much to a teenager's feelings of independence, mobility, and prestige with peers; for the parents it may mean only a feeling of loss, fear for the child's life, and increased insurance payments. Driving is essentially a skill, and many high schools offer courses in how to handle the rather expensive, potentially dangerous vehicle. Thoughts on responsibility, sharing, finances, limits, etc., must be discussed by the parents and the child before misunderstandings arise. There is no one way for parents and child to handle the driving situation; again, the nurse may be able to help by encouraging open communication between them.

Homework sometimes becomes a hassle during these years. Young people can be under tremendous pressures to make good grades so they can get into college. If the parents have had certain ideas about the child's entering a specific career, this may also be a point of dissension. Arguments over homework assignments often indicate other deeper problems and may be only a way to irritate the other party. Discussions on goals, objectives, methods of meeting goals, consequences, ability, etc. may have to be held with the child and the parent rather than just working out a system of dealing with the homework problem.

Sex and all its ramifications can play a major role during these years. With increased exposure to the opposite sex, dating, going steady, constantly being "in love" with someone, and peer pressure, the parents frequently worry about how much their children know, what they do not know, and what they are going to try out. By this stage both boys and girls have some knowledge of sex but the accuracy of this knowledge varies widely. Sex education and prevention of pregnancy are widely debated topics in most communities. Parents frequently feel uncomfortable or inadequate discussing the subject; often it is the school nurse who does much of the counseling. Again there is no set, correct answer. Some children will need basic knowledge of their own anatomy; some need to know the availability of contraception; some need to explore their own attitudes. The wise examiner can comfortably assess the individual situation and help work out solutions before situations deteriorate into unwanted pregnancies, unplanned marriages, and two unhappy teenagers.

Smoking is sometimes a problem for parents. Although this is a society where smoking is fairly common among adults, widely advertised, and commonly discussed, some parents are opposed to their child smoking. Any child can obtain a package of cigarettes, and some children become addicted to the habit by sixth or seventh grade. Today, cigarette smoking may not be as worrisome during the high school years as smoking marijuana, which is illegal. Smoking marijuana may be done for the thrill of doing something wrong or because of peer pressure. Cigarette smoking may begin the same way, but quickly becomes a habit which is difficult to break. Discussions may help, but only a highly motivated person can break the smoking habit, and if the child is uninterested in giving up smoking, little can be done.

There are many more problems, minor and serious, that can erupt during the teen years, and the regular high school nurse is very familiar with them. Most of the problems are irritating to the child and the parents at the time; the sensitive nurse can often initiate the communication between child and adult which will help them work out mutually agreeable solutions.

DANGER SIGNS

This chapter has discussed some of the common problems that appear at different ages and some of the ways of helping parents and children handle these problems. There are many more such problems, and the bibliography lists many good books and articles. However, there are times when a minor problem develops into a major problem, and the nurse should know when to refer the child on for additional help and treatment.

Persistence of a minor problem can indicate more serious troubles. If a child steals once, the nurse can certainly handle that problem with the mother. The child who repeatedly steals and is getting into trouble with the police is not going through a stage of development, but displaying a symptom of much more serious, deeply entangled problems. Management may include everything from consultations to referrals to removal from the home, depending on the situation. Thus any child with minor problems that persist or any child with multiple recurring problems needs careful handling.

Some symptoms should be seen as warning signs as soon as they appear. For example, the child who sets fires, refuses to go to school for weeks, attempts suicide, refuses to eat, or does bodily damage to self or others needs immediate professional help. The nurse may be instrumental in initiating such proceedings and involved in helping to manage such a child, but a team approach is needed with such serious problems.

Part of the excitement, stimulation, and challenge of becoming an excellent clinician is dealing with the common problems that arise as children mature. Truly comprehensive preventive health care involves much more than memorizing a list of recipes to fit a specific complaint; it involves the ability to apply the principles of growth and development by listening carefully and helping each mother and child work out suitable solutions.

BIBLIOGRAPHY

Common Problems

Arnstein, Helene S.: *What to Tell Your Child . . . about Birth, Illness, Death, Divorce and Other Family Crises.*

Aver, William A., and Elliot N. Gale, "Thumb-Sucking Revisited," *American Journal of Orthodontics,* vol. 55, February 1967, pp. 167–170.

———, and ———: "Psychology and Thumbsucking," *Journal of the American Dental Association,* vol. 80, June 1970, pp. 1335–1337.

Beiser, Helen: "Children's Dreams," *Today's Health,* September 1973, pp. 34–40.

Berman, Marvin H.: "Thumbsucking Treatment," *Journal of the American Dental Association,* vol. 81, August 1970, pp. 273.

Better Homes and Gardens: *Baby Book,* New York: Bantam, 1970.

Brazelton, T. Berry: *Infants and Mothers, Differences in Development,* New York: Delacorte Press, 1970.

Crewe, Hilary J.: "Fears and Anxiety in Childhood," *Public Health,* vol. 63, October 1973, pp. 87, 165-171.
Dodson, Fitzhugh: *How to Parent,* New York: Signet Books, 1970.
Epstein, Bruce A.: "The Differential Diagnosis of Breathholding Spells in Children," *Clinical Pediatrics,* vol. 12, no. 12 December 1973, pp. 684-687.
Erickson, Florence: "Viewpoints on Children in Hospitals," *Hospitals, Journal of American Hospital Association,* vol. 37, May 16, 1963, pp. 47-48.
Fraiberg, Selma: *The Magic Years,* New York: Scribner, 1959.
Frankle, Reva T., and F. K. Heussanstamm: "Food Zealotry and Youth," *American Journal of Public Health,* vol. 64, no. 1, January 1974, pp. 11-17.
Fromme, Allen: *The Parents' Handbook: The ABC of Child Care,* New York: Simon & Schuster, 1956.
Gardner, Richard A.: *The Boys and Girls Book about Divorce,* New York: Bantam, 1971, pp. 157.
Gersh, Marvin: *How to Raise Children at Home in Your Spare Time,* Greenwich, Conn.: Fawcett, 1966.
Ginott, Haim G.: *Between Parent and Child,* New York: Macmillan, 1965.
———: *Between Parent and Teenager,* New York: Avon, 1969.
Gregg, Elizabeth M.: *What to Do When "There's Nothing to Do,"* New York: Delacorte Press, 1968.
Hicks, Clifford B.: "'Eat' Says Fat Little Johnny's Mother," *Today's Health,* February 1970, pp. 48-52, 86.
Holt, John: *How Children Fail,* New York: Pitman, 1968.
Homan, William: *Child Sense,* New York: Basic Books, 1969.
Johnson, June: *838 Ways to Amuse a Child,* New York: Gramercy, 1960.
Klein, Ernest T.: "The Thumb-Sucking Habit: Meaningful or Empty?" *American Journal of Orthodontics,* vol. 59, no. 3, March 1971, pp. 283-284.
Klein, Ted: *The Father's Book,* New York: Ace, 1968.
Kliman, Gilbert: *Psychological Emergencies of Childhood,* New York: Grune & Stratton, 1968.
Laird, Constance: "Meeting Parents' Concerns," *Children Today,* May-June, 1973, pp. 2-6.
LaLeche League: *The Womanly Art of Breastfeeding,* Franklin Park, Ill.: LaLeche League, 1958.
LeShan, Eda: "When a Child Bites," *Woman's Day,* October 1971, pp. 48, 118.
———: "The Trouble with Santa Claus," *Woman's Day,* December 1973, pp. 82 and 124.
Lewis, Samuel J.: "Effect of Thumb and Finger Sucking on the Primary Teeth and Dental Arches," *Child Development,* vol. 8, 1937, p. 93.
Long, Barbara: "Sleep," *American Journal of Nursing,* vol. 69, no. 9, September 1969, pp. 1896-1899.
Maternity Center Association: *A Baby Is Born,* New York: Grosset & Dunlap, 1964.
Montessori, Maria: *Dr. Montessori's Own Handbook,* New York: Schocken Books, 1971.
Moss, Sidney, and Miriam Moss: "Separation as a Death Experience," *Child Psychiatry and Human Development,* vol. 3, no. 3 Spring 1973, pp. 187-194.
Oppel, Wallace C., Paul A. Harper, and Rowland V. Rider: "The Age of Attaining Bladder Control," *Pediatrics,* vol. 42, no. 4, October 1968, pp. 614-626.

Patterson, Gerald R., and M. Elizabeth Gullion: *Living with Children,* Champaign, Ill.: Research Press, 1968.

Ribble, Margaret A.: *The Rights of Infants,* New York: Signet Books, 1973.

Rosenthal, M., E. Ni, M. Finkelstein, and G. Berkwitz: "Father-Child Relationships and Children's Problems," *AMA Archives of General Psychiatry,* vol. 7, June 1962, pp. 360-373.

Schulman, Jerome L.: *Management of Emotional Disorders in Pediatric Practice,* Chicago: Year Book, 1967.

Senn, Milton J., and Albert J. Solnit: *Problems in Child Behavior and Development,* Philadelphia: Lea & Febiger, 1968.

Skalka, Patricia: "Solving the Mystery of the Decaying Teeth," *Today's Health,* January 1974, pp. 27-28, 70.

Sparling, Joseph, and Marilyn Sparling: "How to Talk to a Scribbler," *Young Children,* August 1973, pp. 36-42.

Spock, Benjamin: *Feeding Your Baby and Child,* New York: Pocket Books, 1960.

———: *The Common Sense Book of Baby and Child Care,* New York: Pocket Books, 1961.

———: *Dr. Spock Talks with Mothers,* Greenwich, Conn.: Fawcett, 1961.

———: *A Teenager's Guide to Life and Love,* New York: Pocket Books, 1965.

Stehbens, James: "Parental Expectations in Toilet Training," *Pediatrics,* vol. 48, September 1971, pp. 451-454.

Van Wangenen, R. K., Lee Meyerson, Nancy J. Larr, and Kurt Mahoney: "Field Trials of a New Procedure for Toilet Training," *Journal of Experimental Child Psychology,* vol. 8, August 1969, pp. 147-159.

Weinstein, Grace W.: "Making Allowances: A Parents' Guide," *Money,* vol. 1, no. 2, November 1972, pp. 52-58, 62.

———: "How Children Learn about Money," *Money,* vol. 2, no. 2, February 1973, pp. 81-84.

Wolfish, M.: "Adolescent Sexuality," *Clinical Pediatrics,* vol. 12, no. 4, April 1973, pp. 244-247.

APPENDIX A

Certain Nutritional Characteristics of Specific Foods

It is frequently useful for the nurse to be familiar with some of the foods characterized by specific nutritional qualities, such as those high in iron, calcium, and calories and those particularly low in calories. The following is such a list:

Baby foods							
High in iron Milligrams of iron		**High in calories No. of calories**		**Low in calories No. of calories**		**High in calcium Milligrams of calcium (except milk)**	
Beech-Nut (per 100 gm)							
All cereals	50–53	Cereal		Apple juice	46	All cereals	800
Squash in butter sauce	1.32	High-protein	358	Green beans	28	Custard pudding	50
Egg yolks	3.08	Mixed	371	Carrots	35	Chocolate pudding	51
Egg yolks and bacon	3.02	Oatmeal	382	Vegetable soup	39	Caramel pudding	48
Beef	1.56	Rice	371	Vegetable and liver	43	Egg yolks	59
Lamb	1.50	Golden honey mixed	373	Chicken noodle	44	Garden vegetables	46
Vegetables and Liver	1.48	Golden honey oatmeal	383	Garden soup	43	Squash in butter sauce	43
Peas	1.10	Golden honey rice	373	Squash	34	Green beans	42
Chicken	1.27	Assorted fruit-flavored cookies	428	Chicken and vegetables	47	Pineapple dessert	34
Veal	1.16	Honey-flavored teething rings	393	Peas	63	Egg yolks and bacon	38
		Orange-pineapple dessert	120				

Baby foods

High in iron Milligrams of iron		High in calories No. of calories		Low in calories No. of calories		High in calcium Milligrams of calcium (except milk)	
Gerber's (per 100 gm or per can or jar)							
All cereals	100	Animal cookies	439	Green beans	29	All cereals	660
Animal cookies	2.00	Cereal		Squash	27	Teething biscuits	466
Teething biscuits	2.01	Barley	375	Carrots	29	Animal cookies	127
Beef liver	4.43	High-protein	372	Vegetables and chicken	41	Egg yolks	82
Egg yolks	3.18	Mixed	379	Vegetables and turkey	44	Creamed spinach	96+
Egg yolks and ham	2.45	Mixed with bananas	387	Raspberry cobbler	79	Creamed cottage cheese with pineapple	67
Beef with beef heart	2.12	Oatmeal	393	Rice cereal with applesauce and bananas	69	Butterscotch pudding	48
Peas	1.32	Oatmeal with bananas	393	Pears	69	Chocolate custard	58
Chicken with vegetables	1.71	Rice	376	Veal with vegetables	63	Vanilla custard	55
Turkey	1.63	Rice with straw-berries	387	Beets	38	Green beans	38
		Pretzels and biscuits	382				
Heinz (per jar or can)							
Apple-prune juice	0.8	Peaches	160	Orange juice	69	Chicken with chicken broth	58
Lamb with lamb broth	1.7	Apples and cranberries	124	Liver with liver broth	79	Egg yolks	86
High-protein cereal with apples and bananas	7.2	Ham with ham broth	122	Veal and vegetables	84	Chicken and vegetables	89
Pork with pork broth	1.5	Egg yolks	189	Beef with egg noodles	59	Vegetables and beef	50
Chicken soup	1.4	Chicken and vegetables	124	Beef liver soup	57	High-protein cereal with apples and bananas	61
Split peas, vegetables, and bacon	1.5	Ham and Vegetables	124	Tuna and noodles	55	Split peas, vegetables and bacon	59
Mixed cereal with apples and bananas	7.0	High-protein cereal with apples and bananas	132	Vegetables and lamb	56	Creamed spinach	106
Veal and vegetables	1.3	Apricots and tapioca	141	Green beans	37	Apple pie	54
Ham and vegetables	1.1	Pineapple pie	145	Squash	50	Peach pie	61
		Prunes and tapioca	140	Carrots	52		

Junior foods

High in iron Milligrams of iron		High in calories No. of calories		Low in calories No. of calories		High in calcium Milligrams of calcium (except milk)	
Beech-Nut (per 100 gm)							
Peas in butter sauce	1.35	Chicken sticks	204	Vegetable soup	39	Chicken sticks	112
Squash in butter sauce	1.14	Meat sticks	190	Turkey and rice with vegetables	40	Meat sticks	58
Beef	1.43	Pork	111	Squash	33	Macaroni and bacon	52
Chicken	1.42	Apple betty	107	Green beans	27	Custard pudding	56
Meat sticks	1.85	Applesauce and raspberries	109	Carrots	36	Caramel pudding	48
Lamb	1.50	Veal	101	Sweet potatoes	60	Chicken	31
Veal	1.41	Turkey	101	Chicken noodle	44	Green beans in butter sauce	41
Vegetables and liver	1.18	Fruit dessert with tapioca	100	Chicken and vegetables	45	Green beans	35
Peach melba	1.12	Peach melba	112	Vegetables and liver	45	Carrots in butter sauce	32
Chicken sticks	1.20	Lamb	99	Vegetables and lamb	58	Squash in butter sauce	31
Gerber's (per 100 gm or per jar)							
Beef	1.97	Chicken sticks	191	Carrots	30	Chicken sticks	73
Chicken sticks	1.97	Meat sticks	164	Squash	27	Creamed spinach	86
Meat sticks	2.00	Chicken	135	Turkey rice dinner	44	Chicken with vegetables	32
Mixed cereal with applesauce and bananas	3.91	Ham	117	Vegetables and turkey	42	Cream of chicken soup	33
Vegetables and liver with bacon	1.66	Creamed potatoes and ham	106	Carrots and peas	38	Butterscotch pudding	50
Spaghetti with meatballs	.89	Banana pudding	96	Mixed vegetables	40	Chocolate custard	57
Beef with vegetables	.99	Plums with tapioca	99	Creamed corn	62	Vanilla custard	54
Chicken with vegetables	.94	Veal	100	Veal and vegetables	64	Macaroni alphabets and beef casserole	43
Creamed spinach	.80	Turkey	106	Vegetables and lamb	49	Vegetable and turkey casserole	46
Carrots and peas	.85	Pork	114	Vegetables and liver with bacon	49	Meat sticks	35

Heinz (per 1 oz. or per jar)							
Cereals		Peaches	247	Carrots	86	Split peas, vegetables, and bacon	102
Barley	26	Split peas, vegetables, and bacon	213	High-protein cereal	99	Custard pudding	105
High-protein	26	Apricots and tapioca	224	Veal and veal broth	93	Cereals	
Mixed	26	Pineapple pie	237	Lamb and lamb broth	97	Barley	340
Oatmeal	26	Custard pudding	213	Beef and beef broth	99	High-protein	284
Rice	26	Apples and cranberries	191	Chicken sticks	79	Mixed	454
Creamed peas	1.7	Cereal, eggs, and bacon	164	Mixed cereal	100	Oatmeal	312
Cottage cheese with bananas	3.3	Creamed peas	158	Mixed vegetables	100	Rice	340
Split peas, vegetables, and bacon	2.0	Creamed corn	153	Barley cereal	101	Carrots	90
Beef and beef broth	1.5	Apple pie	219	Rice cereal	101	Chicken and vegetables	92
Lamb and lamb broth	1.5					Vegetables and lamb	85

Adult foods (per 100 gm unless otherwise noted)

High in iron Milligrams of iron		High in calories No. of calories		Low in calories No. of calories		High in calcium Milligrams of calcium (except milk)	
Caviar, sturgeon—granular	11.8	Cornmeal, dry—not enriched, (1 cup)	530	Apricots, canned—water-packed with or without artificial sweetener	38	Almond meal, partially defatted	424
Cornflakes with protein concentrate (cosein) and other nutrients added	17.9	Macaroni and cheese—baked, (1 cup)	506	Asparagus—boiled, drained	20	Carrots, dehydrated	256
Egg yolks, dried	10.8	Butter, unsalted	716	Green beans, canned	22	Parmesan cheese	1,140
Fish flour, from whole fish	41.0	American cheddar—grated (1 cup)	458	Cabbage, raw	24	Collard leaves without stems	250
Kidneys, beef—braised	13.1	Baked apple pie (1/6 of 9-in. pie)	410	Celery, raw	17	Egg yolk	275
Liver, hog—fried	29.1	Pecan pie (1/6 of medium pie)	668	Cucumbers, raw	15	Farina, quick-cooking, dry	500
Molasses, blackstrap	16.1	Dried whole eggs (1 cup)	640	Lettuce, raw	14	Filberts (hazelnuts)	209
Potato flour	17.2	Peanut spread	601	Peaches, raw	38	Pancake mix, dry—with enriched flour	450
Wheat bran	14.9	Black walnuts	628	Cantaloupe	30	Rennin tablets (salts, starch, rennin enzyme)	3,510
Sesame seeds, dry, whole	10.5	Potato chips	568	Fruit cocktail—water-packed	37	Whey, dried	646

APPENDIX B

Approximate Daily Dietary Requirements of Children at Different Ages under Ordinary Conditions

	Water		Calories		Protein		Minerals*			Vitamins					
Age	Milligrams per kilogram	Ounces per pound	per kilogram	per pound	Grams per kilogram	Grams per pound	Ca, gm	P, gm	Fe, mg	A, IU	B_1, mg	B_2, mg	Niacin, mg	C, mg	D, IU
3 days	80–100	1.2–1.5													
10 days	125–150	1.9–2.3													
3 months	140–165	2.1–2.5	100–130	45–60	3.5–4	1.8	0.6	1.5	6	1,500	0.3	0.4	3	30	400
6 months	130–155	2–2.3			3.5–4		0.8		6	1,500	0.4	0.7	4	30	
9 months	125–145	1.9–2.2			3.5				6	1,600	0.5	0.9	5	30	
1–3 years	115–135	1.7–2	90–100	41–45	3.5	1.6	1	1.5	8	2,000	0.6	1.0	6	35	400
4–6 years	90–110	1.3–1.7	80–90	36–41	3	1.4	1	1.5	10	2,500	0.8	1.2	8	50	400
7–9 years	70–90	1.1–1.3	70–80	32–36	2.5	1.1	1	1.5	12	3,500	1.0	1.5	10	60	400
10–12 years	60–85	0.9–1.3	60–70	27–32	2	0.9	1+	1.5+	14	4,500	1.3	1.8	12	75	400
13–15 years	50–65	0.75–1	50–60	23–27	1.5	0.7	1+	1.5+	15	5,000	1.6	2.0	14	90	400
Over 15 years	45–55	0.67–0.8	40–50	18–23	1+	0.5+	1+	1.5+	15	5,000	1.9	2.2	16	90	400
Adult	40–50	0.6–0.75	40–45	18–21	1	0.5	1+	1.5+	15	5,000	1.5	2.4	18	75	400

These figures are adapted from recommendations of the Committee on Growth and Development of the White House Conference on Child Health and Protection, the Food and Nutrition Board of the National Research Council, and other sources.

* Other minerals (all ages): magnesium, 200–400 mg/day; potassium, 1–2 gm/day; sodium, 1–2 gm/day; chloride, 2–3 gm/day; iodine, trace.

APPENDIX C

The Caldecott Medal Awards

The Caldecott Medal is a yearly award presented to the illustrator of the best picture book. In general, these books are literary classics and can safely be recommended to mothers as excellent books for preschoolers.

1938 *Animals of the Bible, A Picture Book,* text selected from the King James Bible by Helen Dean Fish, illustrated by Dorothy O. Lathrop, Stokes (Lippincott).

1939 *Mei Li,* Thomas Handforth, Doubleday. *The Forest Pool,* Laura Adams Armer, Longmans.

1940 *Abraham Lincoln,* Ingri d'Aulaire and Edgar P. d'Aulaire, Doubleday.

1941 *They Were Strong and Good,* Robert Lawson, Viking.

1942 *Make Way for Ducklings,* Robert McCloskey, Viking.

1943 *The Little House,* Virginia Lee Burton, Houghton Mifflin.

1944 *Many Moons,* James Thurber, illustrated by Louis Slobodkin, Harcourt, Brace.

1945 *Prayer for a Child,* Rachel Field, pictures by Elizabeth Orton Jones, Macmillan.

1946 *The Rooster Crows,* Maud Petersham and Miska Petersham, Macmillan.

1947 *The Little Island,* Golden MacDonald, illustrated by Leonard Weisgard, Doubleday.

1948 *White Snow, Bright Snow,* Alvin Tresselt, illustrated by Roger Duvoisin, Lothrop.

1949 *The Big Snow,* Berta Hader and Elmer Hader, Macmillan.

1950 *Song of the Swallows,* Leo Politi, Scribner.

1951 *The Egg Tree,* Katherine Milhous, Scribner.

1952 *Finders Keepers,* Will (Lipkind), illustrated by Nicolas (Mordvinoff), Harcourt, Brace.

1953 *The Biggest Bear,* Lynd Ward, Houghton Mifflin.

1954 *Madeline's Rescue,* Ludwig Bemelmans, Viking.

1955 *Cinderella,* Charles Perrault, illustrated by Marcia Brown, Harper.

1956 *Frog Went A-Courtin',* John Langstaff, illustrated by Feodor Rojankovsky, Harcourt, Brace.

1957 *A Tree Is Nice,* Janice May Udry, illustrated by Marc Simont, Harper.

1958 *Time of Wonder,* Robert McCloskey, Viking.

1959 *Chanticleer and the Fox,* edited and illustrated by Barbara Cooney, Crowell.

1960 *Nine Days to Christmas,* Marie Hall Ets and Aurora Labastida, Viking.

1961 *Baboushka and the Three Kings,* Ruth Robbins, illustrated by Nicolas Sidjakov, Parnassus Press.

1962 *Once a Mouse,* Marcia Brown, Scribner.

1963 *The Snowy Day,* Ezra Jack Keats, Viking.

1964 *Where the Wild Things Are,* Maurice Sendak, Harper.

1965 *May I Bring a Friend?* Montresor, Atheneum.

1966 *Always Room for One More,* Hogrogian, Holt.

1967 *Sam, Bangs and Moonshine,* Ness, Holt.

1968 *Drummer Hoff,* Emberley, Prentice-Hall.

1969 *The Fool of the World and the Flying Ship,* Shulevitz, Farrar, Straus, and Giroux.

1970 *Sylvester and the Magic Pebble,* Steig, Windmill/Simon & Schuster.

1971 *A Story - A Story,* Haley, Atheneum.

1972 *One Fine Day,* Hogrogian, Macmillan.

1973 *The Funny Little Woman,* retold by Arlene Mosel, illustrated by Blair Lent, Dutton.

APPENDIX D

The Newbery Medal Awards

The Newbery Medal is an annual award presented to "the author of the most distinguished contribution to American literature for children." This list is an excellent source for recommendations of books to mothers of school-age children.

1922 *The Story of Mankind,* Hendrik Van Loon, Boni & Liveright (Garden City Books).

1923 *The Voyages of Doctor Dolittle,* Hugh Lofting, Stokes (Lippincott).

1924 *The Dark Frigate,* Charles Boardman Hawes, Little, Brown.

1925 *Tales from Silver Lands,* Charles J. Finger, illustrated by Paul Honore, Doubleday, Doran (Doubleday).

1926 *Shen of the Sea,* Arthur Bowie Chrisman, illustrated by Else Hasselriis, Dutton.

1927 *Smoky, the Cowhorse,* Will James, Scribner.

1928 *Gay-Neck,* Dhan Gopal Mukerji, illustrated by Boris Artzybasheff, Dutton.

1929 *Trumpeter of Krakow,* Eric P. Kelly, illustrated by Angela Pruszynska, Macmillan.

1930 *Hitty, Her First Hundred Years,* Rachel Field, illustrated by Dorothy P. Lathrop, Macmillan.

1931 *The Cat Who Went to Heaven,* Elizabeth Coatsworth, illustrated by Lynd Ward, Macmillan.

1932 *Waterless Mountain,* Laura Adams Armer, illustrated by Sidney Armer and the author, Longmans, Green.

1933 *Young Fu of the Upper Yangtze,* Elizabeth Foreman Lewis, illustrated by Kurt Wiese, Winston (Holt).

1934 *Invincible Louisa,* Cornelia Meigs, Little, Brown.

1935 *Dobry,* Monica Shannon, illustrated by Atanas Katchamakoff, Viking.

1936 *Caddie Woodlawn,* Carol Ryrie Brink, illustrated by Kate Seredy, Macmillan.

1937 *Roller Skates,* Ruth Sawyer, illustrated by Valenti Angelo, Viking.

1938 *The White Stag,* Kate Seredy, Viking.

1939 *Thimble Summer,* Elizabeth Enright, Farrar & Rinehart (Holt).

1940 *Daniel Boone,* James H. Daugherty, Viking.

1941 *Call It Courage,* Armstrong Sperry, Macmillan.

1942 *The Matchlock Gun,* Walter D. Edmonds, illustrated by Paul Lantz, Dodd, Mead.

1943 *Adam of the Road,* Elizabeth Janet Gray, illustrated by Robert Lawson, Viking.

1944 *Johnny Tremain,* Esther Forbes, illustrated by Lynd Ward, Houghton Mifflin.

1945 *Rabbit Hill,* Robert Lawson, Viking.

1946 *Strawberry Girl,* Lois Lenski, Lippincott.

1947 *Miss Hickory,* Carolyn Sherwin Bailey, illustrated by Ruth Gannett, Viking.

1948 *The Twenty-One Balloons,* William Pène du Bois, Viking.

1949 *King of the Wind,* Marguerite Henry, illustrated by Wesley Dennis, Rand McNally.

1950 *The Door in the Wall,* Marguerite deAngeli, Doubleday.

1951 *Amos Fortune, Free Man,* Elizabeth Yates, illustrated by Nora Unwin, Aladdin.

1952 *Ginger Pye,* Eleanor Estes, Harcourt, Brace.

1953 *Secret of the Andes,* Ann Nolan Clark, illustrated by Jean Charlot, Viking.

1954 . . . *And Now Miguel,* Joseph Krumgold, illustrated by Jean Charlot, Crowell.

1955 *The Wheel on the School,* Meindert DeJong, illustrated by Maurice Sendak, Harper.

1956 *"Carry on, Mr. Bowditch,"* Jean L. Latham, Houghton Mifflin.

1957 *Miracles on Maple Hill,* Virginia Sorensen, illustrated by Beth and Joe Krush, Harcourt, Brace.

1958 *Rifles for Watie,* Harold Keith, illustrated by Peter Burchard, Thomas Y. Cromwell.

1959 *The Witch of Blackbird Pond,* Elizabeth G. Speare, Houghton.

1960 *Onion John,* Joseph Krumgold, illustrated by Symenon Shimin, Thomas Y. Crowell.

1961 *Island of the Blue Dolphins,* Scott O'Dell, Houghton Mifflin.

1962 *The Bronze Bow,* Elizabeth G. Speare, Houghton Mifflin.

1963 *A Wrinkle in Time,* Madeleine L'Engle, Farrar.

1964 *It's Like This, Cat,* Emily C. Neville, Harper.

1965 *Shadow of a Bull,* Wajciechowska, Atheneum.

1966 *I, Juan De Pareja,* Trevino, Farrar, Straus, and Giroux.

1967 *Up a Road Slowly,* Hunt, Follett.

1968 *From the Mixed-Up Files of Mrs. Basil E. Frankweiler,* Konigsburg, Atheneum.

1969 *The High King,* Alexander, Holt.

1970 *Sounder,* Armstrong, Harper.

1971 *Summer of the Swans,* Byers, Viking.

1972 *Mrs. Frisby and the Rats of Nimh,* Robert C. O'Brien, Atheneum.

1973 *Julie of the Wolves,* Jean Craighead George, Harper.

APPENDIX E

Periodicals for Children and about Children's Literature

The Booklist and Subscription Books Bulletin, American Library Association, 50 E. Huron St., Chicago 60611, Ill. Issued semimonthly. $6.00 per year.

The Bookmark, The New York State Library, Albany, N.Y. Issued five times a year by the University of the State of New York. $1.00 per year. $.10 per copy. Free to libraries of New York State.

The Bulletin of the Center for Children's Books, Graduate Library School, University of Chicago, 5835 Kimbark Ave., Room 206, Chicago 37, Ill. Issued monthly except August. $4.50 per year.

Calendar, Children's Book Council, 175 Fifth Ave., New York, N.Y. 10010. Issued four times a year. Free.

Child Study, Child Study Association of America, 9 E. 89th St., New York, N.Y. 10028. Issued quarterly. $3.00 per year.

Childhood Education, Association for Childhood Education International, 3615 Wisconsin Ave., N.W. Washington, D.C. 20016. Issued monthly from September to May. $4.50 per year.

Elementary English, National Council of Teachers of English, 508 S. 6th St., Champaign, Ill. Issued monthly from October to May. $4.00 per year.

Elementary School Science Bulletin, National Science Teachers Association, 1201 16th St., N.W. Washington, D.C. 20006. Published eight times a year from September to April. $1.00 per year.

The Horn Book, Horn Book, Inc., 585 Boylston St., Boston 16, Mass. Published six times yearly. $4.00 per year.

The Instructor, F. A. Owen Publishing Co., Dansville, N.Y. Ten issues per year. $6.00 per year.

Junior Reviewers, edited by Eleanor Bancroft Trampler, Box 36, Aspen, Colo. Issued bimonthly. $3.50 per year.

Parents Magazine, Parents' Institute, Inc. 52 Vanderbilt Ave. New York, N.Y. 10017. Issued monthly, $3.50 per year.

Publishers' Weekly—Children's Book Number, R. R. Bowker Co., 62 W. 45th St., New York, N.Y. 10036. $11.00 per year.

Saturday Review, 25 W. 45th St., New York, N.Y. 10036. Published weekly. $7.00 per year.

School Library Journal, R. R. Bowker and Co., 62 W. 45th St., New York, N.Y. 10036. Issued monthly from September to May. $3.50 per year.

Wilson Library Bulletin, H. W. Wilson Co., 950-972 University Ave., New York, N.Y. 10052. Issued monthly from September to June. $3.00 per year.

APPENDIX F

References and Book Lists Concerning Children's Literature

REFERENCES

Children's Catalog, compiled by Marion L. McConnell and Dorothy H. West. H. W. Wilson Company, 950-972 University Ave., New York, N.Y. 9th ed., 1956. Sold on service basis. Price on request.

Index to Children's Poetry, compiled by John E. Brewton and Sara W. Brewton. H. W. Wilson Company, 950-972 University Ave., New York, N.Y. 1942, with 1956 supplement. $10.00; supplement, $6.00.

Index to Fairy Tales, Myths and Legends, compiled by Mary Eastman. Faxon, Boston. 1952, with 1954 supplement. $7.00; supplement, $7.50.

Subject and Title Index to Short Stories for Children, compiled by a subcommittee of the American Library Association, 50 E. Huron St., Chicago 60611, Ill. 1955. $5.00.

Subject Index to Books for Intermediate Grades, prepared by Eloise Rue. American Library Association, 50 E. Huron St., Chicago, Ill. 60611. 2d ed., 1950. 493 pp. $6.00.

Subject Index to Books for Primary Grades, prepared by Mary K. Eakin and Eleanor Merritt. American Library Association, 50 E. Huron St., Chicago 60611, Ill. 2d ed., 1961. 176 pp. $4.50.

Subject Index to Children's Magazines, edited by Meribah Hazen. Madison 5, Wis. $7.50 per year.

Subject Index to Poetry for Children and Young People, compiled by Violet Sell et al. American Library Association, 50 E. Huron St., Chicago 60611, Ill., 1957. $9.00.

BOOK LIST—GENERAL

Adventuring with Books, National Council of Teachers of English, 508 S. 6th St., Champaign, Ill., 1960 ed. 146 pp. $.75.

A Basic Book Collection for Elementary Grades, compiled by a subcommittee of the American Library Association, 50 E. Huron St., Chicago 60611, Ill. 7th ed., 1960.

Best Books for Children, offices of *Library Journal* and *Junior Libraries,* 62 W. 45th St., New York, N.Y. 10036. 1961 ed. $3.00 net post paid.

Bibliography of Books for Children, Bulletin of Association for Childhood Education International, 3615 Wisconsin Ave., N.W. Washington, D.C. 20016. 1960 ed. 130 pp. $1.50.

Books for Children: A Selected List, Bank Street College of Education, 69 Bank St., New York, N.Y. 10014. 31 pp. Free.

Books for Elementary Schools, Department of Public Instruction, Indiana. 1959. 18 pp. Free.

Books to Build on, prepared under the direction of Elvajean Hall. R. R. Bowker Co., 62 W. 45th St., New York, N.Y. 10036. 2d ed. 79 pp. $2.00.

Buying List of Books for Small Libraries, compiled by Orilla Blackshear. American Library Association, 50 E. Huron St., Chicago 60611, Ill. 8th ed., 1954. $3.75.

Children's Books . . . for $1.25 or Less, Association for Childhood Education International, 3615 Wisconsin Ave., N.W. Washington, D.C., 20016. 1959. 40 pp. $.75.

Children's Books Too Good To Miss, prepared by May Hill Arbuthnot, et al. Western Reserve University Press, 2040 Adelbert Road, Cleveland 6, Ohio. 2d rev. ed., 1959. 64 pp. $1.25.

Go Exploring in Books, prepared by the Library Extension Service, University of Michigan, Ann Arbor, Mich.

Good Books for Children, edited by Mary K. Eakin. University of Chicago Press, Chicago, Ill. 1959. $5.95.

Growing up with Books, prepared in the offices of the *Library Journal,* 62 W. 45th St., New York, N.Y. 10036. 36 pp. $.10 per copy. $3.35 per 100.

Inexpensive Books for Boys and Girls, compiled by a subcommittee of the American Library Association, 50 E. Huron St., Chicago 60611, Ill., 1953. 33 pp. $.65.

Junior Book Awards, Boy's Clubs of America, 381 Fourth Ave., New York, N.Y. 10016. 1957. 132 pp.

Literature for Children, reprint from *World Book Encyclopedia,* Field Enterprises Educational Corp., Merchandise Mart Plaza, Chicago 54, Ill. 1960. 29 pp. Free.

Recommended Children's Books of 1959-1960, prepared by E. Louise Davis. Reprinted from *Junior Libraries,* 62 W. 45th St., New York, N.Y. 10036. 113 pp. $2.00.

Selected Books of the Year for Children, Child Study Association of America, 9 E. 89th St., New York, N.Y. 10028. $.50.

Seven Stories High—The Child's Own Library, compiled by Anne Carroll Moore. F. E. Compton and Co., 1000 N. Dearborn St., Chicago 10, Ill. Reprint. 15 pp. Free.

Treasure for the Taking, prepared by Anne Thaxter Eaton. The Viking Press, 625 Madison Ave., New York, N.Y. 10022. Rev. ed., 1957. $4.00.

BOOKS LISTS—SPECIFIC

Bible Stories and Books about Religion for Children, selected by the Children's Book Committee of the Child Study Association, 9 E. 89th St., New York, N.Y. 10028. Rev. ed. 1954, with supplement 1954-1956, 22 pp. $.25.

Books about Negro Life for Children, prepared by Augusta Baker. New York Public Library, 5th Ave. at 42d St., New York, N.Y. 10018. 1961 ed. $.25.

Books Are Bridges, American Friends Service Committee (Quakers), 20 S. 12th Street, Philadelphia 7, Penn. and the Anti-Defamation League of B'nai B'rith, 515 Madison Ave., New York, N.Y. 10022. 1957. 64 pp. $.25.

Books Are Vacations!, compiled by Lois R. Markey. Horn Book, Inc., 585 Boylston St., Boston 16, Mass. 1956. 32 pp. $.75.

Character Formation through Books, compiled by Clara J. Kircher. Catholic University of America Press, Washington, D.C. Rev. ed., 1952 (out of print).

Children's Books on Alaska, compiled by Ellen Martin Brinsmade. Secure from Adler's Book Shop, Box 1599, Fairbanks, Alaska. 1956. 32 pp. $1.00.

Children's Literature about Foreign Countries, compiled by Marjorie Scherwitzky. Reprinted from the *Wilson Library Bulletin,* October 1957. 7 pp. $.25.

Christmas Materials in General Children's Books, compiled by Hilda K. Limper. Reprinted from the *Wilson Library Bulletin,* November 1952. 11 pp. $.25.

Good Reading for Poor Readers, compiled by George Spache. The Garrard Press, Champaign, Ill., 1960. 182 pp. $2.50.

Growing up with Science Books, compiled with the assistance of Julius Schwartz and Herman Schneider. *Library Journal,* 62 W. 45th St., New York, N.Y. 10036. 32 pp. $.10 per copy. $3.35 per 100.

Human Relations in the Primary Grades, Mildred Barlow; *Human Relations in the Intermediate Grades,* Ray Schmiedlin; and *Human Relations in the Junior High School,* Irene Harney. National Conference of Christians and Jews, 43 W. 57th St., New York, N.Y. 10019. 8 pp. each. Free.

"I Can Read It Myself!" Some Books for Independent Reading in the Primary Grades, Frieda M. Heller. Center for School Experimentation, The Ohio State University, Columbus 10, Ohio. $1.00.

An Inexpensive Science Library, Hilary J. Deason and Robert W. Lynn. American Association for the Advancement of Science. National Science Foundation, Washington, D.C., 5th ed., 1961, 87 pp. $.25.

Introducing Children to the World in Elementary and Junior High Schools, Leonard Kenworthy. Harper. New York, N.Y. 1956. $3.75.

Latin America in Books for Boys and Girls, compiled by the Children's Book Committee of the Child Study Association, 9 E. 89th St., New York, N.Y. 10028. 1956. 23 pp. $.25.

Light the Candles! compiled by Marcia Dalphin. Horn Books, Inc. 585 Boylston St., Boston 16, Mass. 1953. 24 pp. $.75.

Literature and Music as Resources for Social Studies, Ruth Tooze and Beatrice Krone. Prentice-Hall, Inc. Englewood Cliffs, N.J. 1955. $7.95.

Once Upon a Time, prepared by Augusta Baker and committee. The New York Public Library, 20 W. 53rd St., New York, N.Y. 10019. 1955. 15 pp. $.25.

The Opportunities That Books Offer, prepared by Dorothy M. Broderick. Reprinted from *Junior Libraries,* December 1959. The Children's Book Council, 175 Fifth Ave., New York, N.Y. 10010 (out of print).

Personal Problems of Children, Elvajean Hall. Campbell and Hall, Inc., P.O. Box 350, Boston 17, Mass. 4 pp. $.15.

Reading Ladders for Human Relations, compiled by Margaret M. Heaton and Helen B. Lewis. American Council on Education, 1785 Massachusetts Ave., N.W., Washington, D.C. Rev. ed., 1955. 215 pp. $1.75.

A Selected Bibliography of Books, Films, Filmslides, Records and Exhibitions About Asia, United States National Commission for UNESCO. U.S. Government Printing Office, Washington 25, D.C. 1957. 47 pp. $.25.

Stories: A List of Stories to Tell and to Read Aloud, compiled by Augusta Baker. The New York Public Libraries, 5th Ave. and 42nd St., New York, N.Y. 10018. 1958. 77 pp. $1.00.

Stories to Tell, edited by Isabella Jinnette. Enoch Pratt Free Library, Baltimore 1, Md. 1956. 76 pp. $1.00.

Trade Books for Beginning Readers, Martha Olson Condit. Reprint from the *Wilson Library Bulletin,* December 1959. $.25.

Value Resource Guide, compiled by Mate Graye Hunt for *The Elementary School Teacher.* American Association of Colleges for Teacher Education, Oneonta, N.Y., 1958, 108 pp. $1.00.

World Affairs Book Fair: Political and Cultural, World Affairs Center for the United States, 345 E. 46th St., New York, N.Y. 10017. 1959.

APPENDIX G

Measurement Conversion Tables

APPROXIMATE EQUIVALENTS

Weight—Metric

1,000 milligrams = 1 gram
1,000 grams = 1 kilogram

Weight—Apothecaries'

60 grains = 1 dram
8 drams = 1 ounce
12 ounces = 1 pound

Weight

Metric—Apothecaries'

.1 milligram = 1/600 grain
.2 milligram = 1/300 grain
1 milligram = 1/60 grain
60 milligrams = 1 grain
.06 gram = 1 grain
1 gram = 15 grains
31 grams = 1 ounce
373 grams = 12 ounces (1 pound)

Volume of Liquids—Metric

1 milliliter = 1 cubic centimeter
1,000 cubic centimeters = 1 liter

Volume of Liquids—Apothecaries'

60 minims = 1 dram
8 drams = 1 ounce
16 ounces = 1 pint

Volume of Liquids

Household—Metric—Apothecaries'

1 teaspoon = 5 cubic centimeters = 1⅓ fluid drams
1 dessertspoon = 8 cubic centimeters = 2 fluid drams
1 tablespoon = 15 cubic centimeters = ½ fluid ounce
1 teacup = 120 cubic centimeters = 4 fluid ounces
1 cup = 241 cubic centimeters = 8 fluid ounces
.06 cubic centimeters = 1 minim
1 cubic centimeter = 15 minims
30 cubic centimeters = 1 fluid ounce
500 cubic centimeters = 1 pint+
1 liter = 1 quart+

Gram Equivalents for Pounds and Ounces

Pounds	Ounces															
	0	1	2	3	4	5	6	7	8	9	10	11	12	13	14	15
0	0	28	57	85	113	142	170	198	227	255	284	312	340	369	397	425
1	454	482	510	539	567	595	624	652	680	709	737	765	794	822	851	879
2	907	936	964	992	1,021	1,049	1,077	1,106	1,134	1,162	1,191	1,219	1,247	1,276	1,304	1,332
3	1,361	1,389	1,418	1,446	1,474	1,503	1,531	1,559	1,588	1,616	1,644	1,673	1,701	1,729	1,758	1,786
4	1,814	1,843	1,871	1,899	1,928	1,956	1,985	2,013	2,041	2,070	2,098	2,126	2,155	2,183	2,211	2,240
5	2,268	2,296	2,325	2,353	2,381	2,410	2,438	2,466	2,495	2,523	2,552	2,580	2,608	2,637	2,665	2,693
6	2,722	2,750	2,778	2,807	2,835	2,863	2,892	2,920	2,948	2,977	3,005	3,033	3,062	3,090	3,119	3,147
7	3,175	3,204	3,232	3,260	3,289	3,317	3,345	3,374	3,402	3,430	3,459	3,487	3,515	3,544	3,572	3,600
8	3,629	3,657	3,686	3,714	3,742	3,771	3,799	3,827	3,856	3,884	3,912	3,941	3,969	3,997	4,026	4,054
9	4,082	4,111	4,139	4,167	4,196	4,224	4,253	4,281	4,309	4,338	4,366	4,394	4,423	4,451	4,479	4,508
10	4,536	4,564	4,593	4,621	4,649	4,678	4,706	4,734	4,763	4,791	4,820	4,848	4,876	4,905	4,933	4,961
11	4,990	5,018	5,046	5,075	5,103	5,131	5,160	5,188	5,216	5,245	5,273	5,301	5,330	5,358	5,387	5,415
12	5,443	5,472	5,500	5,528	5,557	5,585	5,613	5,642	5,670	5,698	5,727	5,755	5,783	5,812	5,840	5,868
13	5,897	5,925	5,954	5,982	6,010	6,039	6,067	6,095	6,124	6,152	6,180	6,209	6,237	6,265	6,294	6,322
14	6,350	6,379	6,407	6,435	6,464	6,492	6,521	6,549	6,577	6,606	6,634	6,662	6,691	6,719	6,747	6,776
15	6,804	6,832	6,861	6,889	6,917	6,946	6,974	7,002	7,031	7,059	7,088	7,116	7,144	7,173	7,201	7,229

Example: To find gram equivalent for 7 lbs, 5 oz., read across on 7 and down on 5; the figure where the two meet, 3,317, is the equivalent weight in grams.

Kilogram Equivalents for Pounds

Pounds	Pounds									
	0	1	2	3	4	5	6	7	8	9
0	0.00	0.45	0.90	1.36	1.81	2.27	2.72	3.18	3.63	4.09
10	4.54	4.99	5.45	5.90	6.36	6.81	7.27	7.72	8.18	8.63
20	9.09	9.54	9.99	10.45	10.90	11.36	11.81	12.27	12.72	13.18
30	13.63	14.09	14.54	14.99	15.45	15.90	16.36	16.81	17.27	17.72
40	18.18	18.63	19.09	19.54	19.99	20.45	20.90	21.36	21.81	22.27
50	22.72	23.18	23.63	24.09	24.54	24.99	25.45	25.90	26.36	26.81
60	27.27	27.72	28.18	28.63	29.09	29.54	29.99	30.45	30.90	31.36
70	31.81	32.27	32.72	33.18	33.63	34.09	34.54	34.99	35.45	35.90
80	36.36	36.81	37.27	37.72	38.18	38.63	39.09	39.54	39.99	40.45
90	40.90	41.26	41.81	42.27	42.72	43.18	43.63	44.09	44.54	44.99
100	45.45	45.90	46.36	46.81	47.27	47.72	48.18	48.63	49.09	49.54
110	49.99	50.45	50.90	51.36	51.81	52.27	52.72	53.18	53.63	54.09
120	54.54	54.99	55.45	55.90	56.36	56.81	57.27	57.72	58.18	58.63
130	59.09	59.54	59.99	60.45	60.90	61.36	61.81	62.27	62.72	63.18
140	63.63	64.09	64.54	64.99	65.45	65.90	66.36	66.81	67.27	67.72
150	68.18	68.63	69.09	69.54	69.99	70.45	70.90	71.36	71.81	72.27
160	72.72	73.18	73.63	74.09	74.54	74.99	75.45	75.90	76.36	76.81
170	77.27	77.72	78.18	78.63	79.09	79.54	79.99	80.45	80.90	81.36
180	81.81	82.27	82.72	83.18	83.63	84.09	84.54	84.99	85.45	85.90
190	86.36	86.81	87.27	87.72	88.18	88.63	89.09	89.54	89.99	90.45
200	90.90	91.36	91.81	92.27	92.72	93.18	93.63	94.09	94.54	94.99

Example: To obtain kilogram equivalent for 15 lb, read across on 10 and down on 5; the figure where the two meet, 6.81, is the equivalent weight in kilograms.

Equivalent Temperatures

Degrees Celsius	Degrees Fahrenheit	Degrees Celsius	Degrees Fahrenheit	Degrees Celsius	Degrees Fahrenheit
34.0	93.2	36.4	97.5	38.8	101.8
34.1	93.4	36.5	97.7	38.9	102.0
34.2	93.6	36.6	97.9	39.0	102.2
34.3	93.7	36.7	98.1	39.1	102.4
34.4	93.9	36.8	98.2	39.2	102.6
34.5	94.1	36.9	98.4	39.3	102.7
34.6	94.3	37.0	98.6	39.4	102.9
34.7	94.5	37.1	98.8	39.5	103.1
34.8	94.6	37.2	99.0	39.6	103.3
34.9	94.8	37.3	99.1	39.7	103.5
35.0	95.0	37.4	99.3	39.8	103.6
35.1	95.2	37.5	99.5	39.9	103.8
35.2	95.4	37.6	99.7	40.0	104.0
35.3	95.5	37.7	99.9	40.1	104.2
35.4	95.7	37.8	100.0	40.2	104.4
35.5	95.9	37.9	100.2	40.3	104.5
35.6	96.1	38.0	100.4	40.4	104.7
35.7	96.3	38.1	100.6	40.5	104.9
35.8	96.4	38.2	100.8	40.6	105.1
35.9	96.6	38.3	100.9	40.7	105.3
36.0	96.8	38.4	101.1	40.8	105.4
36.1	97.0	38.5	101.3	40.9	105.6
36.2	97.2	38.6	101.5	41.0	105.8
36.3	97.3	38.7	101.7		

Centimeter Equivalents for Inches

	Inches					
Inches	0	10	20	30	40	50
0	0	25.4	50.8	76.2	101.6	127.0
1	2.5	27.9	53.3	78.7	104.1	129.5
2	5.0	30.4	55.8	81.2	106.6	132.0
3	7.6	33.0	58.4	83.8	109.2	134.6
4	10.1	35.5	60.9	86.3	111.7	137.1
5	12.7	38.1	63.5	88.9	114.3	139.7
6	15.2	40.6	66.0	91.4	116.8	142.2
7	17.7	43.1	68.5	93.9	119.3	144.7
8	20.3	45.7	71.1	96.5	121.9	147.3
9	22.8	48.2	73.6	99.0	124.4	149.8

Example: To obtain centimeter equivalent to 22 inches, read down on 20 and across on the figure where the two meet, 55.8, is the equivalent length in centimeters.

Centimeter Equivalents for Feet and Inches

	Feet					
Inches	**0**	**1**	**2**	**3**	**4**	**5**
0	0	30.4	60.9	91.4	121.9	152.4
1	2.5	33.0	63.5	93.9	124.4	154.9
2	5.0	35.5	66.0	96.5	127.0	157.4
3	7.6	38.1	68.5	99.0	129.5	160.0
4	10.1	40.6	71.1	101.6	132.0	162.5
5	12.7	43.1	73.6	104.1	134.6	165.1
6	15.2	45.7	76.2	106.6	137.1	167.6
7	17.7	48.2	78.7	109.2	139.7	170.1
8	20.3	50.8	81.2	111.7	142.2	172.7
9	22.8	53.3	83.8	114.3	144.7	175.2
10	25.4	55.8	86.3	116.8	147.3	177.8
11	27.9	58.4	88.9	119.3	149.8	180.3

Example: To find centimeter equivalent for 4 ft, 8 in., read across on 4 and down on 8; the figure where the two meet is the equivalent length in centimeters.

APPENDIX H

Free Pamphlets and Other Resources Available for Nurses

The left column lists the publication and the right column the source.

The Skin	Meade Johnson & Co. Evansville, Ind. 47721
The Head	Meade Johnson & Co.
The Eyes	Meade Johnson & Co.
Birthmarks	Meade Johnson & Co.
The Mouth	Meade Johnson & Co.
The External Ear	Meade Johnson & Co.
The Extremities—Part I	Meade Johnson & Co.
The Extremities—Part II	Meade Johnson & Co.
The VD Crisis	Pfizer Laboratories Division Pfizer, Inc., and American Social Health Association 285 E. 42d Street New York, N.Y. 10017

Essentials of the Gynecologic History and Examination	Smith, Kline & French Laboratories 1500 Spring Garden Street Philadelphia, Pa. 19101
A Clinical Review of Concepts and Characteristics in Infant Development	Meade Johnson & Co.
Some Pathological Conditions of the Eye, Ear and Throat (atlas)	Abbott Laboratories Abbott Park North Chicago, Ill. 60064
Common Skin Diseases (atlas)	Abbott Laboratories
Mechanisms and Pathway of Pain and Labor (atlas)	Abbott Laboratories
Cervical Pathology (atlas)	Abbott Laboratories
Human Placenta (atlas)	Abbott Laboratories
Infant Nutrition (book)	Wyeth Laboratories Philadelphia, Pa. 19101
Newer Knowledge of Milk, 3d ed. (book)	National Dairy Council Chicago, Ill. 60606
Newer Knowledge of Cheese (book)	National Dairy Council
Vision Screening of Children (pamphlet)	National Society for the Prevention of Blindness, Inc. 79 Madison Avenue New York, N.Y. 10016
Preschool Vision Screening (pamphlet)	National Society for the Prevention of Blindness, Inc.
A Guide for Eye Inspection and Testing Visual Acuity of Preschool Age Children (pamphlet)	National Society for the Prevention of Blindness, Inc.
Calcium in Nutrition (pamphlet)	National Dairy Council
Milk: Its Food Value (pamphlet)	National Dairy Council
Ice Cream and Similarly Frozen Foods Information Sheet (pamphlet)	National Dairy Council
Obesity Kit	Ross Laboratories Columbus, Ohio 43216
Stethoscopic Heart Sounds (record)	Roerig - Pfizer
Normal and Abnormal Breath Sounds (record)	Roerig - Pfizer

Resource	Source
A. H. Robins GI Series: *Physical Examination of the Abdomen* (book)	A. H. Robins Co. Richmond Va. 23220
Cardiac Auscultation Series (notebook)	Roche Laboratories Division of Hoffman-LaRoche, Inc. Nutley, N.J. 09110
A Child's Cry: A Clue to Diagnosis (record)	Pfizer Laboratories Division
A Breast Check	American Cancer Society (see your local chapter)
Recommendations for Human Blood Pressure Determined by Sphygmomanometers	American Heart Association 44 E. 23d Street New York, N.Y. 10010
Vaginitis—Diagnosis/Treatment	Ortho Pharmaceutical Corp. Raritan, N.J. 08869
Record of Vital Signs	Meade Johnson & Co.
Treatment of Phenylketonuria	Meade Johnson & Co.
Essentials of the Neurological Examination	Smith, Kline & French Laboratories
Oral Contraceptives in the U.S.	Wyeth Laboratories
Neonatal Reflexes: Vol. I Illustrated (slides)	Meade Johnson & Co.
Upper Respiratory Tract	Carnation Co. Medical Marketing Division Los Angeles, Calif. 90036
Enfamil Infant Formula	Meade Johnson & Co.
Estimation of Muscle Tone (poster)	Meade Johnson & Co.
The Moro Reflex (poster)	Meade Johnson & Co.
Starting Point: Primitive Reflexes (poster)	Meade Johnson & Co.
The Premature and the Full-Term Infant (poster)	Meade Johnson & Co.
The Tonic Neck Reflex (poster)	Meade Johnson & Co.
Spinal Related Reflexes (poster)	Meade Johnson & Co.
Food before Six	National Dairy Council
Modern Obstetrics: Pre-Eclampsia-Eclampsia	Ortho Pharmaceutical Corp.
Venereal Disease	Medcom Inc., c/o Pfizer Laboratories Division

Title	Source
Procedure for Fitting the Vaginal Diaphragm	Ortho Pharmaceutical Corp.
Roche Handbook of Differential Diagnosis	Roche Laboratories
Diagnostic Challenges: Pediatrics	Smith, Kline & French Laboratories
Nurses' Handbook on Live Virus Vaccines	Merck, Sharp & Dohme
Diagnostic Challenges: Cardiology	Smith, Kline & French Laboratories
Diagnostic Challenges: Obstetrics	Smith, Kline & French Laboratories
Evaluation & Management of Congenital Cardio Defects	American Heart Association
Facts about Foods	H. J. Heinz Co. Pittsburgh, Pa.
Allergy-free Foods	Gerber Products Co. Fremont, Mich. 49412
Nutrient Values of Gerber Baby Foods	Gerber Products Co.
Nutrient Values of Heinz Baby Foods	H. J. Heinz Co.
Nutrient Values of Beechnut Baby Foods	Beechnut
Examination of the Heart: part I, *History Taking,* part II; part III; part IV	American Heart Association

APPENDIX I

Inexpensive or Free Movies Available for Nurses

The Abdomen in Adults
Time: 33 minutes
Order: CIBA
Division of CIBA Corp.
P.O. Box 195
Summit, N.J. 07901
Cost: $5.00

Abdomen in Infants and Children
Time: 32 minutes
Order: Audio-Visual Utilization Center
Wayne State University
Detroit, Mich. 48202

Allergy
Time: 20 minutes
Color
Order: Audio-Visual Utilization Center
Pediatric Basics Film Series
Wayne State University
Detroit, Mich. 48202

Auscultation of the Heart: Mitral Stenosis
Time: 20 minutes
Color
Order: American Heart Association. See your local chapter.

Bronchitis and Bronchiectasis
Order: Pfizer Laboratories Division Film Library
267 W. 25th Street
New York, N.Y. 10001
Cost: Free

Cancer in Children
Time: 27 minutes
Color
Order: American Cancer Society. See your local chapter.
Cost: Free

Cardiac Arrhythmias
Time: 23 minutes
Color
Order: Abbott Laboratories
Abbott Park
North Chicago, Ill. 60064

The Development of the Immune Capacity in the Newborn
Time: 26 minutes
Order: T' Pfizer Laboratories Division Film Library
267 West 25th Street
New York, N.Y. 10001
Cost: Free

Diagnosis and Management of Acute Abdominal Problems
Time: 55 minutes
Black and white
Order: Upjohn Professional Film Library
7000 Portage Road
Kalamazoo, Mich. 49001
Cost: Free

Diagnosis of Congenital Dislocation of the Hip in the Newborn
Time: 16 minutes
Color
Order: David B. Levine, M.D.
Clinical Associate Professor of Orthopedic Surgery
Hospital for Special Surgery
535 East 70th Street
New York, N.Y. 10021
Cost: Free

Early Diagnosis and Management of Breast Cancer
Time: 19½ minutes
Color
Order: American Cancer Society. See your local chapter.

Errors of Refraction
Time: 21 minutes
Color
Order: Abbott Laboratories
Abbott Park
North Chicago, Ill. 60064
Cost: Free

#3 Examination of the Newborn (videotape)
Time: 19 minutes
Black and White
Order: Ross Laboratories. See your local detail man.
Cost: Free

#5 Examination of the Uncooperative Child (videotape)
Time: 9 minutes
Black and white
Order: Ross Laboratories. See your local detail man.
Cost: Free

The Face - Part I & II
Time: 21 minutes, 33 minutes
Order: CIBA
Division of CIBA Corp.
P.O. Box 195
Summit, N.J. 07901
Cost: $5.00 each

Immunizations against Infectious Diseases
Time: 30 minutes
Order: Lederle Film Library
American Cyanamid Company
1 Casper Street
Danbury, Conn.
Cost: Free

Introduction to Speech Problems
Time: 27 minutes
Order: CIBA
Division of CIBA Corp.
P.O. Box 195
Summit, N.J. 07901
Cost: $5.00

#6 The Measurement of Physical Growth (videotape)
Time: 10 minutes
Black and white
Order: Ross Laboratories. See your local detail man.
Cost: Free

The Neurological Examination of Infants
Time: 26 minutes
Color
Order: Kenny Rehabilitation Institute
1800 Chicago Avenue
Minneapolis, Minn. 55404
Cost: $15.00

Neurological Examination of the Full-Term Newborn
Order: National Medical Audiovisual Center (Annex)
Station K
Atlanta, Ga. 30324

#2 Neurological Examination of the Newborn (videotape)
Time: 20 minutes
Black and White
Order: Ross Laboratories. See your local detail man.
Cost: Free

Oral Lesions in Children and Adults
Time: 28 minutes
Color
Order: Abbott Laboratories
Abbott Park
North Chicago, Ill. 60064

The Otoneurological Examination for Vestibulo-Cerebellar Function
Time: 26 minutes
Color
Order: Abbott Laboratories
Abbott Park
North Chicago, Ill. 60064

Physical Diagnosis: The Neck
Time: 30 minutes
Color
Order: Audio-Visual Utilization Center
Wayne State University
Detroit, Mich. 48202
Cost: $5.00

Physical Examination of the Newborn
Time: 33 minutes
Order: The Pfizer Laboratories Division Film Library
267 West 25th Street
New York, N.Y. 10001
Cost: Free

#1 Physical Examination of the Small Child (videotape)
Time: 12 minutes
Black and White
Order: Ross Laboratories. See your local detail man.
Cost: Free

PKU
Time: 20 minutes
Color
Order: Pediatric Basics Film Series
Audio-Visual Utilization Center
Wayne State University
Detroit, Mich. 48202

The Premature Infant with Esophageal Atresia and Tracheoesophageal Fistula
Time: 20 minutes
Color
Order: Abbott Laboratories
Abbott Park
North Chicago, Ill. 60064
Cost: Free

Proprioceptive and Sensory Systems
Time: 29 minutes
Order: CIBA
Division of CIBA Corp.
P.O. Box 195
Summit, N.J. 07901
Cost: Free

Recognition of Narcotic Withdrawal Symptoms in Newborn Infants
Order: Motion Picture Film Library
American Medical Association
535 North Dearborn Street
Chicago, Ill. 60610
Cost: $3.00

Resuscitation of the Newborn
Time: 30 minutes
Color
Order: Smith, Kline & French Laboratories
1500 Spring Garden Street
Philadelphia, Pa. 19101

The Technique of an Effective Examination
Time: 20 minutes
Color
Order: Audio-Visual Utilization Center
Pediatric Basics Film Series
Wayne State University
Detroit, Mich. 48202

Vitamins and Some Deficiency Diseases
Time: 35 minutes
Order: Lederle Film Library
American Cyanamid Company
1 Casper Street
Danbury, Conn.
Cost: Free

APPENDIX J

Periodicals Containing Useful Information for Nurses

MEDICAL JOURNALS

Acta Paediatrica Academiae Scientiarum Hungaricae
Acta Paediatrica Belgica
Acta Paediatrica Scandinavica
Acta Paediatrica Scandinavica (Supplement)
Advances in Child Development Behavior
Advances in Pediatrics
American Journal of Diseases of Children
American Journal of Public Health
Annales de Pediatrie (Paris)
Archiv fur Kinderheilkunde (Supplement)
Archives of Disease in Childhood
Archives Francaises de Pediatrie
Briefs
Clinical Pediatrics (Philadelphia)
Clinical Proceedings of the Children's Hospital, Washington, D.C.
Current Problems in Pediatrics
Colorado Health

Health Education Journal
Helvetica Paediatrica Acta
Helvetica Paediatrica Acta Supplement
Indian Journal of Pediatrics
Journal of Pediatrics
Journal of Pediatric Ophthalmology
Journal of Reproduction and Fertility
Journal of Reproduction and Fertility Supplement
Journal of Tropical Pediatrics
Journal of Tropical Pediatrics (Supplement)
Minerva Pediatrica
Modern Probelms in Pediatrics
Monographs of the Society for Research in Child Development
Neuropaediatrie
Pediatrie
Pediatric Clinics of North America
Pediatric Digest
Pediatric Herald
Pediatrics
Pediatrics Current
Progress of Gynecology
Public Health (London)
Public Health Monographs
Reprints from the Ross Conference of Pediatric Research
Reprints from the Ross Conference of Pediatric Research (Supplement)
Revue de Pediatrie

NURSING JOURNALS

American Journal of Nursing
Australian Nursing Journal
Bulletin of the American College of Nurse-Midwives
Canadian Nurse
Colorado Nurse
International Journal of Nursing Studies
International Nursing Review
Journal of Continuing Education in Nursing
Journal of Nursing Administration
Journal of Nursing Education
Journal of Psychiatric Nursing and Mental Health Service
New Zealand Nursing Journal
Nursing Clinics of North America
Nursing Forum
Nursing Mirror Midwives Journal
Nursing Outlook
Nursing Research
Nursing Times

Pediatric Nursing Currents
Perspectives in Psychiatric Care
RN
Regan Report on Nursing Law
SA Nursing Journal

NONMEDICAL AND NONNURSING JOURNALS

American Journal of Orthopsychiatry
Child Development
Child Health Investigation
Child Psychiatry and Human Development
Child Welfare
Children
Developmental Psychology
Family Circle
Family Coordinator
Hospitals—Journal of American Hospital Association
Journal of American Diatetic Association
Journal of Health and Social Behavior
Journal of Human Relations
Journal of Comparative Family Studies
Journal of Consulting and Clinical Psychology
Journal of Learning Disabilities
Journal of Marriage and the Family
Journal of Orthopsychiatry
Journal of Social Issues
Merrill Palmer Quarterly
McCall's
Parents' Magazine
Public Health Reports
Scientific American
Redbook
Today's Health
Woman's Day

APPENDIX K

Information for Parents

Nurses working in ambulatory pediatrics will often find it handy to have printed information to give to parents. The authors have used the following material and found it helpful. It may be reprinted in whole or part without permission.

THE NEWBORN

Development

1 Your baby is a unique person—different from you, the father, the sisters, and the brothers. Physically your newborn baby is a completely formed, perfect, tiny human being who is now equipped to live somewhat independently from you. Your newborn no longer needs your blood supply for food or your warmth for shelter. But your baby still needs much help in adjusting to the outside world.

  a Your baby will probably be between 18 and 21 in. in length and 6 and 9 lbs in weight; the newborn will lose several ounces during the first week.

  b The newborn's skin is red, blotchy, dry, scaly, and too big for the body during the first weeks. There may be little white patches or blisters over the nose. These are normal. By the 3d or 4th day the skin may have a slight yellow shade. This is normal and fades in a few days.

c The head may be nice and oval or odd-shaped with ridges owing to shifting during the birth process; the head will regain its oval, smooth look within the first weeks and months of life. The soft spot on top of the head will close by the time the baby is 12 to 18 months old.

d The baby's eyes will remain shut a good deal of the time in the beginning. They may be puffy, swollen, and red for several days.

e On the baby's abdomen will be the cord—a white, elastic-looking tube with a metal or plastic clamp attached. The cord will dry to a black, hard stick and fall off by 1 to 3 weeks.

f Some babies have swollen nipples that ooze small amounts of a white liquid. This is normal and goes away by itself. It is best not to squeeze the nipple.

g The genitalia of boys and girls is often swollen. Little girls often have a white, cloudy discharge for several weeks. This is normal. If your new baby is a boy, you may be asked to decide whether he should be circumcised. We will be glad to discuss this with you.

h Babies frequently hold their legs and arms curled close to their bodies because they have been in that position in your uterus (womb) for 9 months.

2 Your newborn is an individual—different from every other baby you have had or ever will have. From the moment of conception the infant begins to develop a personality. A baby may be active, placid, or unpredictable. Sometimes your baby will be happy and content and at other times unhappy, upset, and crying.

3 While a newborn comes equipped to do some things, like breathe, sleep, and eliminate, many things must be learned and perfected.

a The newborn knows how to suck, but learns how to eat more effectively as each feeding progresses.

b The newborn knows how to breathe with the nose and the chest, but it is not a smooth operation. Sometimes the newborn breathes fast, sometimes slowly, sometimes loudly, and sometimes very softly.

c While newborns can see light and dark, they have difficulty focusing their eyes. The eyes tend to roll around in their sockets in all different directions.

d The newborn can hear and will respond to a sudden loud noise or a bell.

e The newborn can suck, smell, taste, sneeze, cough, hiccough, yawn, and cry.

Discussion

Feeding *When:* Babies will let you know when they are hungry by crying, moving their legs and arms, making sucking noises, and maybe even sucking their fingers. Your baby will probably want to eat every 2 to 4 hours. If your baby wants to eat more frequently or less frequently than this, please discuss it with us.

What: Your baby may be fed formula or breast milk and may need 2 to 4 oz. of water each day; you should offer this amount, but your baby may not take it all.

How: Both you and the baby should enjoy feeding time. Babies like to be held during their feedings. You should sit in a comfortable chair and relax during this time. Burp your baby (by patting the back while the baby is over your shoulder or by propping the baby in a sitting position on your lap and running your fingers up the back) halfway through and at the end of each feeding. Your baby may not have a bubble each time. If the infant is turned on the stomach or side after the feeding, any leftover bubbles will rise by themselves.

Vitamins: Some formulas contain vitamins; others need them added. We will discuss this with you.

Bowels Babies have varying patterns for bowel movements. At first movements may be very frequent—with every feeding, 6 to 8 times a day. But with time they may taper off to one a day or one every 2 to 3 days. The first bowel movements are black and sticky. Within a few days they turn to a light yellow-green and have soft, pasty consistency.

Sleeping Infants usually sleep between 20 and 22 hours a day. This tapers off as they grow older. Some babies seem to need less sleep than others.

The baby may sleep in a bassinet, basket, or crib beside your bed or in a separate room, if you like.

The crib should have a firm mattress and be covered with a waterproof covering. No pillow is needed. In chilly weather it is wise to put the baby in sleepers with feet or in nighties with tied-in bottoms in case the covers are kicked off.

Bathing Until the navel and circumcision are healed the baby needs only a sponge bath. Then the baby may be propped in a small tub of water and washed with a mild soap. Be careful since a wet baby is slippery.

Cord care: The cord will dry and fall off in the first 3 weeks. The cord can be kept dry by dropping 70 percent rubbing alcohol from a cotton ball on the navel 2 or 3 times each day.

Skin care: The skin at the creases may be dry and flaky. This condition usually disappears by itself or with a small application of petroleum jelly or mineral oil. A small amount of baby powder or cornstarch may be applied to the diaper area.

Scalp care: The baby's head should be washed daily. Later with soap, use firm finger pressure over the entire scalp (including the soft spot) and rinse. If you wish to use oil, apply it right before the baby's bath; comb the hair with a fine baby comb and wash.

Circumcision care: Circumcision is the removal of extra skin from the end of the penis. Some doctors leave a small plastic ring around the penis. This will fall off by itself after several days. The penis is frequently red and swollen for a day or two. Frequently the diaper will show a trace of blood. The area should be kept clean and as dry as possible. Sometimes a small amount of petroleum jelly also helps.

Clothing Keep it comfortable and simple. In summer, remember babies get warm, too.

Washing: Diapers and clothes should be washed in Ivory soap, rinsed well, and if possible, hung in the sun to dry. Avoid detergents, water softeners, and presoaks. They cause rashes. Diapers may be soaked in a solution of borax (½ cup to 1 gallon of water) while awaiting washing. Additional rinses (or a final vinegar rinse) also help.

Safety Support the head when picking the baby up or holding the baby. Do not leave the baby unattended on the bed, sofa, or sink. Do not use a pillow in the crib. Always test the bath water before placing the baby in the tub. This can be done by dipping the wrist or elbow in the water to make certain it is not too hot.

Suggested Reading For further information on the newborn, we suggest:

Infants and Mothers, Differences in Development, by T. Berry Brazelton, chapters 1 and 2.

Baby and Child Care, by Benjamin Spock.

THE 1-MONTH-OLD

Development

1 Physically your baby will change a good deal within the first 4 to 5 weeks.

- **a** Your baby will gain between 1½ to 2 lbs in weight.
- **b** The skin will be prettier, begin to look pink and smooth and not so large on the frame.
- **c** The head will continue to be flat and funny-shaped.
- **d** The eyes will no longer be puffy and red. Your baby will be keeping them open for longer times and looking at you.
- **e** The navel and circumcision will be completely healed.

f When lying on their stomachs, babies will be able to lift their heads off the bed.

2 By now you will know if your baby is very active, very placid and quiet, or different each day.

a Your baby may begin to have preferences when awake—prefer being held upright over your shoulder or on one side, or on the stomach.

b You will begin to see quick smiles that do not always happen while the baby is asleep.

c Now the baby will watch your face for a few seconds at a time and may even follow a toy for a short distance.

Discussion

Feeding By now you and the baby have a schedule or routine that is generally followed. You know that the baby usually eats every 3 to 4 hours and will fuss right up to the time the nipple slides past the lips. If babies are hungry, they cannot wait a minute. By this time some babies give up one bottle at night; others require one or two bottles at night to make it through.

Bowels The baby may still be having a bowel movement with each feeding, or the movements may begin to be less frequent. The bowel movements should be yellow and have a soft, pasty consistency, but the baby may grunt and make facial grimaces while having a bowel movement.

Sleeping The baby is still sleeping most of the 24 hours, but during the waking hours is definitely awake and beginning to notice the surroundings.

Bathing By now the baby can be propped in a small tub of water for the bath. The baby does not enjoy the bath and cries through most of it. Be certain to wash the head well with each bath to avoid cradle cap.

Play It is important to play with your baby. Much of babies' pleasure comes from people doing things with them. You both will enjoy it if you hold, rock, sing to, and talk to your baby.

Safety Outside air is good for the baby, but do not leave the baby in direct sunshine. Babies' tender skin burns easily and quickly. Keep plastic bags, safety pins, and buttons out of the crib. Avoid propping the bottle; the baby can spit up milk and inhale it.

Suggested Reading For further information on the 1-month-old, we suggest:

Infants and Mothers, Differences in Development, by T. Berry Brazelton, chap. 3.

THE 2-MONTH-OLD

Development

1 Physically, by 2 months your baby is beginning to look like the magazine pictures of newborns. The body is filling out and looking a little chubby. The skin is pink, smooth, and soft, and the eyes are settling on a color.

   a The baby is still gaining weight, and the slight plumpness and lovely skin come from getting enough fluids to fill out the tissues.

   b While the eyes will still cross or one eye may roll to the outer socket area, the baby can for short periods of time focus both eyes on one object. Your baby will gaze at your face for long moments. If a bright toy is carried past the baby's face, the baby will follow it, sometimes to 180°.

   c If placed on the stomach, the baby will hold the head up 90° and look around.

   d When held on your lap, the baby is beginning to now hold the head more steady above the shoulders.

   e The hands still have a good tight grasp, and if a rattle is placed in the palm, the baby will hold it and wave it for a moment or so.

2 The baby is rapidly becoming a social being.

   a If someone talks or looks at the baby, the baby will coo and gurgle back.

   b The baby likes to smile and will do so if anyone approaches.

   c Babies now definitely prefer being held upright or being propped upright so they can view their world. They can become quite vocal about being laid in bed away from all activity.

Discussion

Feeding By 2 months, feeding is usually going smoothly. Babies may be very hungry for some feedings and refuse others because they are uninterested.

Around 6 weeks, babies sometimes have a sudden jump in appetite. For the formula baby this just requires adding another ounce to each bottle. For the breastfed baby this means a day or two of extra feedings until mother's body can produce the extra milk. Then she can return to the usual 3- to 4-hour schedule.

Bowels If new foods are being added to the diet, the bowel patterns, consistency, and color will change.

Sleeping During this period babies frequently go to bed with little fuss and may be sleeping through the night. They may also be shortening morning and afternoon nap times and so are awake more during the day.

Bathing By now they may begin to enjoy the bath—splashing, cooing, enjoying the water, and playing.

Play Your baby and you should enjoy playing. Let the baby listen to the radio. Let the baby kick with no clothing on. Put up a bright-colored mobile or bright-colored picture by the crib. Let the baby look out the window at the bright lights.

Safety Always check the bath water before placing the baby in the tub. The baby may be traveling more with the family by now and should have a car bed or be held. Never place the baby on the seat without securing.

Suggested Reading For further information on the 2-month-old, we suggest:

Infants and Mothers, Differences in Development, by T. Berry Brazelton, chap. 4.

THE 3-MONTH-OLD

Development

1 Physically the 3-month-old is getting cuter all the time as the body continues to fill out and get rounder.

- **a** The baby will continue to gain weight by 1 or 2 lbs a month.
- **b** With the possible exceptions of diaper rash, prickly heat, or cradle cap, the skin is soft, smooth, and pink.
- **c** The eyes still wander in different directions, but they focus for longer periods of time.
- **d** The saliva glands in the mouth begin producing saliva. The baby does not know how to swallow this and so begins to drool.
- **e** Babies may have discovered their fingers, and frequently stick them in their mouths and suck for pleasure and contentment.

2 Babies of this age are becoming more sociable all the time.

- **a** They like to laugh and squeal and make little noises. They will do this by themselves for their own entertainment, or if someone will talk with them.
- **b** They like to look at bright objects—mobiles over the bed, bright curtains, bright pillows.

Discussion

Feeding By this time the formula routine is well established. The baby may be ready to try new textures and tastes in some solid foods. The tongue-thrusting movement should be gone, making spoon eating much more enjoyable for the baby and you.

Bowels Most bowel patterns will have tapered off to one or two movements per day or one every other day. Babies who are on breast only may be having one bowel movement every few days.

Sleeping The baby should be sleeping more at night and less during the day. However, some babies that have been sleeping through the night may have a period of waking during the night, crying, and wanting an extra bottle. This can be very disturbing if you have just adjusted to sleeping through the night. Usually it corrects itself in several weeks. If the baby has been sleeping in your room, now is a good time to consider a separate room. The cry is certainly loud enough to let you know if the baby needs you.

Bathing The baby should be enjoying the bath and splashing and water play.

Play This is an important activity for your baby. Let the baby splash and kick in the bath. Talk and sing to the baby; let the baby listen to the radio. Let the baby hold a rattle, shake it, and drop it.

Safety Never leave your baby unattended. The only safe place to leave your baby is in the crib with the rails up, on the floor, or in the playpen. A baby can scoot off the sofa or bed in a second.

THE 4-MONTH-OLD

Development

1 Physically the 4-month-old is round and firm. The baby is not fat, but just well built and looking like the babies in advertisements.

- **a** At this age babies may like movement—being bounced on a lap or held in a standing position on their own wobbly legs.
- **b** They have tried rolling over and probably done it once or twice to their own surprise.
- **c** If placed on their tummies, they will rise up on their elbows for a better look at the world, or they may arch their backs and move their arms and legs as if swimming. This becomes a type of play.
- **d** They are now able to focus on some object in front of them and reach for it. If the object is big, they may be able to grasp it with a wide scoop of the arm and hand.
- **e** They discover that they have hands and may spend long minutes looking at their hands and touching them.

2 Socially they are developing into noticeable members of the family.
   a They love to squeal, coo, laugh, and babble—either to themselves or for someone else's enjoyment.
   b They recognize family members with their verbal noises, but are willing to go to almost anyone who will hold them and give them some attention.
   c They like attention and being with the family and are likely to protest when placed in a room by themselves.
   d They definitely like the sitting position and need to be propped with pillows on the floor, seated in a little infant seat, or held some of each day.

Discussion

Feeding Feedings should be going smoothly, and the baby can be eased toward a schedule of three meals and a bedtime snack. The baby should not be taking more than 32 oz. of formula each day (four 8-oz. bottles). But if the baby is taking this and asking for more, try increasing the solid foods. The baby will probably be drooling all the time and need a bib and frequent dabs at the chin. If the baby gets a rash, a little petroleum jelly sometimes helps to protect the skin.

Bowels Bowel movements may change consistency with more solid foods. Green vegetables may give looser, green stools, while red vegetables may give red stools.

Sleeping The baby may sleep through the night.

Play At this age babies are more fun to play with all the time. They are now learning to entertain themselves for short periods. Place your baby on the stomach on the floor and put bright objects (rattle, plastic cup, spoon, blocks) where the baby can see and reach for them.

Give your baby time lying down to do the rocking, swimming movements. Prop your baby up in the room with the family to watch the activity and have time to explore his or her own hands.

Safety Since babies at this age are now reaching, avoid hanging strings or mobiles that your baby can touch.

Babies are now strong enough to tip an infant seat to the side. The seat can be used if placed on the floor.

Always keep a hand on your baby in the tub—babies slip easily. Be watchful of safety pins, buttons, coins, and small objects which the baby could swallow.

Suggested Reading For further information on the 4-month-old, we suggest:

Infants and Mothers, Differences in Development, by T. Berry Brazelton, chaps. 5 and 6.

Better Homes and Gardens Baby Book, by the editors of *Better Homes and Gardens,* chaps. 10 and 11.

A Doctor Discusses the Care and Development of Your Baby, by May Guy and Miriam Gilbert, chap. 7.

THE 5-MONTH-OLD

Development

1 Physically the 5-month-old is a bundle of activity and movement.

- **a** The eyes focus most of the time except when the baby is tired.
- **b** Babies can now coordinate their eyes, fingers, and mouths for exploring their world, and when this fails they show their frustration.
- **c** They will sit erect with some support.
- **d** They reach for everything they can see and put everything they can reach in their mouths.
- **e** They will transfer a toy from one hand to the other.

2 The 5-month-old is a very social being.

- **a** At this age babies babble to themselves or anyone who will listen. They soon discover several consonants and vowels and find that combinations of "Dadadada" or "Babababa" bring great rewards from the family.
- **b** The span of attention is longer. Babies may be content to play in a chair or propped up for 30 to 60 minutes with only occasional help from the family.
- **c** They may hold out their arms to their mothers when they want to be picked up.

Discussion

Feeding Eating is messy because babies of this age like to help. They like to hold their own bottles, grab for spoons, and feel the food squeeze through their fingers. They also learn to blow bubbles with a mouthful—usually of spinach or beets or something highly colored.

Bowels The bowel movements will change as the food changes.

Sleeping Babies now generally sleep through the night, but may begin to waken early because there is so much to be done in one day. They may waken and play quietly in the crib for awhile, or they may waken and let the whole household know they are ready to go.

Playing They like to play—with their hands and feet, their food, and their toys. They like to watch and reach for bright objects (rattles, blocks, plastic spoons, metal cups).

They like to make noise—bang two blocks together, bang a spoon on the table.

Safety Keep all small objects—safety pins, buttons, coins, beads—out of sight. If you must leave your baby alone, the only safe places are in the crib, on the floor, or in a playpen. The infant seat will tip very easily with your baby's constant twistings and turning; it is best to avoid using it.

THE 6-MONTH-OLD

Development

1 A good deal of control has been gained by the time a baby is 6 months old.

- **a** Babies can now hold their heads in line when they are pulled to a sitting position; they can reach for objects, roll over, scoot around, and sit up by themselves.
- **b** The eyes almost never cross or wander as they focus on the surrounding world.
- **c** Babies like activity and are in constant motion during most of the day and often even in sleep.
- **d** Placed in a bouncing seat, they will stand for moments with support.
- **e** Your baby may be getting the first tooth.
- **f** Everything goes in the mouth, including the feet.

2 Babies are learning control in social behavior during this time.

- **a** They learn that some sounds, like "Mamamama" may bring mother on the run.
- **b** Separation anxiety begins, and they cry when left alone in the room.
- **c** They like talking to themselves or anyone who will listen.

Discussion

Feeding Feeding is still messy since the 6-month-old likes to help and actively participate in the process. If they are getting teeth or getting ready to get teeth, they like chewing. They can handle pretzels, zwieback, crisp toast, crackers, or items for just biting, like teething rings, cold toys, spoons.

Bowels If this is the time whole milk is introduced, the bowel movements may change (become softer, firmer; more frequent, less frequent).

Since the 6-month-old is such a bundle of activity, changing the diapers often becomes a hassle because the baby will not lie still long enough. Speed always helps, but sometimes a toy or extra talking to during the process will help.

Sleeping Some babies are so active that they seem to practice their new motor activities even in their sleep. They may be so tired they fall asleep sitting up, but protest every time they are laid horizontal. Gentle, firm help into bed usually makes them relax for a moment—long enough for sleep to come. They generally need a nap.

Playing At this stage babies play and work all day long. The days are not long enough. They like to bounce in a bounce chair or swing and try standing, and they like to reach, pick up, bang and drop objects—rattles, blocks, metal cups, metal spoons, balls, pans, and lids.

Safety With the sudden motor activity, it is time to look around the house and see what your baby can get into. If you cannot watch your baby, the floor, full-sized bed, and yard are unsafe. Do not leave your baby for a second in the bath, and do make certain the faucets stay out of reach. Check toys to be certain that dropping will not split them or leave sharp edges. Keep all small objects—buttons, pins, coins, peanuts—out of reach. Do not hold your baby while you smoke cigarettes or drink hot liquids, since a sudden movement may cause you to burn the baby.

Suggested Reading For further information on the 6-month-old, we suggest:

Infants and Mothers, Differences in Development, by T. Berry Brazelton, chap. 7.

The Magic Years, by Selma Fraiberg, chap. 2, pp. 35–56.

A Doctor Discusses the Care and Development of Your Baby, by May Guy and Miriam Bilbert, chap. 8.

THE 7- TO 9-MONTH OLD

Development

1 Physically these will be happy contented months of concentrated learning of motor activities.

- **a** Some babies scoot backward and forward; others actually master the art of crawling. This gives them instant mobility, and they can move with real speed.
- **b** Babies will work on moving around more quickly and more smoothly and will cover more territory. They may crawl, scoot, or just roll over and over, but they will learn to cover a lot of ground in a hurry.
- **c** They reach for all objects and can transfer an item from one hand to the other.

d They learn to pick up tiny objects with their thumbs and forefingers.

e Using their new-found hand coordination, they learn to pull themselves to standing and find they take many bumps when their hands and legs suddenly give out and they sit very abruptly.

2 This period is also a busy time for social adjustments.

a Their increased ability to sit up and a need to be with the family may make this the time to try a high chair. Even if babies are not eating, they may want to join the family at mealtimes, and a high chair in the kitchen may keep them out from under foot during meal preparation.

b Babies chew on everything—fingers, toes, toys, crackers.

c They touch everything—including their own bodies. As they discovered their hands earlier, they now discover their genitalia and may play with the area at every diaper change and bath. With time, the novelty wears off, and they move on to play with other things.

d They go through a period of definitely knowing Mommy and preferring her to anyone else. Babies cry whenever anyone else picks them up. This is called stranger anxiety. Some babies barely show this stage, and others very definitely demonstrate their anxiety. It usually passes with time.

e A playpen will contain babies of this age for only so long before they cry to get out.

f They may show an interest in something for as long as 20 minutes. That means the mother's day is divided into 20-minute sections.

g They like to babble and seem to carry on entire conversations with no words.

Discussion

Feeding Babies of this age have definite likes and dislikes and let you know with a shake of the head, clenched mouth, and dumped food. They like to help feed themselves, and finger foods work best—crackers, toast, hot dogs, banana pieces, dry cereals.

Bowels Bowel movements should be firmer and less frequent and may have a routine pattern. Babies may verbally fuss with a wet or dirty diaper.

Sleeping At this age babies will sleep through the night, but it is sometimes a chore to get them to bed, since they do not want to stop whatever they are doing. They may take two or three naps per day, or they may begin balking at the morning nap. The crib will still contain them at this stage, but they can rock it with violent movements when they want to. If they have several teeth, they may learn to grind them, which is always annoying. Sometimes they will do it just as they are going to sleep. This habit usually passes with time.

Playing Let your baby practice finger control. Put half a dozen flakes of cereal on the tray of the high chair and let the baby push them around, pick them up, and drop them. Babies love to drop things, hear them hit, and then have someone pick them up. That may be okay for a while. Then tie several items to the high chair, and show the baby how to retrieve them.

Babies like to be destructive; let your baby crumple wax paper or tissue paper or shred an old magazine. They like to make noise; let your baby play with the metal pots and pans, spoons, measuring cups. They like to take things apart; give your baby a metal coffee pot, a set of measuring cups. They will stack, drop, and chew on blocks.

Safety At this stage, babies are beginning to learn the meaning of the word "no," but they cannot be trusted to always obey. Say the word and remove your child from the danger. This will have to be repeated *many* times.

With your baby's greater mobility, you need to look around the house for new dangers. Electrical sockets need to be covered with safety plugs. Remove breakables from low tables and remove hanging tablecloths. Use guards to protect your baby from floor and wall heaters, stairs, and fireplaces. Do not iron when the baby is crawling around the floor. Do not leave peanuts, popcorn, small pieces of carrots around—your baby can choke on them. Never leave your baby alone in the house, and do not turn your back on the baby in the kitchen unless he is in the high chair. Use the strap on the high chair so the baby will not slip or crawl out.

Suggested Reading For further information on the 7- to 9-month-old, we suggest:

Infants and Mothers, Differences in Development, by T. Berry Brazelton, chaps. 9, 10, 11.

Better Homes and Gardens Baby Book, by the editors of *Better Homes and Gardens,* chap. 12.

THE 10- TO 12-MONTH-OLD

Development

1 Physically the last 2 months of the 1st year are used to polish up some of the activities the baby tried earlier but did not do very well.

- **a** At this age, babies are very good at crawling or scooting around and soon discover they can walk holding onto the furniture.
- **b** They may try letting go and just standing and then taking the first shaky steps, or they may wait until after their first birthday.
- **c** By this time some babies begin to perceive heights and will test for distance (like backing off the sofa to see if their feet will touch the

ground, and, if not, scrambling back up the sofa), while others are in such a hurry they do not bother.

2 The baby's integration into the social world continues rapidly.

- **a** Babies of this age will display definite moods with some days being "good days" and others a pain for mother and child.
- **b** They learn to like music and may rock with it when they are sitting or standing.
- **c** They understand simple directions and sometimes will carry them out and other times ignore them.
- **d** When they want to, they can help in dressing by sticking out arms or legs. Other times you can dress them if you can catch them.
- **e** They learn to wave good-bye and may do so on command.
- **f** They learn how to separate from their mothers. They may play peek-a-boo or crawl around a corner and then peek back to see if mother is still there. By a year the baby can lose a toy and go hunt for it instead of just forgetting it.
- **g** They may have special blankets or toys that go to bed with them and are dragged all other places.
- **h** They have simple vocabularies of "Mamma," "DaDa," "no," and several other words.

Discussion

Feeding Their likes and dislikes continue, but they may change their minds from week to week. Table foods may be more appealing, especially if they have several teeth. They like to feed themselves and are best with the finger foods, but they try spoons and cups. This can be messy.

They may show signs of giving up the bottle, or they may still cling to it. Usually the last bottle to go is the night bottle. Since the baby has teeth, the bottle should contain only water because the milk sugar dripping over the teeth all night will rot the front teeth.

At about 1 year the appetite may drop sharply. The baby will eat one good meal and refuse all others. The baby is not growing as rapidly and is too busy to eat.

Bowels Bowel movements may be coming in routine patterns, and the baby may let you know when the diaper needs changing. But the baby probably will not be interested in toilet training. If you are, it can be done, but it is much easier if you can wait until the child is ready.

Sleeping Some babies go to bed very peacefully; others fight every night to stay up. Your baby may be able to crawl out of the crib, even with the rails up, and can make a great deal of racket in bed by screaming, rocking, and shaking the entire bed.

Playing At this stage babies like to play with someone—peek-a-boo, pat-a-cake, bye-bye. Their increased coordination makes nesting toys fascinating—a set of measuring cups, stacked blocks, graduated rings on a stand. They like to put things into containers and take them out—old-fashioned clothespins in metal bread pans, all the paper out of the wastebasket, spoons in a pan.

Babies like to touch and feel things. A texture box is fun—put pieces of velvet, silk, fur, and sandpaper in a box, and let the baby feel the different textures.

Safety Check the kitchen; remove from under the sink all detergents, cleaners, solvents, and poisonous liquids. Put them up high or get rid of them. When the stove or electrical appliances (coffee pot, toaster) are being used, put your baby in the high chair. In the bathroom, lock up all medicines, drain cleaners, and soaps or get rid of them. Guard the stairs with railings and gates. If you take your baby bicycle riding, check to see that the child's feet cannot reach the spokes.

Suggested Reading For further information on the 10- to 12-month old, we suggest:

Infants and Mothers, Differences in Development, by T. Berry Brazelton, chaps. 12, 13, 14.

The Magic Years, by Selma Fraiberg, chap. 3.

Better Homes and Gardens Baby Book, by the editors of *Better Homes and Gardens,* chap. 13.

THE 13- TO 16-MONTH-OLD

Development

1 Physically babies will not be changing as much as they did earlier.

- **a** The weight tends to become more stable. They do not gain as much each month.
- **b** They work on walking more smoothly and with more balance.
- **c** They may learn to climb. Then they will climb everything in sight.
- **d** Their small muscles become more controlled. They learn to hold a cup, stack one block on top of another, and get food on a spoon and to their mouths.
- **e** In their rush to perfect their motor skills, they try many times and fail, but this does not bother them. They are often clumsy and fall frequently but get right up and try again.

2 Socially they are much more mature and generally fun to have around. Civilization moves in to socialize them.

a They learn about independence and want to do things for themselves and have a choice in matters. They learn to say "no," but that is not what they may mean.

b They become explorers with real zeal—they want to look into everything, touch everything, and try everything, and they will protest if stopped.

c They like other children but play alone.

d The vocabulary increases to four to eight words, and they babble a lot to themselves or anyone who will listen.

e In their drive for independence they may discover the temper tantrum and use it effectively if mother does not catch on to the act.

f Despite their growing independence, they will have days of dependence when they want to be with Mommy all day, do not want to venture out, or become suddenly shy of any new idea or face.

Discussion

Feeding The appetite may be appreciably less since they seem to eat and run. They like table foods and really need to have only meat cut in small bites. Make servings small so your baby has the satisfaction of finishing. Give your baby easy-to-handle utensils—nonbreakable dishes, small forks and knives.

Mealtime should be happy—babies of this age can be allowed to eat with the family as long as they do not have to sit through an entire meal. A sturdy, comfortable chair that places the baby at the table level is handy.

Bowels Now babies may let you know when they have a bowel movement, but they mention it after the fact. Your baby may show a passing interest in a potty chair, but toilet training is easier if you can wait a little longer.

Sleeping Some babies take one morning and one afternoon nap, and some protest the morning one and take a longer afternoon nap. They still cling to their "security" blankets and may insist on taking all their favorite toys to bed with them. They may be very pleasant up to bedtime and then struggle. Usually it is best to decide how much you will give in, and then be firm.

Playing At this age, babies are active and on the run all the time. They like to play in the water—tub, sink, toilet bowl, hose—but they need supervision in any of these areas. They like soft, cuddly toys—dolls, teddy bears, stuffed animals. They like to help their mothers with work—dusting, wiping dishes, picking up, sweeping. They like pull-push toys—a wagon, duck on a string, push balls on a stick. They like balls—big ones, little ones.

Safety If babies are to play outside, they need a fenced yard and constant watching. Streets are a big danger, as are driveways. Check the garage and basement for kerosine, cleaners, paints, solvents. Either lock them up or discard them. Check the kitchen for knives, scissors, matches, lighters. Do not leave the baby alone—in the house, in the bathtub, or in the yard.

Suggested Reading For further information on the 13- to 16-month old, we suggest:

Baby and Child Care, by Benjamin Spock.

FEEDING—FORMULA FEEDING

Feeding your baby a formula is one of the nicest and best ways of loving him. Your baby may take a prepared formula or a milk formula (using evaporated milk, sugar, and water). The following are some hints that may make the feeding more efficient and a happy time for you and the baby.

Preparation

Formula Prepared formulas can be purchased ready-to-feed, concentrated (equal parts of water are added), or powdered (1 scoop of powder to 2 oz. of water).

Evaporated milk is usually mixed 13 oz. of canned milk to 19 oz. of water and 2 tablespoons of sugar.

When the baby first comes home from the hospital, the formula may be divided into bottles as it is made or kept in a large container and poured into a bottle with each feeding. Each bottle generally contains the following amounts: newborn to 1 month: 2 to 3 oz.; 1 to 2 months: 3 to 4 oz.; 3 to 4 months: 4 to 5 oz.; 4 to 5 months: 5 to 6 oz. or more as the infant seems hungry.

Equipment

8 bottles and nipples
1 bottle brush
1 measuring cup
1 measuring spoon
1 sterilizing kettle
1 pair tongs

Sterilization As long as your have clean hands, clean equipment, and a good water supply, there is no need to sterilize bottles. However, if you wish to sterilize, we recommend the terminal sterilization method:

Wash hands.
Wash equipment and bottles with good soap and hot water.
Prepare formula and divide into bottles—place the nipple on loosely.
Place the bottles in a large kettle, add 2 in. of water.
Cover.
Once the water boils, boil for 20 minutes.
Let cool with the lid on.
Tighten the caps and nipples.
Refrigerate.

The Feeding

1 Your baby enjoys being held during feeding. It is good for you to take a break. Find a comfortable chair, put your feet up, and enjoy this time with your baby.

2 Hold the bottle at such an angle that the nipple is always filled with milk. This allows less air to get in the baby's stomach.

3 Use an extra diaper for a burping cloth and to wipe at the baby's chin. The baby should be burped half way through the bottle and after finishing or whenever it seems necessary.

4 Within 1 or 2 weeks a routine will be established, and the baby will probably be hungry every 3 to 4 hours.

5 If some formula is left in the bottle after the feeding, return it to the refrigerator. Formula left out over 1 hour needs to be discarded.

FEEDING—BREAST FEEDING

Breast feeding is one of the nicest ways you can feed your baby. The following are some hints that may make the feedings more comfortable and happier for you and the baby.

Your Health

1 You may eat most foods while you are nursing, and you should try to get some of the basic four each day: meat and eggs, fruits and vegetables, dairy products, and cereals. Onions, chocolates, and cabbage sometimes irritate babies and should be tried with caution. However, many babies have no trouble with these foods.

2 Some medicines are passed through the milk. Check with your doctor about specific medications.

3 Do drink plenty of liquids: water, juice, beer, milk, coffee, tea.

4 Do try to get enough rest.

5 Nipple care: Nipples need no extra bathing other than during your regular bath. If you wish, the nipples may be washed with clean water and wiped dry with a cotton ball before the feeding. For mild tenderness to the nipple, a thin coating of ointment can be applied after each nursing: A&D ointment, pure lanolin, or petroleum jelly is good for this. Expose your nipples to the air either by going topless for a brief period of time or by inserting small tea strainers (with handles removed) in each bra cup.

The Feeding

1 Make yourself comfortable—after all, this is your time with the baby. Try lying down, sitting, holding the baby in different positions. Put your feet up.

2 Begin slowly. Some babies are eager; some are procrastinators; some need coaxing; and some are too sleepy to care about anything the first few days. The baby has to get used to feeding, and your nipples have to get used to the sucking and pulling.

3 Start on one side for 1 minute and then go to the other side. The time may be increased each day to about 10 minutes a side. Usually you start on one side, burp the baby, and finish on the opposite side. The last breast should be completely emptied. At the next feeding start with the last breast. Most babies get 90 percent of the milk within the first 7 minutes of nursing, but many enjoy and need the extra sucking and may suck for as long as 20 minutes on the last breast. For a baby who needs extra sucking, a pacifier may help.

4 The more you nurse, the more milk you will have. It takes several days to 2 weeks to get the routine established. Once the routine is established, your baby will probably be hungry every 3 to 4 hours. Sometimes in establishing the milk, the breasts are full before the baby is hungry, and the nipples will drip milk. Additional absorbent shields for the bra will avoid any embarrassment of wet clothing. To increase the milk production, put the baby to breast more frequently and for longer periods. Usually this will increase the flow within 1 or 2 days.

5 Supplemental feeding. We feel your baby should know how to use a baby bottle in case you wish to go out for an evening. This can be accomplished by offering water from a bottle.

Suggested Reading For further information on breast feeding, we suggest:

The Womanly Art of Breastfeeding, by the La Leche League.
Baby and Child Care, by Benjamin Spock.
If you need someone to talk to or have more questions, answered, please call us.

FEEDING—BEGINNING SOLIDS

Your baby can grow and be perfectly happy on formula for the first 6 months of life. However, many mothers feel their babies are hungrier and would like to try solid foods before then. There is a large selection of commercially prepared baby foods on the market.

The Method

Babies have to become accustomed to new tastes and textures. During the first 6 to 8 weeks of life the infant's tongue is well adapted for sucking a nipple but not for taking food from a spoon. The infant has a tendency to push all solid food out of the mouth; therefore the spoon must be placed far enough back on the tongue so the baby can swallow the food but not choke on it. This procedure is much easier once the baby loses the tongue-thrusting movement.

As with any new thing, start slowly—one new food per week.

A Sample Schedule

Day 1: Mix 1 teaspoon of cereal with a little formula. Use a small spoon and place the food toward the back of the mouth. Try feeding the new food when you both have time to enjoy it—not at a time when the baby is crying for milk. Sometimes giving an ounce of milk first takes the edge off the hunger and enables the baby to try something new. But do not give the whole bottle, or the baby will be too worn out and full to try the new solid food.

Day 2: If the baby took the food well (did not develop a rash or diarrhea), you can increase the food to 2 teaspoons.

Day 3: Increase the food to 3 teaspoons.

Day 4: Try 3 teaspoons of food for several days, and then increase to a small bowl as the baby's appetite increases.

Infants begin eating every 4 hours, but the general goal is for the child to have three meals a day.

Birth to 2 months: six feedings (about 6 A.M., 10 A.M., 2 P.M., 6 P.M., 10 P.M., and 2 A.M.)

4 to 6 months: four feedings (breakfast, lunch, supper, and bedtime)

The Foods

There are many ways of starting new foods. But the following schedule usually works well. We will discuss times to begin these.

Cereal: Start with rice, barley, or oatmeal. Whole wheat and mixed cereal can be tried after 6 months.

Fruits: Start with applesauce, pears, peaches, bananas, plums, prunes, or cherries. Apricots can be tried later.

Vegetables: Start with carrots, squash, sweet potatoes, spinach, peas, or beets.

Meats: Start with beef, chicken, and lamb. Pork, veal, and ham can be tried later.

Some General Guides

1 It is generally best to try a new food by itself. Do not try mixed fruits until you are certain the baby can tolerate all the fruits alone.

2 Generally orange juice, wheat cereal, and egg yolks are started after the baby is 6 months old because after that age the baby is less likely to be allergic to these foods.

3 Around 6 months some babies like foods to chew on—teething biscuits, plain cookies, zweiback.

4 Some babies will take pureed foods and then junior baby and then table foods. Others prefer pureed and table foods.

5 Commercial baby foods come in all varieties. A jar of baby meat is all meat. A jar of meat-vegetable dinner has more meat than vegetables. A jar of vegetable-meat dinner has nearly all vegetables and very little meat.

6 Around 6 to 8 months babies can have juices (apple, grape, cherry). These can be bought in small cans or in large containers for the entire family. There is no nutritional advantage to baby cans, but they may be more convenient.

7 Mothers with blenders often prefer to prepare their own pureed food. Some foods, like bananas, can be mashed with a fork.

Weaning

1 Babies usually stay on formula or breast milk until they are between 4 and 8 months old.

2 If it is easier for the family routine, a bottle-fed baby can be switched to whole milk or 2 percent milk around 4 to 6 months.

3 Some mothers prefer to leave the baby on formula for 8 to 12 months and then switch to whole milk and a cup.

4 If the baby is ready, giving up the bottle or breast is usually very simple. If the baby is not ready, weaning may be a struggle.

5 Weaning (either from breast to bottle or cup or from bottle to cup) should be a gradual process. Let us discuss with you some ways of making it more comfortable for you and the baby.

COLIC

No one really knows what colic is, and there is no fast cure for it. But it happens with a lot of babies and is most upsetting to the baby and the parents. It does go away after awhile.

Signs of Colic

Crying—sometimes for short periods, sometimes for long periods. The crying may seem to happen at the same time every day—every morning at 10 o'clock, or every evening at 5 P.M. as you are trying to get dinner ready.

Fussing and irritability—the baby just does not seem comfortable in any position.

Drawing the legs up to the stomach as if in pain.

Passing gas.

What You Can Do

Check to see whether the baby is hungry, is wet, has an open safety pin sticking him, is lying in an uncomfortable position, or has a bubble. If none of the above conditions is causing the crying, try some of the following:

Change the baby's position, e.g., from stomach to side or back.
Hold the baby—often over the shoulder seems to help.
Rock the baby.
Walk with the baby.
Prop the baby up in a sitting position.
Place a *warm* water bottle on the baby's tummy.
Try a little sugar water.
Try a pacifier.
Try some kind of monotonous, soothing noise—music, a metronome, a loud clock.

When to Call for Help

Seek help if you have tried all the above without success or if you think the baby is sick, that is, has fever, is not eating as usual, has diarrhea, or has vomiting.

Suggested Reading

For further information on colic, we suggest:

Baby and Child Care, by Benjamin Spock.

IMMUNIZATIONS

Your baby will have a series of shots for protection from certain diseases. You should keep a record of which shots your baby receives and when they are given so that the series can be continued and not have to be restarted.

What Your Baby Will Get

DPT: This is a series of three shots plus a booster. This protects your baby against diptheria, whooping cough, and tetanus.

Polio: These are not shots, but drops on the tongue. Your baby will get a series of three plus a booster.

Measles: This is one shot and protects your baby against "hard" measles.

Rubella: This is one shot and protects your baby against German measles.

Mumps: This is one shot. Sometimes mumps, rubella, and measles are combined into a single shot.

Tine test: This is not a shot at all, but a small prick that tells whether the child has been exposed to tuberculosis. This test should be done around 6 to 9 months of age and every 2 years thereafter.

Schedule of Shots

DPT and polio
DPT and polio (usually 8 weeks later)
DPT and polio (8 weeks later)

Tine test (around 6 to 9 months of age)
DPT and polio boosters (around 18 months)
Measles, rubella, mumps (around 1 year)

Reaction to Shots

Many babies show no reaction to their shots.

Some babies become fretful and irritable for 24 hours after the shot, show a fever of 101 to 103°F for 24 hours, and show a hard, reddened, or swollen injection site.

A few babies develop a fine red rash over their bodies 1 to 2 weeks after receiving a measles shot.

What You Can Do

For fretfulness—extra holding, rocking, and loving

For a fever—a lukewarm bath and one dose of Tempra, Tylenol, or baby aspirin (ask us about the dose)

For a swollen injection site—a warm, wet washcloth applied several times to the site

When to Call Us

Call us if your baby is fretful and irritable for more than 24 hours, if your baby's fever is higher than 103°F or stays longer than 24 hours, or if your baby develops vomiting or diarrhea.

DIAPER RASHES

Most babies will have a diaper rash sometime during their diaper-wearing days.

Prevention of Diaper Rash

1 Change the diaper as soon as it is wet, if possible.
2 When changing the diaper, wash the area with clear water (soap if soiled), and dry between the skin folds.
3 A thin layer of lubrication can be applied—A&D ointment, Desitin, Vaseline, or Diaperene.
4 Limit plastic pants to outings and special occasions.
5 Try disposable diapers with caution. They can be very handy for babies when traveling, but they do tend to hold the warm, wet urine close to the skin and allow diaper rashes to get worse. Some babies can tolerate diapers very well.
6 Launder diapers with care.
    a Soiled diapers should be soaked in a solution of borax (½ cup to 1 gallon of water) while awaiting washing.
    b Diapers should be washed with a mild soap, such as Ivory. Avoid detergents, water softeners, and some presoaks.

c Diapers should be thoroughly rinsed and vinegar (½ cup) added to the last rinse.

d If possible, hang the diapers to dry in the sun.

Symptoms of a Diaper Rash

1 At first, slightly reddened skin in the area covered by the diaper—may be just in the front or just in the back

2 Later, red bumps that look painful

What You Can Do

1 Leave the diaper off during nap times. Turn the baby on the stomach, place the diaper under the buttock area, and leave the buttocks exposed.

2 Change the diaper as soon as it is wet.

3 Take special care to wash with mild soap and dry the diaper area when changing the diaper.

4 Apply a thin layer of lubrication after each change of diaper.

5 Avoid plastic pants and disposable diapers for several days.

6 Check laundering of diapers with above list.

When To Call the Doctor

Call the doctor if the diaper rash does not seem to improve or if the area looks infected.

SAFETY

Accidents kill more children in the United States than all diseases put together. Many children are also crippled by accidents. Most accidents in young children can be anticipated and prevented. During the 1st year of life, preventing your baby from having an accident is 100 percent your job. You must control the baby's environment totally. By school age, the child can share the responsibility for preventing an accident.

To Help Your Child Learn Self-Protection

Watch your vocabulary. Keep your words simple: "no," "watch out," "stop."

Ration your demands. A child who hears "no" at every turn soon learns to tune it out. Instead of offering a negative command (such as "No, Johnnie, don't sit on that chair") give a positive statement ("Johnnie, come sit on this stool").

Carry out your promises. If you promise to spank a child if she does something once more, you have to spank her when she does it. Then she knows you mean business.

Be consistent. Do not let a child play on the steps today and spank him for it tomorrow.

House Check for Safety

Kitchen A heated stove (either the oven or the burners) can burn. Always turn pot handles toward the back of the stove.

Do not let electrical appliance cords dangle where babies can pull them and get a burn from hot metal and hot food.

Low cabinets and shelves are not the place for detergents, bleaches, cleansers, insect killers, ammonia, furniture polish, and drain uncloggers. Canned goods and pots and pans are safe to play with and can be kept at this low level.

Keep knives, forks, and other cooking tools out of reach. Matches should be kept in a tight-fitting container out of reach. Broken glass, dishes, and tin cases should not be put in the wastebasket if the child has a tendency to remove the contents.

Living Room The child must be watched around the hot pipes, hot radiators, and heaters.

Matches, cigarettes, ash trays, and lighters should be moved to higher levels.

Cords from lamps, radios, and clocks should be well hidden, and sockets should have heavy furniture in front of them or socket covers put over them.

Doors should have screens with locks, and stairs should have protective gates.

Firearms and ammunition should be locked up.

Never iron when the child is awake and crawling around; if you must iron, put the child in the crib or playpen.

Bathroom All medicines should be locked up. Find a high shelf for cosmetics, razor blades, mouth wash, perfumes, shoe polish, and toilet bowl cleaners.

Never leave the child in the tub alone—even for 1 second.

Bedroom Do not keep cosmetics, deodorants, or cleaners in an easily accessible place. Keep sewing baskets, needles, pins, and buttons out of the bedroom. Lock them up out of reach.

Leave the baby only in the crib with the rails pulled up. Babies learn to scoot very early and can move rapidly from the center of a full-size bed to the floor.

Cover all plugs with socket covers.

Do not cover the mattress with plastic or use a plastic clothes bag. Babies can easily remove the sheets and suffocate. Avoid hanging clothes in plastic covers from cleaners.

Garage, Basement, Outdoors Remove to a locked cabinet all rodent and insect killers, kerosine, gasoline, and paint equipment. Store all rakes, hoes, sharp tools, and nails out of reach.

Check the yard and neighborhood for cisterns, wells, swimming pools, ponds, streams, and old refrigerators.

Look before you back the car out of the garage; do not risk running over your own child.

Remove all skates, tricycles, scooters, and rolling equipment from sidewalks and stairs at evening.

Until the child learns to cross the street, do not leave him unattended in the front yard.

Traveling Insist that the child be buckled into the seat with the regular seat belt, a car chair, or a car bed. Never let the child sit in your lap while you are driving. Never let the child stand on the back seat or in the front seat.

Lock all doors before starting the motor.

Do not let the child stick hands or head out of an open window.

Never leave the child alone in a car.

Make certain the child climbs out of the car on the curb side.

If you must reprimand the child while traveling, stop the car first. Do not hit at the child from the front seat while trying to watch traffic.

What to Do in Case of Poisoning

1 Call your doctor and tell him what you think your child has swallowed and how much. Your doctor will advise you what to do.

2 If you have ipecac, your doctor may have you give a dose with water.

3 Keep the jar, bottle, or can that contained the swallowed substance. Your doctor may want to examine it.

SIBLING RIVALRY

Jealousy is a feeling that everyone experiences sometime. The arrival of a new baby in a family gives many chances for jealousy to appear. A child's first experience with jealousy may be the arrival of a new baby and the lesson of having to learn to share the mother and father.

Some Things to Do before the Baby Comes

Make any room changes before the baby comes so that the older child does not feel pushed out.

If the child is getting an adult-sized bed, move him into it before the baby comes so that he does not feel as if the baby is sleeping in *his* crib.

If the child is about to go to nursery school, get him settled and happy in nursery school before the baby comes. Otherwise he will think he is being pushed out of the house so Mommy and the baby can be alone.

Let the child know a baby is coming. For the younger child, the last few months are soon enough; older children may be told earlier and will understand the time lag. Say it will be a baby, not a playmate.

Let the child help you get ready for the baby—pick out new garments, fold clothing, fix the room, the crib, etc.

What to Expect When You Return from the Hospital

For a few hours or days the older child will be interested in the new baby and then will ignore the baby and you or comment that the baby can now return to the hospital.

The older child may make sudden demands for attention. As you sit down to feed the baby, the child may demand a glass of water or do something across the room that requires you to stop the feeding and go to him.

If the child was toilet-trained, he may now suddenly revert to wetting and soiling the pants.

The older child may request a bottle or ask to sit in your lap and try breast feeding.

The older child may begin whining.

Love pats to the baby may become slaps.

What You Can Do

Remember that jealousy is normal, even among adults.

When you are in the hospital, make some contact (a telephone call or small gift) to let the child know you have not forgotten him or her.

On returning from the hospital, let someone else carry in the new baby while you focus your attention on the older child.

Bring a gift home to the older child "from the new baby."

Buy the older child a doll which can be diapered and fed at the same time you diaper and feed the infant.

If the child shows an interest, let him help with the baby by bringing the washcloth, carrying the diapers, etc.

During the first few weeks the new baby will not need your undivided attention, so play down the new arrival and plan on doing things with the older child, emphasizing how nice it is to be big. Talk about the advantages the baby does not have, like staying up later, taking a walk, helping Mommy, etc.

Say as little as possible about the panty wetting and soiling; it will pass.

If the older child wants a bottle, let him have it.

Avoid leaving the two alone.

Help friends and relatives who come to call notice the older child.

Suggested Reading For further information on sibling rivalry, we suggest:

Baby and Child Care, by Benjamin Spock.
The ABC of Child Care, by Allan Fromme, pp. 268–274.
Child Sense, by William Homan, pp. 13–24, 168–174.

TOILET TRAINING

Mothers always feel it is an important milestone once a child is able to go to the bathroom alone. Most children will train themselves if they are showing signs of being ready and they have a little encouragement from their mothers. Usually bowel control comes first (around 1½ to 3 years) and then bladder control (around 2 to 3 years) and finally control at night.

Signs That Your Child Is Ready for Toilet Training

The child is showing some independence—likes to take off some clothing, make a choice of whether to eat a cookie or not, likes to do some things unaided.

The child is pretty good at walking—the same muscles that help a child to walk, climb, stoop, and sit also help relax and tighten the muscles around the rectum.

The child is talking—likes to control the situation by saying "no," is trying new words, and has a small vocabulary.

The child likes to please you and knows how—and sometimes how to annoy you.

The bowel movements come in some routine pattern—the child has a bowel movement every morning at the same time, or every other day after supper, etc.

The child is showing some interest in imitating others—has an interest in knowing what Daddy does in the bathroom or going with Mommy every time she goes.

Making It Easier

Put a potty chair in the bathroom and let the child get used to it. The large toilet seat is too high and may be frightening.

Give the child some opportunities to watch Mommy, Daddy, sisters, brothers in the bathroom.

Put the child in some cotton training pants. It is too time-consuming to undo a diaper and go. Pants can be pulled down and pulled up, and the child soon learns to do it alone.

Problems

The child lets you know he has to go—after he has gone. He did not do it on purpose; he just is not quite ready yet.

The child has a lot of accidents. This is normal.

The child is trained; the new baby arrives, and the older child wets and soils. This will pass.

If things are not going smoothly, let us discuss them with you.

Suggested Reading For further information on toilet training, we suggest:

Baby and Child Care, by Benjamin Spock.
Child Sense, by William Homan, pp. 108-114.
Between Parent and Child, by Haim G. Ginott, pp. 149-151.

THUMB SUCKING AND PACIFIERS

Babies are born with the ability to suck and soon discover that sucking brings them a lot of pleasure—food, warmth, love. Some babies seem to have a great need to suck—much more than what they can get from nursing or taking a bottle. Some people feel that if the baby satisfies the need to suck in the early months, there will be less need to suck a thumb or a pacifier later. Thumb sucking is frequently used as a means of reducing tension and bringing comfort and a general sense of well-being.

Most dentists do not worry about infant thumb sucking. The thumb in the mouth does little damage until the child is 5 or 6 years old. Then it may push the teeth out of line. Left alone, most children will give up the habit by the time they are of school age.

Thumb or Pacifier?

The thumb is always handy and present.

The newborn cannot get the thumb into the mouth and can become frustrated in trying.

The pacifier can be used during the early months before the child has control to move the thumb to the mouth.

The pacifier is something extra to carry along—just in case.

It is easier to remove the pacifier than to remove the thumb when you decide it is time to give up sucking.

Your Attitude

Thumb sucking will be a problem immediately if you do not want the child to suck anything but the bottle, because the infant will soon discover the thumb and suck it. Please discuss this with us.

For the older child (2 to 4 years), try not to make an issue of the thumb sucking. Do not scold, bribe, punish, or shame. Try to ignore it. When you see the thumb going into the mouth, give the child something to do with his hands; help the child begin some activity.

Tying the arms down or applying splints, mittens, nasty-tasting stuff on the thumb, or metal hooks in the mouth are cruel, hurt the child, and do not usually stop the thumb sucking. If you are worried about thumb sucking and pacifiers, please discuss it with us.

Suggested Reading For further information on thumb sucking and pacifiers, we suggest:

Baby and Child Care, by Benjamin Spock.
Child Sense, by William Homan, pp. 104-108.
The ABC of Child Care, by Allen Fromme, pp. 293-297.
The Magic Years, by Selma Fraiberg, pp. 68-72.

PLAY

It has been said that the child "manifests in every way an eagerness, a curiosity, a great love of life that thrills and delights him in its simplest pleasures. Normally, a child loves growing up and strives for it constantly—sometimes out-reaching himself in his eagerness. He is both humble and proud, courageous and afraid, dominant and submissive, curious and satisfied, eager and indifferent. He hates and loves and fights and makes peace, is delightfully happy and despairingly sad."

A child does not distinguish between work and play. A child works hard all day at play, and it is a serious business.

Often it is not the expensive, store-bought toy that really sparks the child, but some simple household gadget that occupies the attention for hours.

Suggested Reading

Play Therapy, by Virginia M. Axline, p. 12.

Some Activities for Different Ages

From Birth to 2 Months

Likes to grasp a rattle
Will look at a mobile over the bed
Will look at pictures on the walls
Likes to kick, twist, squirm

From 2 to 6 Months

Will listen to music
Will look at mobile over the bed
Will reach for blocks
Likes to squeeze toys and cuddle toys
May like biting toys—teething rings, crackers, spoons
Will play with hands—pat-a-cake, hug-a-toy

From 6 to 12 Months

Prefers sitting up to lying down
Prefers mother to others
Will play ball, rolling it back and forth
Likes put-in-take-out toys—removing all the paper from the wastepaper basket, taking all the clothespins from a pan, removing the inside of a coffee pot
Likes to make noise—shred paper, bang blocks and pans, yell
Will stack objects—graduated measuring cups, plastic doughnuts on a pole

From 12 to 24 Months

Likes push-pull toys
Likes noise makers
Will stack and throw blocks
Likes containers that can be opened, object removed and top put back on
Likes balls, big and little
Likes floating bath toys
Will turn the pages of a book, but can be rough (cloth books sometimes last longer)
Enjoys singing, rhythms
Likes being read to, but span of attention very short and may sit for only 1 to 5 minutes for a story

Household Items to Save and Use in Play

First year

Elastic, for dangle toys, wrist bells
Plastic salt shakers, for rattles
Plastic cleanser containers—two rammed together will make a rattle
Plastic napkin rings, for dangle toys, teething rings
Plastic measuring spoons, for noise makers, sand play
Plastic cups, for nesting toys, water play
Foam sponges, for bath toys, water play
Small metal pie tins, for nesting toys, noise makers
Wooden spoons, for banging toys
Plastic bracelets, for dangle toys, toys for handling, mouthing
Cotton socks, for balls, dolls, broom horsie
Pictures from magazines, for crib and wall decorations

Second year

Plastic jars with screw tops, for storage of small items and for practice in twisting motion of wrist
Pieces of silk, velvet, bright colors, for a touching box and sorting games
Clothespins (the old-fashioned kind), for manipulation play

Wrapping paper, for drawings, painting, hats, masks
Grocery shopping bags, for drawing, painting
Showlaces for stringing beads and practicing tying bows
Old gloves, for puppet heads, dress-up dolls
Cold cream, for messy play
Scotch tape, for manipulation play, pictures, scrapbooks
Big cardboard grocery cartons, for doll houses, airplanes, and boats, and for crawling in and out of

Some Activities for Fun

A dab of honey and a feather for the child sitting in a high chair
Drawing on a steamy, winter window
A trip to the grocery store—feeling how heavy a 5-lb sack of sugar is, how cold a can of juice is, the tickle of a feather duster
A jar of bubble-blowing liquid and a circle ring for blowing endless bubbles and watching them float to the ground

Suggested Reading For further information on play and fun, we suggest:

What to Do When "There's Nothing to Do," by Elizabeth Gregg.
The Magic Years, by Selma Fraiberg.

DIARRHEA

Diarrhea—loose and frequent stooling—is a common symptom of many different disorders or diseases. Mild cases often end without specific treatment, but severe cases may be very serious and even require hospitalization.

It is important to know just what diarrhea is because stooling patterns in young infants change frequently in the first 4 to 8 months of life. It is normal in the first 1 to 3 months for your baby to have soft, mushy stools six to eight times daily (with every feeding). With breast feeding or when new foods, especially vegetables, are introduced, the baby's stools may even become watery. In general, when stools become liquid (more watery than mushy), green, change in odor, and more frequent than six times daily, these are signs of diarrhea in the young infant under 3 months old. Often there will be lumps of mucus or faint streaks of blood in the diaper.

After 4 months most babies begin having more regular bowel movements (three or four times daily). The consistency often remains mushy up to 10 or 12 months of age. Diarrhea is recognized because the frequence of stooling increases (from three to six stools per day) and the consistency becomes more loose than usual. After the first year diarrhea is usually easy to identify by simply noting a change to more frequent and looser stooling.

Some of the many causes of diarrhea include a change of diet or drinking water, food allergies, and infections of all kinds (sore throat, ear infections, gastroenteritis, stomach flu, urinary tract infections).

There are several danger signs seen in serious cases of diarrhea, and you should call your doctor if any of these are noted:

1 Diarrhea and fever (higher than 101.5°F rectal)
2 Blood and mucus present
3 Distension of stomach
4 Excessive water loss in the stool (diaper will be soaked)
5 Diarrhea in a child that is weak, is very sleepy (will not take a bottle), or has dry eyes and mouth

If none of these signs are present in a baby that has diarrhea, you may want to correct the problem at home.

1 First, stop all milk and solid foods.
2 Offer the child clear liquids (water, sugar water, Kool-aid, weak tea, etc.) for 12 to 18 hours. Begin by giving 2 or 3 oz. every 2 to 3 hours and work up to 4 or 5 ounces every 4 to 6 hours.
3 If the condition has improved, you may then begin to use half strength of your baby's usual formula or skim milk, again increasing the volume slowly over 12 to 18 hours.
4 Finally, you may return to the usual formula, and if all goes well, return to solids the following day.

Sometimes during this program, the baby's diarrhea will return. If this occurs, you should return to clear liquids and advance more slowly (using 24-hour intervals).

If this fails, you should contact your doctor.

THE COMMON COLD

Most children will develop between two and eight colds each year. Some children seem to have "bad" years (continuous colds) and "good" years (one or two colds).

Symptoms of a Cold

The first sign is usually a clear, watery discharge from the nose. This is followed by sneezing, watery eyes, and a scratchy throat. Night may bring a dry, tickling cough. There may be a slight fever (99 to 100°F) during the first 3 days. By the 4th and 5th days:

The base of the nose may be red and raw.
The discharge may be yellow and thick.
The cough may be present all day and night.
The nose may be stuffy.
The appetite may be poor.
The child may be tired.

Most symptoms last 7 to 14 days.

What You Can Do

There are no drugs or medicines to cure a cold, but there are several ways of making the child more comfortable during the cold.

1 Offer extra liquids (juice, pop, water, weak tea) and do not worry if the child does not seem to want to eat.

2 Allow extra time for naps or rest periods.

3 At night use a vaporizer near the child's bed. Cold vapor is best, but hot vapor will also help. *Use caution* in setting up a hot vaporizer. Do not set it in the bed or on the floor where you will trip on it or an older child will fall on it and be burned during a trip to check on the ill child.

4 For infants who cannot blow their noses, a nose syringe can be purchased at the drug store and used to remove some of the discharge at the edge of the nose. Compress the bulb, gently insert it into the nostril, and slowly release.

5 For raw noses, use a dab of petroleum jelly or mentholated ointment at the base of the nose. Spread it thinly so it will not be inhaled.

6 For a slight fever, let the child play in a lukewarm bath for 20 minutes, encourage extra fluids, and give Tempra, Tylenol, or children's aspirin as directed.

When to Call the Doctor

Call the doctor if you are worried about your child or any of the following occur:

1 The cold symptoms continue too long.

2 The fever persists over 101°F.

3 The child complains of a sore throat or an earache, or pulls at the ears.

4 The child stops drinking fluids.

5 The child starts vomiting or having diarrhea.

6 The child seems different.

URINARY TRACT INFECTIONS

Urinary tract infections (UTIs) are common, second only to respiratory infections. UTIs occur in the child's kidney, bladder, or urethra.

We are not certain why these infections occur, but believe poor voiding habits and germs entering into the urethra play an important role. Abnormalities in the bladder, kidneys, and their draining tubes (urethra and ureter) are another important cause of UTIs. For this reason, we often request x-rays of the kidneys and bladder.

These infections can be very dangerous if not treated, for they may damage the kidneys and cause lifelong problems. However, if they are properly treated, most children recover completely from a UTI. Despite initial

Common Medications

Condition	Drug	Frequency	Dosage at 3 months	Dosage at 6 months	Dosage at 1 year	Dosage at 2 years	Dosage at 3 years	Dosage at 5 years	Dosage at 8 years	Dosage at 12 years
Fever	Tempra or Tylanol drops	May be given every 4 hours as long as child is drinking fluids and not vomiting.	0.15 ml	0.3 ml	0.6 ml	1.2 ml				
	Tempra or Tylanol syrup		Do not give	Do not give	1 tsp	1 tsp	2 tsp	3 tsp		
	children's aspirin		¼ tablet	½ tablet	1 tablet	2 tablets	3 tablets			
	adult aspirin		Do not give	Do not give	Do not give	Do not give	Do not give	1 tablet	1½ tablets	2 tablets
Congestion	Normal saline nose drops	Make by mixing ½ tsp salt in 8 oz. of water. Place child on back on the bed with head hanging over the side of the bed. Place 2–3 drops of saline in each nostril. Wait 1 minute and then use a bulb syringe to gently suction the loosened mucus. Infants may have the bulb syringe used on their noses before each feeding.								
	Sudafed	Given by mouth. Ask us for directions.								
Cough	Honey and lemon	May be given every 3–4 hours.	Place honey on teaspoon and drop 1–2 drops of lemon juice on spoon.							
	Robitussin cough syrup	May be given every 4 hours	Do not give	⅓ tsp	½ tsp	1 tsp				
Poisoning	Ipecac causes vomiting and can be used when children swallow certain substances. If your child swallows something that should not be swallowed, *call us.* We *may* tell you to give 1 Tbs ipecac with several glasses of water. Have the child walk around. Wait 20 minutes. Vomiting will occur.									

good treatment, over half of all children who have had one UTI will develop a second infection within a year.

Many children do not complain of pain, going to the bathroom too often, or any of the usual warning signs seen with UTIs. Therefore, one of the most important parts of treatment is frequent examination of the urine. That is why we want to see your child again and again after the first UTI.

There are additional measures that may prevent further UTIs in your child:

1 Girls should learn to wipe themselves from front to back after using the toilet.

2 Girls should avoid taking baths (showers are preferable).

3 Girls should avoid having large, hard (constipated) stools.

4 If a girl is frequently scratching between her legs, ask your doctor to check her for pinworms.

5 Both boys and girls should drink plenty of fluids (ask your doctor for the right amount, which varies with your child's age).

6 Both boys and girls should be encouraged to void frequently with complete emptying.

ANTIALLERGY REGIME IN INFANTS

1 Avoid overheating and sudden chills.

2 No pets; if there are pets, keep them away from the baby.

3 No whole milk.

4 No egg, chocolate, wheat, or citrus fruits the 1st year.

5 Use wetproof mattress covers even after the baby does not need them.

6 Keep stuffed animals and toys made of fabric away from the baby. Plastic, metal, and wooden toys and animals stuffed with foam rubber are okay.

7 Use a damp cloth on baby's face; do not use soap.

8 During pollen season, keep baby away from high-pollen-count areas. When driving in the country, keep windows closed.

9 No bubblebath, bath oils, or afterbath lotion.

10 Keep baby away from high concentrations of dust.

11 No mixed cereals. One type of grain at a time. Do not add new cereal for at least one week.

12 No wool clothing the 1st year.

13 Wash new clothes before allowing the baby to wear them.

INDEX